LUMBAR DISC HERNIATION

LUMBAR DISC HERNIATION

Edited by

Robert Gunzburg, M.D., Ph.D.
Senior Consultant
Department of Orthopedics
Centenary Clinic
Antwerp, Belgium

Marek Szpalski, M.D.
Senior Consultant and Associate Professor
Department of Orthopedics
Centre Hospitalier Molière Longchamp
Teaching Hospital of the Free University of Brussels
Brussels, Belgium

LIPPINCOTT WILLIAMS & WILKINS
A **Wolters Kluwer** Company
Philadelphia · Baltimore · New York · London
Buenos Aires · Hong Kong · Sydney · Tokyo

Acquisitions Editor: Robert Hurley
Developmental Editor: Jenny Kim
Production Editor: W. Christopher Granville
Manufacturing Manager: Colin Warnock
Cover Designer: Mark Lerner
Compositor: Lippincott Williams & Wilkins Desktop Division
Printer: Edwards Brothers

© 2002 by LIPPINCOTT WILLIAMS & WILKINS
530 Walnut Street
Philadelphia, PA 19106 USA
LWW.com

Printed in the USA

Library of Congress Cataloging-in-Publication Data

Lumbar disc herniation / edited by Robert Gunzburg, Marek Szpalski.
   p. cm.
  Includes bibliographical references and index.
  ISBN 0-7817-3600-5
    1. Intervertebral disc—Hernia. 2. Lumbar vertebrae—Wounds and injuries.
  I. Gunzburg, Robert. II. Szpalski, Marek.
RD771.I6 L854 2001
617.5'6044—dc21

                                          2001038454

10 9 8 7 6 5 4 3 2 1

Contents

Section 3. Diagnosis

Section 4. Conservative Treatment Modalities

Section 5. Surgical Treatment Modalities

Section 6. New Treatment Modalities and Results

Section 7. Economic and Ethical Considerations in the Management of Spinal Stenosis

Contributing Authors

Dieter Adelt, M.D., *Department of Neurosurgery, Osteeklinik Damp, Damp, Germany*

Max Aebi, M.D., F.R.C.S.C. *Professor and Chairman, Division of Orthopaedic Surgery, McGill University; Chief, Department of Orthopedics, Royal Victoria Hospital, Montreal, Quebec, Canada*

Mauro Alini, Ph.D. *Head, Biochemistry Unit, Orthopaedic Research Laboratory, McGill University, Montreal, Quebec, Canada; Head, Biochemistry and Cell Biology Group, AO Research Institute, Davos, Switzerland*

Gunnar B. J. Andersson, M.D., Ph.D. *Senior Attending, Department of Orthopaedic Surgery, Rush-Presbyterian-St. Luke's Medical Center; Professor and Chairman, Department of Orthopedic Surgery, Rush Medical College, Chicago, Illinois*

J. Assheuer, M.D. *Attending Physician, Department of Neuroanatomy, University of Dusseldorf, Dusseldorf, Germany*

L.E. Augustinsson, M.D. *Department of Neurosurgery, Linkoping University Hospital, Linkoping, Sweden*

Federico Balagué, M.D. *Vice Head, Rheumatology Physical Medicine and Rehabilitation, Cantonal Hospital, Fribourg, Switzerland; Adjunct Associate Professor, Department of Orthopedic Surgery, New York University School of Medicine, New York, New York*

Michel Benoist, M.D. *Consultant Rheumatologist of Paris Hospitals, University of Paris, Paris, France*

Nick Boeree, M.D. *Southampton General Hospital, Shirley, Southampton, United Kingdom*

Norbert Boos, M.D. *Chief of Spinal Surgery, Orthopaedic University Hospital Balgrist, Zurich, Switzerland*

M. Brayda-Bruno, M.D. *Spine Surgery Center-Galeazzi Institute, San Donato Hospital Group, Milan, Italy*

Helena Brisby, M.D., Ph.D. *Department of Orthopaedics, Göteborg University, Sahlgrenska University Hospital, Göthenburg, Sweden*

A. Kim Burton, Ph.D. *Director, Spinal Research Unit, University of Huddersfield, Huddersfield, United Kingdom*

Marco Campello, M.D. *Associate Clinical Director, Occupational and Industrial Orthopaedic Center, Hospital for Joint Diseases, Mount Sinai/New York University Health, New York, New York*

Nan Clausen, B.A. *Raymedica, Inc., Bloomington, Minnesota*

John Cleary, M.D.   *Department of Orthopaedics, Huddersfield Royal Infirmary, Huddersfield, United Kingdom*

Henry V. Crock, M.D., F.R.C.S., F.R.A.C.S.   *Consultant Spinal Surgeon, Spinal Disorders Unit, Cromwell Hospital, London, United Kingdom*

M. Carmel Crock   *Spinal Disorders Unit, Cromwell Hospital, London, United Kingdom*

Thierry David, M.D.   *Spine Surgery Unit, Polyclinique De Bois, Bernard, France*

Robert Deutman, M.D., Ph.D.   *Department of Orthopedics, Martini Hospital, Groningen, The Netherlands*

Peter Donceel, M.D., Ph.D.   *Professor, Department of Occupational and Insurance Medicine, School of Public Health, Kathoieke Universiteit Leuven, Leuven, Belgium*

Marc Du Bois, M.D.   *Research Fellow, Department of Occupational and Insurance Medicine, School of Public Health, Kathoieke Universiteit Leuven, Leuven, Belgium*

Jiri Dvorak, M.D.   *Chief of Neurology, Schulthess Hospital Spine Unit, Zürich, Switzerland*

Gordon Findlay, M.D., M.B., Ch.B., F.R.C.S.   *Consultant Neurosurgeon, Walton Centre for Neurology & Neurosurgery, Liverpool, United Kingdom*

Alastair Gibson, M.D., F.R.C.S., Orth.   *Consultant Spinal Surgeon, Department of Orthopedic Surgery, The Royal Infirmary of Edinburgh, Edinburgh, United Kingdom*

C. G. Greenough, M.D., M.chir., F.R.C.S.   *Middlesborough General Hospital, Middlesborough, Cleveland, United Kingdom*

Robert Gunzburg, M.D., Ph.D.   *Senior Consultant, Department of Orthopedics, Centenary Clinic, Antwerp, Belgium*

Keita Ito, M.D., Sc.D.   *Head, Cartilage Biomechanics Group, AO Research Institute, Davos, Switzerland*

André J. Kaelin, M.D.   *Chief, Pediatric Orthopedic Unit, Children's Hospital; Charge de Cours, Department of Surgery, Medical School, University of Geneva, Geneva, Switzerland*

Stephen D. Kuslich, M.D.   *Spinology Inc., Stillwater, Minnesota*

Bengt Lind, M.D., Ph.D.   *Department of Orthopaedics, Göteborg University, Sahlgrenska University Hospital, Göthenburg, Sweden*

Christian Mélot, M.D., Ph.D., M.Sci., Biostat.   *Associate Professor, Department of Intensive Care, Erasme University Hospital; Professor of Biostatistics, Faculty of Medicine, Free University of Brussels, Brussels, Belgium*

Elizabeth Smith Mikkelsen, B.S., B.A., C.C.R.A.   *Raymedica, Inc., Bloomington, Minnesota*

Margareta Nordin, Dr. Sci., P.T., Ci.E.   *Director, Occupational and Industrial Orthopedic Center, Hospital for Joint Diseases, Mount Sinai/New York University Health; Research Professor, Departments of Orthopedic Surgery and Environmental Health Sciences, New York University School of Medicine, New York, New York*

Britt K. Norton, B.S.Chem.E., M.B.A.   *Vice President, Research, Raymedica, Inc., Bloomington, Minnesota*

Kjell Olmarker M.D., Ph.D.   *Associate Professor, Department of Orthopedics, Göteborg University, Sahlgrenska University Hospital, Göthenburg, Sweden*

Malcolm H. Pope, Dr.Med.Sc., Ph.D.   *Professor, Department of Occupational and Environmental Medicine, King's College, University of Aberdeen, Aberdeen, Scotland, United Kingdom*

Charles D. Ray, M.D., F.A.C.S., F.R.S.H.   *President, American College of Spine Surgery; Former President, North American Spine Society, Williamsburg, Virginia*

Björn Rydevik, M.D., Ph.D.   *Professor and Chairman, Department of Orthopedics, Göteborg University, Sahlgrenska University Hospital, Göthenburg, Sweden*

Barton L. Sachs, M.D.   *Texas Back Institute, Plano, Texas*

Dietrich Schlenzka, M.D., Ph.D.   *Department Head, Children's Department, ORTON Orthopedic Hospital, Invalid Foundation, Helsinki, Finland*

Ali Sheikhzadeh, Ph.D.   *Occupational and Industrial Orthopedic Center, Hospital for Joint Diseases, Mount Sinai/New York University Health, New York, New York*

Michael Sullivan, M.D.   *Consultant Surgeon, Department of Orthopedics, Royal National Orthopedic Hospital; Senior Lecturer, Department of Orthopedics, London University, London, United Kingdom*

Marek Szpalski, M.D.   *Senior Consultant and Associate Professor, Department of Orthopedics, Centre Hospitalier Molière Longchamp, Teaching Hospital of the Free University of Brussels, Brussels, Belgium*

K. Malcolm Tillotson, C. Stat.   *Statistician, Spinal Research Unit, University of Huddersfield, Huddersfield, United Kingdom*

Jill P.G. Urban   *Physiology Laboratory, Oxford University, Oxford, United Kingdom*

Gordon Waddell, D.Sc., M.D., F.R.C.S.   *Orthopedic Surgeon, Glasgow Nuffield Hospital, Glasgow, United Kingdom*

Preface

Ever since Mixter and Barr first described lumbar disc herniation in 1934, the understanding of its etiopathogenesis has been the subject of much controversy. Sciatica is a household name in the spine patient community and lumbar discectomy is probably the most common spinal surgical procedure performed throughout the world. This book brings a "state of the art" review of the current knowledge on this topic.

Through the study of biomechanics and physiology we try to understand the etiopathology and thus also the clinical presentation of lumbar disc herniation and its natural history, as well as the back and leg pain it can cause. The aging and degeneration processes of the disc are reviewed and the lesser–known subject of disc herniation in children and adolescents is thoroughly covered. This brings us towards clinical practice with a review of the diagnostic modalities covering imaging and electrophysiological exams. The importance of specificity and sensitivity of diagnostic tests, a major measure of their true value, is discussed.

Although Mixter and Barr made their discovery while performing surgery, there remains a large array of conservative treatment modalities for this condition. These different conservative approaches are analyzed in separate chapters and cover rheumatologic and physical medicine treatments, manipulation, global pain clinic approaches, and chemonucleolysis.

Surgery is still the golden standard approach if conservative treatment fails. However, there is currently a range of diversely invasive treatment modalities being proposed such as microdiscectomy, percutaneous approaches, and disc prosthesis. Many of these treatments still have to pass the test of proven efficacy through randomized controlled prospective trials. In a world leaning more and more towards evidence-based medicine, it is important to consider if all new techniques are really new advances. Chapters in this book also cover other areas of controversy such as silent herniations, recurrent herniations, and the prevention of fibrosis after surgery.

The importance of the financial aspect of health care is a growing concern. The economic and outcome measure issues surrounding the diagnosis and treatment of lumbar disc herniation are covered in Section VII of this book.

This book will be of interest to a wide range of practitioners including primary care physicians involved in back treatment, rheumatologists, physiatrists, neurologists, orthopedic and neurosurgeons, as well as basic researchers in spinal pathologies and health policy analysts.

Robert Gunzburg, M.D., Ph.D.
Marek Szpalski, M.D.

SECTION 1

Basics

1

Disc Biomechanics and Herniation

Malcolm H. Pope

This chapter is a synthesis of the literature on disc biomechanics taking into account biomechanical, biochemical, and morphologic considerations. Discs exhibit time-dependent deformations (creep) when subjected to load variations. These deformations are caused by fluid flow and viscoelastic deformation of the annulus fibrosus (AF). The fluid flow is caused by differences between mechanical and osmotic pressure. There is a diurnal pattern of standing heights. The majority of this diurnal height change can be accounted for by height loss within the disc, which bulges radially with loading. The disc is very vulnerable to factors influencing nutrition. Motion aids nutrition and even respiration plays an important role in the normal nutrition of the functional spinal unit (FSU). Our knowledge of spine loading is based on the pioneering intradiscal pressure (IDP) measurements recorded by Nachemson, but recent work by Wilke disputes some of those findings. The central region of the disc acts like a hydrostatic cushion between adjacent vertebrae. However, this property depends on the water content of the tissues and may be diminished after creep. Diurnal changes in the loads acting on the spine affect the water content and height of the intervertebral discs. Disc protrusions are a necessary step in the events leading to a disc prolapse and herniation. Disc protrusion and prolapse are commonly present without symptoms, but degenerated discs have a net reduction of flexibility. The cause of disc pathology leading to protrusion of the nucleus pulposus (NP) is not fully understood. The segment can usually accommodate a disc cleavage but when a fragment develops from a double cleavage there is potential for protrusion under minimal load.

The intervertebral disc is a vital part of the spinal system. Indeed the kinematics are determined by the three-joint system of disc and facets. Weightlessness and bed rest, an analog for weightlessness, reduce the mechanical loading on the musculoskeletal system. When unloaded, discs will expand, increasing the nutritional diffusion distance and altering the mechanical properties of the spine. Unfortunately, due to the combined effects of aging and degeneration, the disc may be disrupted when exposed to excessive or repetitive loads. Disc protrusions, prolapse and herniation are a continuum of degenerative failure. Age and gender influence the prevalence of this pathology. Disc protrusion and prolapse are commonly present without symptoms, being recognized in 30% to 70% of the asymptomatic population (30). Spangfort (97) finds that the mean age for disc herniation surgery is 40.8 years. Kelsey and Ostfeld (48), Lawrence (55), and Spangfort (97) report disc surgery is performed twice as often in men than in women. This is probably because more men work in occupations requiring physical labor. Valkenburg and Haanen (103) report that men in physically demanding jobs have more than a fourfold increase of symptomatic disc prolapse than men in "white collar" professions.

MECHANICS OF THE DISC
Disc as a Structure

Burton and colleagues (18) find reduced lumbar flexibility is due to decreasing disc height together with increasing age, weight, and back pain frequency. Pearcy and Tibrewal (83) have measured deformations of the anterior and posterior margins of the annulus fibrosus (AF) and the interspinous ligaments in flexion–extension lumbar radiographs of healthy men. The anterior and posterior disc heights compressed and extended up to 35% and 60%, respectively, while the interspinous distance extended up to 369%. These deformations implied that the soft-tissue elements were lax or in compression during part of the range of motion. Adams and associates (4) find the bending strength of lumbar discs decrease with age. Disc failure in bending occurs through overstretching the outer AF in the vertical direction. Reducing intradiscal pressure (IDP) does not affect strength. Mimura and others (69) have determined the relationship between disc degeneration and flexibility of lumbar FSUs under pure moments. The neutral zone (NZ), range of motion (ROM), and neutral zone ratio (NZR = NZ/ROM) were measured. In flexion–extension, the ROM decreased and the NZR increased with degeneration. In axial rotation, NZ and NZR increased with degeneration. In lateral bending, the ROM decreased and the NZR increased with degeneration. In all three loading directions the NZR increased, indicating greater joint laxity with degeneration.

Panjabi and coworkers (81) find that the coupling patterns under pure axial or lateral bending movements change with level. Panjabi and others (82) also find that motions are nonlinear as well as coupled. Panjabi and coworkers (81) suggest that abnormal coupling patterns in the lumbar spine may be an indicator of low back pain (LBP). Panjabi and associates (80) find that an injury to the AF and a removal of the nucleus pulposus (NP) altered the main and coupled motions and resulted in asymmetric facet joint movements.

Adams and colleagues (3) used inclinometers to show that the range of motion (ROM) increased by 5 degrees during the day. FSUs were creep loaded to simulate a day's activity and it was found that it reduces the spine's resistance to bending and increases the ROM. Thus, forward flexion causes higher bending stresses in the early morning than later in the day (about 300% for the discs and 80% for the ligaments of the neural arch), leading to a greater risk of injury in the early morning. Previous studies have indicated an increased risk of LBP with bending forward in the early morning. Snook and others (96) show that control of lumbar flexion in the early morning will significantly reduce chronic LBP.

Stokes (98) used photogrammetry to establish that AF strains are 6% or less under physiologic conditions, which suggests fluid loss or endplate deformation. A mathematical model showed that disc strain is very sensitive to disc height/diameter and to fluid loss from the disc but is less sensitive to the helix angle of the fibers. Koeller and associates (52) have found that mean disc height and cross-sectional area increases caudally but the water content is constant. Axial deformation and ventral bulging increases down the spine due to increasing disc height. Creep is smallest between T10-T11 to L1-L2 and increases above and below this level. The increase below L1-L2 is mainly due to the increasing disc height; the increase above T10-T11 occurs because the thoracic discs behave in a more viscous manner than the lumbar discs.

Disc Components

The behavior of the disc as a structure is dependent on the properties of its component tissues. Marchand and Ahmed (64) find that the AF consists of 15 to 25 distinct layers.

In any 20-degree circumferential sector, nearly half of the layers terminate or originate, causing local irregularities. Iatridis and coworkers (41) have tested samples from the anterior outer AF of L2-L3 discs. Degeneration affected compressive stiffness due to water loss. Neither degeneration nor orientation affected the strain-dependent permeability. Degeneration shifts loads from fluid pressurization and swelling pressure to deformation of the solid matrix of the AF. Iatridis and colleagues (42) find that the AF in torsional shear is less stiff and more dissipative at larger shear–strain amplitudes, stiffer at higher frequencies of oscillation, and stiffer and less dissipative at larger axial compressive stresses. Shear behavior was predominantly elastic. Iatridis and associates (40) used torsional shear to determine viscoelastic shear properties of cylindric samples of NP. A significant increase in the shear moduli and decreased capacity for the NP to dissipate energy is found with increasing age and degeneration. The NP undergoes a transition from fluid-like behavior to more solid-like behavior with aging and degeneration. Iatridis and others (39) also find that under transient conditions, the NP stress is indicative of fluid-like behavior while under dynamic conditions it was more viscoelastic. Fujita and colleagues (29) find that the radial tensile properties of the AF are nonlinear. Specimens from the middle layers were stiffer and failed at smaller strains than those from the inner or outer AF. Degenerated discs had a 30% decrease in ultimate stress. Krismer and associates (54) find that the AF restricts axial rotation more than the facets.

The tensile behavior of single- and multiple-layer samples of AF has been shown to vary with specimen orientation, position in the disc, and environmental conditions. Ebara and coworkers (26) find that the anterior AF has a larger tensile modulus and failure stresses than the posterolateral AF. The outer AF has greater modulus and failure stresses and lower failure strains than the inner. Strain energy density did not vary significantly with region. Best and others (13) have determined that the AF is nonhomogeneous, with regional and radial variations in both material properties and biochemical composition. Skaggs and colleagues (95) find the anterior AF stiffer than the posterolateral, and the outer stiffer than the inner. The regional differences in tensile properties may result from structural rather than compositional variations and may contribute to AF failure in the posterolateral region.

Bone affects the disc and vice versa. Keller and coworkers (45) find that trabecular compressive strength and stiffness increase with increasing bone density. For normal discs, the ratio of strength of bone overlying the NP to bone overlying the AF was 1.25, decreasing to 1.0 for moderately degenerated discs. These results suggest that an interdependency of trabecular bone properties and disc properties exists.

DISC CHANGES

Disc Changes with Age

The aging of the disc is well documented. Marchand and Ahmed (64) find that increased age reduces the number of distinct layers, increases the thickness of individual layers, and increases the interbundle spacing within an individual layer. The reduction in the number of distinct layers in older discs is related to both the thickening of the transition zone and gradual loss of organized fiber structures of the inner layers. The net width of the annulus is not reduced because of a concomitant increase in the thickness of the remaining layers. Increasing age also causes more irregular distribution of bundles within a layer. Bernick and associates (12) report that the AF from individuals less than age 40 consists of obliquely oriented collagen fibers in a pennate arrangement. From middle age there is a progressive degeneration of the laminae (fraying, splitting, and loss of collagen fibers). Johnson and others (43) find that approximately 10% of the matrix of the AF consists of elastic fibers and their numbers decrease slightly with increased age. Yasuma and associates (109) find that after age 60 that the AF inner fiber bundles orientation is reversed, so that they bulge inward. The reversal is due to degeneration of the middle AF fibers, (where the stresses are highest), NP atrophy, and disc-space narrowing.

Umehara and colleagues (101) have studied the local elastic modulus of the disc by indentation tests on L3-L4 and L4-L5 discs with various degrees of degeneration. The distribution of elastic modulus in normal discs is symmetric about the midsagittal plane. The elastic modulus of the degenerated NP shows an irregular distribution of elastic modulus but is higher than those in normal discs.

Sether and coworkers (89) find there is a decrease in magnetic resonance image (MRI) signal intensity of 6% in 80 years. The decrease in signal intensity is related to decreases in water and chondroitin sulfate and increases in collagen according to Chiang (21) and Cole and associates (22). The water content of the NP ranges from 90% at birth to 70% at age 60. The decrease is most pronounced in the second to fourth decade, according to Koeller and others (53). Peereboom (84) report that these changes lead to decreased viscosity of both the AF and NP. Biochemical changes are crucial to the mechanical behavior due to the osmotic balance of the disc. The water content decreases in a nonlinear fashion with increasing age. Urban and McMullin (102) report that the water content of the NP decreases as pressure increases, but the level of equilibrium hydration depends on the relative amounts of collagen and proteoglycan in the tissue. Discs in older individuals have a low proteoglycan-to-collagen ratio and their equilibrium hydration is also low. A far larger proportion of the total water is associated with the collagen in the discs of older individuals than in younger people.

Gross Structural Changes with Age

Koeller and colleagues (53) and De Candido and colleagues (25) found that degeneration increased with age until the fifth decade of life, after which it remained unchanged. There was a positive relationship between disc degeneration and prolapse or herniation. De Candido and colleagues (25) and Butler and colleagues (19) report that degeneration is more prevalent at the lower lumbar levels and that both disc degeneration and facet osteoarthritis increase with increasing age. Disc degeneration generally occurs before facet joint osteoarthritis, which may be secondary to mechanical changes in facet loading. The cross-section of the vertebrae increases with age, the lumbar being larger than the thoracic. The increase after age 70 is mainly due to osteophytes. Amonoo-Kuofi (7) finds an overall increase in the disc dimensions with age and alternating periods of overgrowth and thinning. After age 50 there is a marked loss of disc height. Twomey and Taylor (100) report that the actual average disc height actually increases with age as the discs "sink" into the vertebrae. The loss of transverse trabeculae of lumbar vertebrae is primarily responsible for the change in shape of both vertebrae and discs in older adults.

Aoki and associates (8), Peereboom (84), and Van den Hoof (104) show that, in aging lumbar spines, the cartilaginous endplates are degenerated and are replaced by subchondral bone proliferation. The endplate change is positively correlated with disc-space narrowing and NP degeneration. Harris and McNab (32) report that the nucleus becomes fibrotic and slows chondroid changes and diffuse calcification. Obviously such changes can be expected to have major effects on the mechanical behavior of the disc and subsequently of the FSU.

Mechanical Changes with Age

Plutte and coworkers (85) find no variation of disc compressive strength and elastic modulus with age. Likewise, Berkson (11) and Nachemson and coworkers (73) find no significant influence of age in either flexion, extension, or lateral bending. However, Umeeehara and colleagues (101) report that there is an irregular distribution of the elastic modulus in degenerative discs. Farfan and associates (28) find that the average failure torque was 25% higher for nondegenerated versus degenerated discs.

Koeller and coworkers (53) find that from the first to the third decade, axial deformability decreases in the thoracic region and remains constant in the lumbar spine. Afterward, axial deformability remains unchanged with age. Creep decreases in both regions with age up to the third decade. From the middle of the third decade to the beginning of the sixth decade, creep remains fairly constant within the lumbar spine. After the sixth decade, increased disc bulge with age is reported by Hirsch and Nachemson, (37), Lin and associates (57), and Reuber and associates (86).

Virgin (106) reports that hysteresis is highest in discs of young people, less the degenerated discs of older people, and least in discs of middle-aged people. This is of particular importance when we consider the high instance of disc protrusion in middle age. Hysteresis is a measure of energy absorption and, thus, may have implications in injury under impact loading. Twomey and Taylor (99) report a marked decrease of initial flexion deformation, and a slight increase of the flexion creep deformation in older individuals. Kazarian (44), however, finds that degenerated discs creep more than young discs under compressive or cyclic compressive load. Mimmou and colleagues (70) find that the neutral zone, a measure of laxity, increases with degeneration.

Disc Degeneration

Haughton and associates (34) find that AF tears increase the motion under applied torque. Radial and transverse tears of the AF have a greater effect on motions produced by an axial rotation than on those produced by flexion, extension, or lateral bending torque. Age-related disc degeneration begins early in adulthood, and progresses thereafter, altering disc morphology and mechanical properties that predispose to disc herniation. Disc degeneration results in abnormal motions of the spine. Haughton and coworkers (33) have correlated MRI appearance to disc stiffness. Stiffness averaged 7.0 nm per degree for the normal group; 1.9 nm per degree for the discs with concentric or transverse tears; 1.7 nm per degree for discs with radial tears; and 3.1 nm per degree for discs with advanced degeneration. Concentric, transverse, and radial tears of the disc indicate reduced stiffness of the disc and increased motions under applied torque. The most severely reduced stiffness was found in discs with radial tears of the AF. With collapse of the disc space, the stiffness increases.

Nachemson (71) proposes that in a young disc with a fluid NP, compressive stresses are resisted by the hydrostatic pressure in the NP, whereas high hoop stresses are present in the AF. In degenerate discs, the measured swelling pressures decrease with severity of degeneration, and approach zero in degenerated discs. Shirazi-Adl and colleagues' (91) finite element model (FEM) demonstrates that in degenerated discs the endplates are subjected to less pressure in the center, and loads are distributed around the periphery. The axial stress is compressive and the circumferential stress close to zero. Horst and Brinckmann (38) show that the AF in a mature disc resists compressive stresses perpendicular to the endplates. Thus, the degenerate disc behaves like a thick-walled cylinder rather than a pressurized vessel. Seroussi and colleagues (88) implanted markers in the disc. For

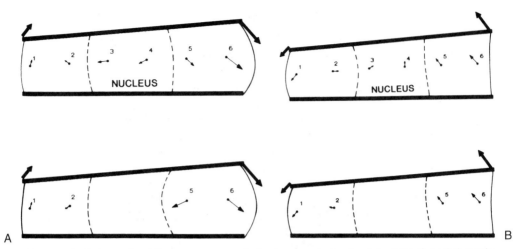

FIG. 1.1. A: Schematic of the average row 2 displacements for the intact **(top)** and denucleated **(bottom)** discs: flexion. **B:** Schematic of the average row 2 displacements for the intact **(top)** and denucleated **(bottom)** discs: extension.

intact discs, in compression, the marker displacements were predominantly anterior. In flexion, the beads in the center of the disc moved posteriorly whereas the beads closer to the periphery of the disc moved anteriorly. In extension, the central beads moved anteriorly and the beads closer to the disc periphery moved posteriorly. Denucleation, an analog of degeneration, resulted in an inward bulge of the AF under load whereas the intact disc AF bulged outward under load (Fig. 1.1). Once a disc has bulged inward a defect is present. The increased compressive stresses cause the disc to narrow with time. Asymmetries appear, probably due to defects caused by the inward bulging.

McNally and Adams (66) used a pressure transducer to determine a pressure profile representing vertical and horizontal components of compressive stresses. In the young disc the vertical and horizontal stress is uniform across the NP and inner AF. In the degenerate disc the pressure profile is disrupted, usually on one side. Adams and associates (5) show that age-related degenerative changes reduce the diameter of the central hydrostatic region of each disc by 50%, and the pressure within this region falls by 30%. The width of the functional AF increases by 80% and the height of compressive "stress peaks" within it by 160%. The effects of age and degeneration are greater at L4-L5 than at L2-L3, and the posterior AF is affected more than the anterior. Age and degeneration are themselves closely related, but the stage of degeneration has the greater effect on stress distributions. This work shows that structural changes within the AF and endplate lead to load transfer from the NP to the posterior AF. It also shows that the mechanical behavior of individual disc tissues is dependent not only on its location, but also on the loading history of the disc. As the disc narrows, the vertical cleavage probably forms the focus for a horizontal cleavage tear. Once formed, the cleavage tear can propagate. Shepherd (90) has shown that such horizontal cleavage tears markedly change the kinematics.

DISC HERNIATION

Discs do not herniate due to a pure compressive load. McNally and coworkers (67) tested FSUs in combined compression and anterolateral bending. Failure occurred in the vertebral body in half the specimens and in the posterolateral AF in the remainder. The latter group showed a significantly greater incidence of stress concentrations in the posterior AF when loaded in compression and bending. It was concluded that some discs are predisposed to prolapse because of damaging, localized concentrations of stress in the posterior AF in combined anterolateral bending and compression.

Failure of the aging disc is a complex phenomenon influenced by asymmetric force distributors. Early in life the NP and AF are strong, and disc protrusion or prolapse is infrequent. Yasuma and others (110) find that only when a large asymmetric force is applied to a healthy young disc can a disc protrusion or prolapse occur. Acute trauma may produce disc herniation whether or not there is degeneration, but disc herniation in the absence of acute injury requires the presence of preexisting degenerative changes. Schmorl and Junghanns (87) note clefts extending from the NP into the AF with NP desiccation that they associate with prolapse.

Coventry and colleagues (23) describe concentric fissuring during the third decade of life that precedes NP changes. Vernon-Roberts (105) reports that radial tears usually appear by the fourth or fifth decades, and affect the posterolateral disc. Circumferential clefts occur generally in the fourth decade, again posterolaterally. Rim lesions are common in the fifth decade and beyond. When failure occurs in the aging disc it appears to be a complex phenomenon influenced by asymmetric forces. Harada and Nakahara (31) report that in 70% of discs from patients between the age of 60 and 69, and in 80% of discs from patients over 70, herniated disc fragments are composed of the AF and cartilaginous endplate. The cartilaginous endplate had avulsed from the vertebra and had herniated with the AF. This type of herniation is common in older adults because of advanced disc degeneration.

Adams and Hutton (1) fatigue-loaded FSUs in compression and bending. The NP was stained with blue dye and radiopaque solution. A gradual prolapse started with the lamellae of the AF being distorted to form radial fissures and then nuclear pulp was extruded from the disc. Discs most commonly affected were from the lower lumbar spine of young cadavers. Older discs with preexisting ruptures were stable and did not leak NP.

The Disc Fragment

Brinckmann and Porter (16) find that introducing a fragment into an intact disc results in rapid failure of the disc under loads. Aspden and Porter (9) estimate the stresses generated in the AF by a loose fragment prove that a fragment can generate stress concentrations in a disc that could lead to progression of a fissure. A fragment is formed first and that prolapse is the final event of a chronic process of fissuring and premature failure. Brinckmann and Porter (16) created a radial AF fissure and fragmented tissue pieces that resembled those retrieved at surgery for prolapse which were created in the center of the disc. The discs exhibited prolapse at loads in the physiologic range. Adams and associates (2) state that a loose fragment begins to develop as a cleavage tear bifurcates. A semi-loose fragment becomes mobile as it begins to separate, forming the basis for a herniation. In the absence of a fragment, degenerative discs with simple cleavage tears do not necessarily protrude or prolapse. Loading the spine after an experimental disc cleavage has been created will not cause a protrusion (1). These studies support the hypothesis that disc prolapse, aside from the hyperflexion trauma described in the literature, has to be preceded by generation of radial fissures and tissue fragmentation within the disc. Thus, prolapse appears to be a late event during the course of a long-term degenerative process.

TABLE 1.1. *In vivo measurements of IDP*

Activity	Pressure
lying prone	0.10 Mpa
lying laterally	0.12 Mpa
relaxed standing	0.50 Mpa
standing flexed forward	1.1 Mpa
sitting unsupported	0.46 Mpa
sitting with maximum flexion	0.83 Mpa
free sitting	0.3 Mpa
lifting 20-kg weight, round flexed back	2.3 Mpa
lifting a 20-kg weight, flexed knees	1.7 Mpa
lifting 20-kg weight close to the body	1.1 Mpa

INTRADISCAL PRESSURE

Loading of the spine has become somewhat controversial. Pioneering intradiscal pressure (IDP) measurements were made by Nachemson during the 1960s. Since that time, there have been few data to corroborate or dispute those findings. Wilke and others (108) recently made *in vivo* measurements of IDP with one subject doing various activities (Table 1.1). Good correlation was found with much of Nachemson's data, with the exception of the comparison of standing and sitting or of the various lying positions (Fig. 1.2). It was suggested that this was due to an artifact in Nachemson's data. It was concluded that the IDP during sitting may be less than that in erect standing, that muscle activity increases IDP, that constantly changing position is important to promote flow of fluid to the disc, and that many physiotherapy methods should be reevaluated. Wilke and colleagues (107) also determined the effect of muscle forces on the IDP. Simulated muscle activity strongly influenced load pressure characteristics, especially for the multifidus.

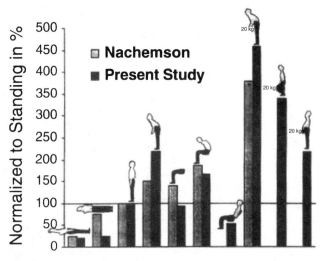

FIG. 1.2. A comparison between data of Nachemson and those of the Wilke study (108) (both for 70-kg individuals) regarding intradiscal pressure in common postures and activities, normalized to standing. Lifting weight is 20 kg in the current study. Lifting weight was 10 kg in Nachemson study.

Without muscle forces active, pressure increased proportionately with increasing movement. With five pairs of symmetric constant muscle forces active (80 N per pair), the pressure increased more than 200% in a neutral position and did not increase with increasing movement. The pressure without muscle forces and without axial preload was 0.12 MPa, which is about the same found in *in vivo* studies of anesthetized subjects in the prone position. With simulated muscle forces, the pressure was 0.39 MPa and in the range found for nonanesthetized subjects.

Case and colleagues (20) measured the *in vitro* change of IDP while the volume of the NP was increased by the infusion of saline colored with methylene blue. In both loaded and unloaded discs the IDP rose linearly. The intact NP therefore has the properties of a tight hydraulic space in which a large pressure rise will result from a small increase in volume.

VISCOSITY

The Disc Osmotic System

The disc is an osmotic system for the exchange of ions and fluid. The macromolecules in the disc interior have such a high hydroscopic capacity that they can take up fluid even when under pressure. Osmotic fluid flow occurs until the osmotic pressure and loading pressure are in equilibrium.

Creep

Both disc height and overall body height decrease with applied loads. Under prolonged loading the disc will continue to lose height after an initial deformation immediately after the load is applied. The height and area of the disc varies within the disc itself, between levels, between people, between genders, with aging, and during the day. Changes in body height occur after different stress environments including vibration, gravity inversion, space flight, traction, and increased loading. Alterations in spinal height are dependent on body forces, externally applied forces, and disc properties.

Adams and associates (5) have determined profiles of vertical and horizontal compressive stress after specimens were creep loaded in compression for 2 to 6 hours. Creep reduced the hydrostatic pressure in the nucleus by 13% to 36%. Compressive stresses in the AF were only slightly affected when the profiles were measured at 1 kN, but at 2 kN, localized peaks of compressive stress appeared in the posterior AF after creep. Increased loading of the facet joints caused an overall reduction in intradiscal stresses after creep. In addition, water loss from the nucleus caused a transfer of load from NP to AF.

Broberg (17) used a model of the disc to calculate both the extent of fluid flow and its implications for disc height as well as the role played by AF viscoelastic deformation. The normal diurnal fluid flow was found to be about ± 40% of the disc fluid content late in the evening. Viscoelastic deformation of AF contributes one-fourth of the height change obtained after several hours of normal activity, but dominates during the first hour.

Keller and coworkers (46) performed *in vivo* creep-recovery and IDP measurements on the lumbar spine of immature and mature swine. Creep rate, modulus, and viscosity were computed using a three-parameter solid rheologic analysis of the response recorded during the application of a 300-N load. The adult FSU tended to be stiffer, deform or creep more slowly, and had a significantly higher viscosity than the FSU of immature pigs.

Disc injury produced changed stiffness, viscosity, and creep rate analogous to that of aging, and it was found that a small AF defect is as bad as a large defect. The results indicate that respiration plays an important role in the normal, *in vivo* mechanical and nutritional behavior of the porcine FSU.

Adams and others (3) subjected cadaveric lumbar spines to periods of creep loading to show a disc height change similar to the physiologic change. As a result discs bulged more, became stiffer in compression, and were more flexible in bending. Disc tissue becomes more elastic as its water content falls. Disc prolapse becomes more difficult. The neural arch and associated ligaments resist an increasing proportion of the compressive and bending stresses acting on the spine.

Panagiotacopulos and coworkers (77, 78) measured stress-relaxation using AF specimens at various strain levels. Synthesis of experimental data into a master relaxation curve allows prediction of specimen response over time intervals not readily accessible experimentally. Panagiotacopulos and coworkers (77, 78) also performed tension–relaxation experiments on disc lamellae specimens. The water content was found to affect the viscoelastic behavior and a master relaxation curve was constructed from the experimental data. The water content of disc phantoms was measured by MRI and was used to compare discs of different ages. Panagiotacopulos and others (79) performed stress relaxation experiments on specimens from NP and from the external AF in two different orientations. Tests were run with varying moisture content so as to develop a relaxation master curve. A model was developed based on the experimental data. It was found that the short-term master curve for the lamellae of AF and NP are similar, whereas the long-term rubbery plateau is different. The master curves for different lamellae and the NP were shifted relative to each other in the time domain due to changes in water content. The average relaxation modulus of the whole disc was obtained by averaging the properties between the AF and NP.

Eklund and Corlett (27) used a stadiometer (a device to measure the overall height of a subject) to show diurnal shrinkage during a working day and how rapid recovery is achieved when lying down. Other experiments demonstrate how the rate of shrinkage is a function of the load on the spine. Shrinkage when sitting in different chairs was compared, and the results were in agreement with the IDP measurements of Nachemson (71). Magnusson and colleagues (61) determined the effect of hyperextension in rehydration of the disc. Hyperextension for 20 minutes in a prone posture was compared with the prone posture alone for 20 minutes. The stadiometer measurement was made after the subject was exposed to 10 kg of loading applied to the shoulders for 5 minutes and after each of the recovery postures. Hyperextension gave a significantly increased height recovery compared with the prone posture. In other experiments (62) it was found that even hyperextension stretches caused a reversal of height loss and some recovery (Fig. 1.3).

Malko and associates (63) used MRI to measure the changes in volume of the lumbar disc *in vivo* during a load cycle and related these changes to changes in fluid content. The experiment was designed to simulate a diurnal load cycle, but over less time. The load cycle consisted of bed rest, followed by walking with a 20-kg backpack for 3 hours, followed by bed rest for 3 hours. The average volume increase 3 hours after removing a highly compressive load was 5.4%. The water content of the NP and AF in a young disc was 80% and 70%, respectively. If the disc gained 5.4% of its initial total volume, and assuming that the initial fluid content was 75%, then it gained approximately 7% (i.e., 5.4% per 75%) of its fluid. Botsford and coworkers (14) measured *in vivo* diurnal variation in disc volume and morphology. In one protocol, the subjects were in the supine

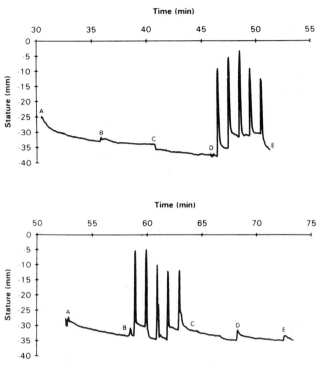

FIG. 1.3. Typical height change curves. *A and B:* Loaded sitting period. *B and C:* Unloaded sitting/hyperextension. *C and D:* Loaded sitting. *D and E:* Hyperextension/unloaded sitting.

position for 6 hours before MRI scanning. In another, the subjects spent 4 hours standing and 3 hours sitting before MRI scanning. Volume, height, and AP diameter of the lumbar discs decreased significantly. The mean decrease in disc volume after standing was 21.1% at L3-L4, 18.7% at L4-L5, and 21.6% at L5-S1. Most of the disc height loss was due to volume loss and the effect of radial bulging was minimal. LeBlanc and coworkers (56) measured disc cross-sectional area and transverse relaxation time (T2) from MRI after an overnight rest; before, during, and after 5 or 17 weeks of bed rest; and before and after 8 days of weightlessness. Overnight or longer bed rest caused expansion of disc area, which reached an equilibrium value of about 22% above baseline within 4 days. Increases in disc area were associated with modest increases in disc T2. During bed rest, disc height increased approximately 1 mm. After 5 weeks of bed rest, disc area returned to baseline within a few days of ambulation, whereas after 17 weeks, disc area remained above baseline 6 weeks after reambulation. After 8 days of weightlessness, T2, disc area, and lumbar length were not significantly different from baseline values 24 hours after landing. Significant adaptive changes in the discs can be expected during weightlessness or bed rest.

INSIGHT FROM MODELS

Various types of models exist, some with simple construction and others with marked analytical complexity. Klisch and Lotz (50) present a model for the AF as an isotropic ground substance reinforced with collagen fibers. Two strain energy functions for the AF are used to derive the constitutive equations. Keller and Nathan (47) present a sagittal plane, viscoelastic model of the spine composed of rigid vertebral bodies and deformable discs that demonstrate an instantaneous loss in height of 11.7 mm (0.67% of body height) and a loss of height of 19.6 mm (1.1% of body height) at the end of 8 hours. Changes in sagittal profile contributed to 12% of the overall height loss after 8 hours. Discs in the lumbar region lost the most height, but the contribution of the lumbar region to the total height loss was 32%. The height loss contribution of the thoracic region was higher (57%) because of the increased number of discs contributing to the total height loss in this region. For degenerated discs, the model predicted a similar instantaneous height loss but a 28% greater height loss after 8 hours. These results suggest that the majority of spinal height loss is a direct result of disc deformation, and about two-thirds of the total height loss occurs immediately on axial loading of the spine. McNally and Arridge (68) modeled the disc as an axially symmetric structure comprising a fluid-filled center, retained by a thin, fiber-reinforced membrane under tensile stress. The AF consists of two lamellae reinforced by oppositely oriented collagen fibers that are free to follow defined paths.

Natarajan and Andersson (76) used an FEM (Fig. 1.4) to establish that discs with a smaller ratio of disc area to disc height are more prone to larger motion, higher AF

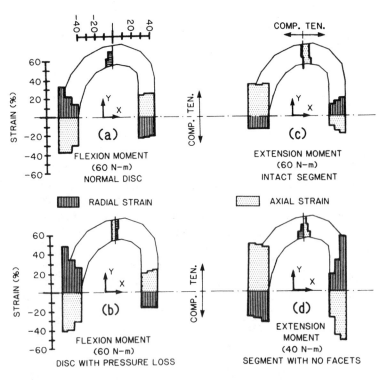

FIG. 1.4. Variation of the predicted radial and axial strains along the thickness of the annulus bulk at the mid-height section (z = 0) for the anterior, lateral, and posterior locations under the maximum values of loadings. **a and b:** In flexion for segments with a normal disc and a disc with pressure loss, respectively. **c and d:** In extension for an intact segment and a segment with no facet joints, respectively.

stresses, and larger disc bulge. When the disc height alone was increased, its flexibility also increased. Discs with the most height and smallest area are exposed to much higher risk of failure. Lu and others (60) presented a viscoelastic FEM and found that: (a) the viscoelastic behavior of the disc depends on the rate of fluid loss; the intrinsic properties of disc tissue play a role only at the early stage of compressive loading; (b) the axial strain increases, whereas the IDP and the posterior radial disc bulge decrease with increasing fluid loss; (c) a decreasing fluid loss rate from the NP with a total fluid loss of 10% to 20% occurs during the first hour of compressive loading. Martinez and colleagues (65) presented an axisymmetric FEM based on Biot's theory of coupled solid–fluid interaction and the disc modeled as an anisotropic, nonlinear poroelastic solid. Upon loading, the disc develops a maximum hydrostatic excess pore pressure that gradually decays as water is exuded from the matrix. During decay process, the applied load is transferred to the solid components of the matrix until the load is borne fully by the solid. AF disruptions result in an increase in the NP principal stresses suggesting that disrupted regions of the AF play a reduced role in load bearing. Lu and coworkers (58, 59) used the FEM to find variations in disc height have a significant influence on the axial displacement, the posterolateral disc bulge, and the tensile stress in the peripheral AF, but the effect on the IDP and the longitudinal stress distribution at the endplate–vertebra interface is minimal.

Lu and coworkers (58) used a viscoelastic FEM of a lumbar FSU to compute tensile stresses in the AF to determine the steps required to create a fissure in the disc. Of three models tested, the first to fail was a saturated disc under compression, bending, and twisting. This was the disc failure mechanism found in the laboratory. As loading rate increased, AF failure started at a lower value of compressive load. An increasing compressive load applied to a flexed, twisted, and saturated disc resulted in progressive fissure propagation starting at the posterior inner AF at the junction of the disc and the endplate. The results suggest that there are several key factors involved in the initiation and propagation of acute AF failure: axial compressive load, bending and twisting, and disc saturation. If one of these is lacking, AF failure is harder to achieve. Natarajan and associates (75) used an FEM of an FSU without posterior elements to show that failure always started at the endplates, indicating that they are the weak link. AF injuries are unlikely to be produced by pure compressive loads, a point borne out by experimental studies. The FEM predicted that it would require a larger extension movement as compared to flexion movement to initiate and propagate failure in an FSU, meaning that the FSU is stiffer in extension. The FEM also suggested that discrete peripheral tears in the AF may have a role in the formation of concentric AF tears and in accelerating disc degeneration. Shirazi-Adl (93) used a three-dimensional, nonlinear FEM to predict large tensile strains of about 10% in the AF under the maximum loads simulating symmetric lifting. Addition of lateral bending and twisting increases the maximum fiber strain to more than 20% which occurs in the innermost AF layer at the posterolateral location. Loss of IDP diminishes the magnitude of maximum fiber strain predicted under flexion loading. Failure analysis shows that rupture initiates in the fibers in the innermost layer at the posterolateral location. With a slight load increase, rupture progresses radially to the adjacent outer layer. Further progress of rupture in the fibers toward the AF outer periphery results in complete radial fissure; disc prolapse requires additional load increase. In the presence of large IDP, the generated partial or complete radial fissure is likely to result in AF protrusion or disc herniation, respectively.

Shirazi-Adl and colleagues (92) present an FEM subjected to pure moments in which they demonstrate the radial and axial strains in the AF (Fig. 1.4). Shirazi-Adl (94) also presents an FEM in which various combined loads are applied on the FSU and are then kept constant while the fluid is changed incrementally to a maximum of 12% gain or loss in its original volume. Loss of fluid increased the contact forces on the facets and diminished tensile forces in the AF, with the inner AF layers more affected than the outer. Reverse trends were computed when the fluid content was increased. Loss of fluid caused inward bulge at the inner AF layers and altered the stress distribution in the vertebral bodies. A loss in fluid predisposed the AF to lateral instability, disintegration, and degeneration; facets were subjected to significant additional loads; and vertebral bodies underwent a markedly different stress distribution.

SURGERY

Cunningham and coworkers (24) measured IDP changes at three adjacent disc levels (L2-L3, proximal; L3-L4, operative; and L4-L5, distal) under four conditions of spinal stability: intact, destabilized, laminar hook, and pedicle screw reconstructions. With destabilization and instrumentation, proximal IDP increased 45%, and operative IDP decreased 41% to 55%. Ahlgren and others (6) used a sheep model to biomechanically analyze the healing strength of the AF after two types of incisions, a full thickness removal of an AF box and a full thickness straight transverse AF slit were made in the discs. The box-incised discs showed a significantly greater loss in strength during the early healing phase (2 to 4 weeks) and a longer response before recovering AF strength. The type of incision also affected the multidirectional flexibility of the FSU. Larger amounts of motion were seen with the box incision when compared with the slit incision at all time periods and in all pure moments. Brinckmann and Grootenboer (15) performed a partial discectomy on lumbar discs. The changes in disc height, radial disc bulge, and IDP were measured in relation to the mass of central disc tissue excised. Disc height decreases and radial disc bulge increases approximately in proportion with the mass of the tissue excised. At the same time, IDP decreases. On average, removal of 1 g of disc tissue results in a height decrease of 0.8 mm and a radial bulge increase of 0.2 mm. Removal of 3 g of central disc tissue lowers the IDP to approximately 40% of its initial value. A high IDP is a prerequisite for the mechanical function of the disc under physiologic conditions.

POSTURE

Hedman and Fernie (36) used *in vitro* force and deformation measurements for determinate, quasistatic analysis of principal forces in the seated lumbar spine. Lumbar spines (L1-S1) were loaded while in simulated flexed and extended seated postures. Time-dependent forces were measured in the anterior column at the L4 and L5 superior endplates and in the facets. The remaining principal joint forces, including ligament, disc shear, and facet impingement forces were computed. The vertical creep displacement was greater in the extended seated posture but the escalation of forces was more severe in the flexed posture. The results suggest flexed postures produce large increases to the tensile forces in the region of the posterior AF. Hedman and Fernie (35) used the MRI to establish that creep, while in an extended posture, is greater than creep while in a flexed posture. Adams and Hutton (1) compared postures that flatten the lumbar spine with those that preserve the lumbar lordosis. Flexed postures have several advantages: flexion improves the transport of metabolites in the discs, reduces the stresses on the facets and on the posterior AF, and gives the spine a high compressive strength. Flexion also has disadvantages: it increases the stress on the anterior AF and increases the hydrostatic pressure in the NP. The disadvantages are not of much significance and we conclude that it is mechanically and nutritionally advantageous to flatten the lumbar spine when sitting and when lifting heavy weights. However, Magnusson and colleagues (61) have determined that hyperextension results in a significantly increased height recovery compared with the prone posture.

DISCUSSION

The disc is an osmotic system that allows for the exchange of ions and fluid. The macromolecules in the disc interior have a high hydroscopic capacity so that osmotic fluid flow occurs until the osmotic pressure and loading pressure are in equilibrium. The disc affects the overall disc kinematics. Reduced lumbar flexibility occurs due to decreasing disc height together with increasing age, weight, and back pain frequency. There is greater joint laxity with degeneration. Motions of the FSU are nonlinear and coupled and are affected by injury to the AF and NP. The ROM increases during the day and control of lumbar flexion in the early morning reduces chronic LBP.

Discs strain under load and disc strain is sensitive to disc height/diameter and to fluid loss from the disc but is less sensitive to the helix angle of the fibers. The behavior of the disc as a structure is dependent on the properties of its component tissues. The AF consists of 15 to 25 distinct layers but nearly half of the layers terminate or originate in the AF, causing local irregularities. There are regional variations; the anterior AF has a larger tensile modulus and failure stresses than the posterolateral AF. The outer AF has greater modulus and failure stresses and lower failure strains than the inner AF.

Age-related disc degeneration begins early in adulthood, altering disc morphology and mechanical properties that predispose to herniation. Degeneration and age cause a water loss. There is a decrease in MRI signal intensity with age related to decreases in water and chondroitin sulfate and increases in collagen. A significant increase of stiffness and a decreased capacity to dissipate energy occurs with increasing age and degeneration. The NP changes from fluid-like behavior to more solid-like behavior with aging and degeneration. Increased age changes the morphology of the AF with a reduced number of distinct layers, increased thickness of individual layers, and increased interbundle spacing within an individual layer.

After the age of 60, the orientation of the AF inner fiber bundles is reversed and they bulge inward due to degeneration of the middle AF fibers. The mechanism of disc protrusion has its genesis in vertebral endplate and disc nutrition. The segment can usually accommodate a disc cleavage but when a fragment develops from a double cleavage there is a potential for protrusion under minimal load. Torsion and forward bending or torsion and compression are likely to cause AF damage. A degenerate disc, even with a simple cleavage tear, does not usually protrude or prolapse. It will however lose height and produce a posterior annular bulge. The regional differences in tensile properties may contribute to AF failure in the posterolateral region. When a cleavage tear has been produced, the disc does not protrude when loaded. However, if a fragment of disc from another disc is introduced into the cleavage, then with minimal load the posterior AF will bulge and sometimes rupture.

Changes in segmental IDP levels occur after spinal destabilization and instrumentation. Since IDP differentials drive the metabolic production and exchange of disc substances, spinal instrumentation may serve as the impetus for altered metabolic exchange and predispose operative and adjacent levels to disc degeneration. In addition stresses may be shifted to adjacent levels, thus increasing the rate of disc degeneration.

New data cause us to reevaluate disc loading. IDP during sitting may in fact be less than that in erect standing. These data show that muscle activity increases IDP, that constantly changing position is important to promote flow of fluid to the disc, and that many physiotherapy methods should be reevaluated.

Disc height and overall body height decrease with externally applied loads. Under prolonged mechanical loading a disc will continue to lose height after an initial deformation after the load is applied. Changes in body height occur after different stress environments including vibration, gravity inversion, space flight, traction, and increased loading, while hyperextension can restore height.

REFERENCES

1. Adams MA, Hutton WC. The effect of posture on the lumbar spine. *J Bone Joint Surg [Br]* 1985;67(4): 625–629.
2. Adams MA, Dolan P, Hutton WC. The stages of disc degeneration as revealed by discograms. *J Bone Joint Surg* 1986;68:B:36–41.
3. Adams MA, Dolan P, Hutton WC, et al. Diurnal changes in spinal mechanics and their clinical significance. *J Bone Joint Surg [Br]* 1990;72(2):266–270.
4. Adams MA, Green TP, Dolan P. The strength in anterior bending of lumbar intervertebral discs. *Spine* 1994;19(19):2197–2203.
5. Adams MA, McMillan DW, Green TP, et al. Sustained loading generates stress concentrations in lumbar intervertebral discs. *Spine* 1996;15(4):434–482.
6. Ahlgren BD, Vasavada A, Brower RS, et al. Annular incision technique on the strength and multidirectional flexibility of the healing intervertebral disc. *Spine* 1994;19(8):948–954.
7. Amonoo-Kuofi HS. Morphometric changes in the heights and anteroposterior diameters of the lumbar intervertebral discs with age. *J Anat* 1991;175:159–168.
8. Aoki J, Tamamoto I, Kitamura N, et al. End plate of the discovertebral joint: degenerative changes in the elderly adult. *Radiology* 1987;164(2):411–414.
9. Aspden RM, Porter RW. Localized stresses in the intervertebral disc resulting from a loose fragment. A theory for fissure and fragment. *Spine* 1999,1;24(21):2214–2218.
10. Benini A. *Ischias ohne bandscheibenvorfall.* Bern: Huber, 1976.
11. Berkson MH. Mechanical properties of the human lumbar spine. Flexibilities, intradiscal pressure, posterior element influences. *Proc Inst Med Chicago* 1977;31:138–143.
12. Bernick S, Walker JM, Paule WJ. Age changes to the annulus fibrosus in human intervertebral discs. *Spine* 1991;16(5):520–524.
13. Best BA, Guilak F, Setton LA, et al. Compressive mechanical properties of the human annulus fibrosus and their relationship to biochemical composition. *Spine* 1994;19(2):212–221.
14. Botsford DJ, Esses SI, Ogilvie-Harris DJ. In vivo diurnal variation in intervertebral disc volume and morphology. *Spine* 1994;19(8):935–940.
15. Brinckmann P, Grootenboer H. Change of disc height, radial disc bulge, and intradiscal pressure from discectomy. An in vitro investigation on human lumbar discs. *Spine* 1991;16(6):641–646.
16. Brinkmann P, Porter RW. A laboratory model of lumbar disc protrusion: fissure and fragment. *Spine* 1994; 19:228–235.
17. Broberg KB. Slow deformation of intervertebral discs. *J Biomech* 1993;26(4–5):501–512.
18. Burton AK, Battie MC, Gibbons L, et al. Lumbar disc degeneration and sagittal flexibility. *J Spinal Disord* 1996;9(5):418–424.
19. Butler D, Trafimow JH, Andersson GB, et al. Discs degenerate before facets. *Spine* 1990;15(2):111–113.
20. Case RB, Choy DS, Altman P. Change of intradiscal pressure versus volume change. *J Clin Laser Med Surg* 1995,13(3):143–147.
21. Chiang YL. A study on topographical change of proteoglycans in human lumbar disc. *Nippon Seikeigeka Gakkai Zasshi* 1983;57(5)539–551.
22. Cole TC, Ghosh P, Taylor TKF. Variations of the proteoglycans of the canine intervertebral disc with aging. *Biochim Biophys Acta* 1986;880:209–219.
23. Coventry MB, Ghormley RK, Kernohan JW. The intervertebral disc: its microscopic anatomy and pathology. III. Pathological changes in the intervertebral disc. *J Bone Joint Surg* 1945;27:460.
24. Cunningham BW, Kotani Y, McNulty PS, et al. The effect of spinal destabilization and instrumentation on lumbar intradiscal pressure: an in vitro biomechanical analysis. *Spine* 1997;22(22):2655–2663.
25. De Candido P, Reinig JW, Dwyer AJ, et al. Magnetic resonance assessment of the distribution of lumbar spine disc degenerative changes. *J Spinal Disord* 1988;1(1):9–15.
26. Ebara S, Iatridis JC, Setton LA, et al. Tensile properties of nondegenerate human lumbar annulus fibrosus. *Spine* 1996,15;21(4):452–461.

27. Eklund JA, Corlett EN. Shrinkage as a measure of the effect of load on the spine. *Spine* 1984;9(2):189–194.
28. Farfan HF, Cossett JW, Robertson GH, et al. The effect of torsion on the lumbar intervertebral joints. *J Bone Joint Surg* 1970;52A:468–478.
29. Fujita Y, Duncan NA, Lotz JC. Radial tensile properties of the lumbar annulus fibrosus are site and degeneration dependent. *J Orthop Res* 1997;15(6):814–819.
30. Garfin SR, Herkowitz HN. The intervertebral disc: disc disease-does it exist? In: Weinstein JN, Wiesel S, eds. *The lumbar spine*. Philadelphia: WB Saunders, 1990:369–380.
31. Harada Y, Nakahara S. A pathologic study of lumbar disc herniation in the elderly. *Spine* 1989;14(9): 1020–1024.
32. Harris RI, McNab I. Structural changes in the lumbar intervertebral disc. *J Bone Joint Surg* 1954;36B:304–322.
33. Haughton VM, Lim TH, An H. Intervertebral disk appearance correlated with stiffness of lumbar spinal motion segments. *AJNR Am J Neuroradiol* 1999;20(6):1161–1165.
34. Haughton VM, Schmidt TA, Keele K, et al. Flexibility of lumbar spinal motion segments correlated to type of tears in the annulus fibrosus. *J Neurosurg* 2000;92[1 Suppl]:81–86.
35. Hedman TP, Fernie GR. In vivo measurement of lumbar spinal creep in two seated postures using magnetic resonance imaging. *Spine* 1995;20(2):178–183.
36. Hedman TP, Fernie GR. Mechanical response of the lumbar spine to seated postural loads. *Spine* 1997; 1;22(7): 734–743.
37. Hirsch C, Nachemson A. New observations on the mechanical behavior of lumbar discs. *Acta Orthop Scand* 1954;23:254–283.
38. Horst M, Brinckman P. Measurement of the distribution of axial stress on the end-plate of the vertebral body. *Spine* 1981;6:217–232.
39. Iatridis JC, Weidenbaum M, Setton LA, et al. Is the nucleus pulposus a solid or a fluid? Mechanical behaviors of the nucleus pulposus of the human intervertebral disc. *Spine* 1996; 21(10):1174–1184.
40. Iatridis JC, Setton LA, Weidenbaum M, et al. Alterations in the mechanical behavior of the human lumbar nucleus pulposus with degeneration and aging. *J Orthop Res* 1997;15(2):318–322.
41. Iatridis JC, Setton LA, Foster RJ, et al. Degeneration affects the anisotropic and nonlinear behaviors of human annulus fibrosus in compression. *J Biomech* 1998;31(6):535–544.
42. Iatridis JC, Kumar S, Foster RJ, et al. Shear mechanical properties of human lumbar annulus fibrosus. J Orthop Res 1999;17(5):732–737.
43. Johnson EF, Berryman H, Mitchell R, et al. Elastic fibres in the annulus fibrosus of the adult human lumbar intervertebral disc. A preliminary report. *J Anat* 1985;153:57–63.
44. Kazarian LE. Creep characteristics of the human spinal column. *Orthop Clin North Am* 1975;6:3–18.
45. Keller TS, Hansson TH, Abram AC, et al. Regional variations in the compressive properties of lumbar vertebral trabeculae. Effects of disc degeneration. *Spine* 1989;14(9):1012–1019.
46. Keller TS, Holm SH, Hansson TH, et al. The dependence of intervertebral disc. Mechanical properties on physiologic conditions. *Spine* 1990;15(8):751–761.
47. Keller TS, Nathan M. Height change caused by creep in intervertebral discs: a sagittal plane model. *J Spinal Disord* 1999;12(4):313–324.
48. Kelsey JL, Ostfeld AM. Demographic characteristics of persons with acute herniated lumbar intervertebral disc. *J Chronic Dis* 1975;28:37.
49. Kelsey JL. Epidemiology of radiculopathies. *Adv Neural* 1978;19:385.
50. Klisch SM, Lotz JC. Application of a fiber-reinforced continuum theory to multiple deformations of the annulus fibrosus. *J Biomech* 1999;32(10):1027–1036.
51. Knutsson F. The instability associated with disc degeneration in the lumbar spine. *Acta Radiol* 1944;25: 593–609.
52. Koeller W, Meier W, Hartmann F. Biomechanical properties of human intervertebral discs subjected to axial dynamic compression. A comparison of lumbar and thoracic discs. *Spine* 1984;9(7):725–733.
53. Koeller W, Muehlhaus S, Meier W, et al. Biomechanical properties of human intervertebral discs subjected to axial dynamic compression–influence of age and degeneration. *J Biomech* 1986;19(10):807–816.
54. Krismer M, Haid C, Rabl W. The contribution of annulus fibers to torque resistance. *Spine* 1996;15(22): 2551–2557.
55. Lawrence JS. Disc degeneration: its frequency and relationship to symptoms. *Am Rheum Dis* 1969;28:121.
56. LeBlanc AD, Evans HJ, Schneider VS, et al. Changes in intervertebral disc crosssectional area with bed rest and space flight. *Spine* 1994;19(7):812–817.
57. Lin HS, Liu YK, Adams KH. Mechanical response of the lumbar intervertebral joint under physiological (complex) loading. *J Bone Joint Surg* 1978;60A:41–55.
58. Lu YM, Hutton WC, Gharpuray VM. Do bending, twisting, and diurnal fluid changes in the disc affect the propensity to prolapse? A viscoelastic finite element model. *Spine* 1996;21(22):2570–2579.
59. Lu YM, Hutton WC, Gharpuray VM. Can variations in intervertebral disc height affect the mechanical function of the disc? *Spine* 1996;21(19):2208–2216.
60. Lu YM, Hutton WC, Gharpuray VM, The effect of fluid loss on the viscoelastic behavior of the lumbar intervertebral disc in compression. *J Biomech Eng* 1998;120(1):48–54.
61. Magnusson ML, Pope MH, Hansson T. Does hyperextension have an unloading effect on the intervertebral disc? *Scand J Rehabil Med* 1995;27(1):5–9.

62. Magnusson ML, Pope MH. Body height changes with hyperextension. *Clin Biomech* 1996;11(4):236–238.

63. Malko JA, Hutton WC, Fajman WA. An in vivo magnetic resonance imaging study of changes in the volume (and fluid content) of the lumbar intervertebral discs during a simulated diurnal load cycle. *Spine* 1999;24(10): 1015–1022.

64. Marchand F, Ahmed AM. Investigation of the laminate structure of lumbar disc annulus fibrosus. *Spine* 1990;15(5):402–410.

65. Martinez JB, Oloyede VO, Broom ND. Biomechanics of loadbearing of the intervertebral disc: an experimental and finite element model. *Med Eng Phys* 1997;19(2):145–156.

66. McNally DS, Adams MA. Internal intervertebral disc mechanics as revealed by stress profilometry. *Spine* 1992;17:66–73.

67. McNally DS, Adams MA, Goodship AE. Can intervertebral disc prolapse be predicted by disc mechanics? *Spine* 1993;18(11):1525–1530.

68. McNally DS, Arridge RG. An analytical model of intervertebral disc mechanics. *J Biomech* 1995;28(1):53–68.

69. Mimura M, Panjabi MM, Oxland TR, et al. Disc degeneration affects the multidirectional flexibility of the lumbar spine. *Spine* 1994;19(12):1371–1380.

70. Mimmou M, Panjabi MM, Oxland TR, et al. Disc degeneration affects the multidirectional flexibility of the lumbar spine. *Spine* 1994;19:12:1371–1380.

71. Nachemson AL. Lumbar intradiscal pressure. *Acta Orthop Scand* 1960;43[Suppl]:1–104.

72. Nachemson A, Lewin T, Maroudas A, et al. In-vitro diffusion of dyes through the end plates and the annulus fibrosus of human intervertebral disc. *Acta Orthop Scand* 1970;41:589–607.

73. Nachemson A, Schultz AB, Berkson MH. Mechanical properties of human lumbar spine motion segments. Influences of age, sex, disc level, and degeneration. *Spine* 1979;4:1–8.

74. Nakamura S, Takahashi K, Takahashi Y, et al. The afferent pathways of discogenic low-back pain. *J Bone Joint Surg* 1996;78-B:606–612.

75. Natarajan RN, Ke JH, Andersson. A model to study the disc degeneration process. *Spine* 1994;19(3):259–265.

76. Natarajan RN, Andersson GB. The influence of lumbar disc height and cross-sectional area on the mechanical response of the disc to physiologic loading. *Spine* 1999;24(18):1873–1881.

77. Panagiotacopulos ND, Pope MH, Bloch R, et al. Water content in human intervertebral discs. Part II. Viscoelastic behavior. *Spine* 1987;12(9):918–924.

78. Panagiotacopulos ND, Pope MH, Krag MH, et al. Water content in human intervertebral discs. Part I. Measurement by magnetic resonance imaging. *Spine* 1987;12(9):912–917.

79. Panagiotacopulos ND, Pope NIH, Krag MH, et al. A mechanical model for the human intervertebral disc. *J Biomech* 1987;20(9):839–850.

80. Panjabi MM, Krag MH, Chung TQ. Effects of disc injury on mechanical behavior of the human spine. *Spine* 1984;9(7):707–713.

81. Panjabi M, Yamamoto I, Oxland T, et al. How does posture affect coupling in the lumbar spine? *Spine* 1989; 14(9):1002–1011.

82. Panjabi MM, Oxland TR, Yamamoto L, et al. Mechanical behavior of the human lumbar and lumbosacral spine as shown by three-dimensional load-displacement curves. *J Bone Joint Surg Am* 1994;76(3):413–424.

83. Pearcy MJ, Tibrewal SB. Lumbar intervertebral disc and ligament deformations measured in vivo. *Clin Orthop* 1984;(191):281–286.

84. Peereboom JWC. Some biochemical and histochemical properties for the age pigment in the human intervertebral disc. *Histochemie* 1973;37:119–130.

85. Platte R, Gerner HJ, Salditt R. Das elasto-mechanische verhalten menschlicher bandscheiben unter statischem druck. *Arch Orthop Unfallchir* 1974;79:139–148.

86. Reuber M, Schultz A, Denis F, et al. Bulging of lumbar intervertebral discs. *J Biomech Eng* 1982;104:187–192.

87. Schmorl G, Junghanns H. *The human spine in health and disease*, 2nd [Am] ed. New York: Grune & Stratton, 1971.

88. Seroussi RE, Krag MH, Muller DL, et al. Internal deformations of intact and denucleated human lumbar discs subjected to compression, flexion, and extension loads. *J Orthop Res* 1989;7:122–131.

89. Sether LA, Yu S, Haughton VM, et al. Intervertebral disk: normal age-related changes in the MR signal intensity. *Radiology* 1990;177(2):385–388.

90. Shepperd JAN. Pathological changes contributing to back pain and sciatica. In: Aspden RM, Porter RW, eds. *Lumbar spine disorders*. Singapore: World Scientific Co, 1995:105–114.

91. Shirazi-Adl SA, Shrivastava SC, Ahmed AM. Stress analysis of the lumbar disc body unit in compression: a three-dimensional non-linear finite element study. *Spine* 1984;9(2):120–126.

92. Shirazi-Adl SA, Ahmed AM, Shrivastava SC. A finite element study of a lumbar motion segment subjected to pure sagittal plane moments. *J Biomech* 1986;19(4):331–350.

93. Shirazi-Adl A. Strain in fibers of a lumbar disc. Analysis of the role of lifting in producing disc prolapse. *Spine* 1989;14(1):96–103.

94. Shirazi-Adl A. Finite-element simulation of changes in the fluid content of human lumbar discs. Mechanical and clinical implications. *Spine* 1992;17(2):206–212.

95. Skaggs DL, Weidenbaum M, Iatridis JC, et al. Regional variation in tensile properties and biochemical composition of the human lumbar annulus fibrosus. *Spine* 1994;19(12):1310–1319.

96. Snook SH, Webster BS, McGorry RW, et al. The reduction of chronic nonspecific low back pain through the control of early morning lumbar flexion. A randomized controlled trial. *Spine* 1998 1;23(23):2601–2607.
97. Spangfort EV. The lumbar disc herniation. *Acta Orthop Scand* 1972;142[Suppl]:1.
98. Stokes IA. Surface strain on human intervertebral discs. *J Orthop Res* 1987;5(3):348–355.
99. Twomey L, Taylor J. Flexion creep deformation and hysteresis in the lumbar vertebral column. *Spine* 1982;7:1 16–122.
100. Twomey L, Taylor J. Age changes in lumbar intervertebral discs. *Acta Orthop Scand* 1985;56(6):496–499.
101. Umehara S, Tadano S, Abumi K, et al. Effects of degeneration on the elastic modulus distribution in the lumbar intervertebral disc. *Spine* 1996;21:811–820.
102. Urban JP, McMullin JF. Swelling pressure of the intervertebral disc: influence of proteoglycan and collagen contents. *Biorheology* 1985;22(2):145–157.
103. Valkenburg HA, Haanen HCM. The epidemiology of low back pain. In: White AA III, Gordon SL, eds. *Symposium on idiopathic low back pain*. St. Louis: Mosby-Year Book, 1982:9–22.
104. Van den Hoof A. Histological changes in the annulus fibrosus of the human intervertebral disc. *Gerontologia* 1964;9:136–149.
105. Vernon-Roberts B. The normal aging of the spine: degeneration and arthritis. In: Andersson GBJ, McNeill TW, eds. *Lumbar spinal stenosis*. St. Louis: Mosby-Year Book, 1992:57–75.
106. Virgin WJ. Experimental investigations into physical properties of the intervertebral disc. *J Bone Joint Surg* 1951;33B:607–611.
107. Wilke HJ, Wolf S, Claes LE, et al. Influence of varying muscle forces on lumbar intradiscal pressure: an in vitro study. J Biomech 1996;29(4):549–555.
108. Wilke HJ, Neef P, Caimi M, et al. New in vivo measurements of pressures in the intervertebral disc in daily life. *Spine* 1999;24(8):755–762.
109. Yasuma T, Koh S, Okamura T, et al. Histological changes in aging lumbar intervertebral discs. Their role in protrusions and prolapses. *J Bone Joint Surg [Am]* 1990;72:220–229.
110. Yasuma T, Makino E, Saito S, et al. Clinico-pathological study on lumbar intervertebral disc herniation. 1. Changes in the intervertebral disc relation with age including Schmorl's node. *Seikei Saigaigeka* 1986;29: 1565–1578.

SUGGESTED READING

Adams MA, Dolan P, Hutton WC. Diurnal variations in the stresses on the lumbar spine. *Spine* 1987;12(2):130–137.
Adams MA, Hutton WC. Gradual disc prolapse. *Spine* 1985;10(6):524–531.
Adams MA, McNally DS, Dolan P. 'Stress' distributions inside intervertebral discs. The effects of age and degeneration. *J Bone Joint Surg [Br]* 1996;78(6):965–972.
Natali AN. A hyperelastic and almost incompressible material model as an approach to intervertebral disc analysis. *J Biomed Eng* 1991;13(2):163–168.
Oloyede A, Broom ND, Martinez JB. Experimental factors governing the internal stress state of the intervertebral disc. *Med Eng Phys* 1998;20(8):631–637.
Pereboom JWC. Age dependent changes in the human intervertebral disc. *Gerontologia* 1971;17:236–252.
Pooley J, Pooley JE, Stevens J. Evidence for an intraosseous arteriovenous shunt operating in long bones during exercise conditions. *J Bone Joint Surg* 1985;67:B:319.
Schmidt TA, An HS, Lim TH, et al. The stiffness of lumbar spinal motion segments with a high-intensity zone in the annulus fibrosus. *Spine* 1998;23(20):2167–2173.
Yingling VR, McGill SM. Mechanical properties and failure mechanics of the spine under posterior shear load: observations from a porcine model. *J Spinal Disord* 1999;12(6):501–508.
Ziran BH, Pineda S, Pokharna H, et al. Biomechanical, radiologic, and histopathologic correlations in the pathogenesis of experimental intervertebral disc disease. *Spine* 1994;19(19):2159–2163.

2

The Physiology of the Intervertebral Disc

Jill P.G. Urban

The discs are the joints of the spinal column and their major functional role is mechanical. The ability of the discs to support compressive loads and allow flexion, bending, and torsion, depends on the organization and composition of the major macromolecules that make up this tissue. Collagen provides mechanical strength and anchors the disc to the bone, while proteoglycans impart a high swelling pressure to the disc enabling it to maintain hydration even under high compressive loads. These macromolecules are made by the disc's cells; cellular function ultimately determines the disc's composition. This chapter discusses the functional roles of collagen and proteoglycans, and also how factors such as nutrient supply and mechanical load affect cellular activity.

FUNCTIONAL PROPERTIES OF COLLAGEN AND AGGRECAN

Composition and Organization

The three major constituents of the disc are water, fibrillar collagens, and aggrecan—the large aggregating proteoglycan. The organization of these components varies considerably with position across the disc. The outer region of the disc, the annulus fibrosus, is made up of concentric collagenous lamellae. These consist of bundles of collagen fibers running obliquely from one vertebral body to the next and firmly anchoring the disc to the bone or the cartilaginous endplate. The angle of the collagen bundles alternates between successive lamellae thus forming a crosswoven and reinforced structure (21). The collagen fibrils of the nucleus, in contrast, are finer and form a loose, randomly organized network. Composition also varies across the disc. Collagen content is highest in the outer annulus and falls toward the nucleus. Aggrecan, in contrast, has its highest concentration in the nucleus and lowest in the outer annulus and endplate. With age, aggrecan in the nucleus falls steeply as does water, while collagen rises; a similar change is seen with degeneration (42). The mechanism for these proportional changes appears to be loss of aggrecan rather than an increase in the amount of collagen that is produced and laid down.

Swelling Pressure, Mechanical Load, and Hydration

The mechanical role of collagen and aggrecan are understood to some extent and can be explained using a model suggested initially by Szirmai (50) and built by Broom and Marra (5). The model consists of a string network filled with balloons. The balloons inflate the network, putting the string under tension while the string holds the balloons in place. Neither component on its own is able to support load; the string would collapse and the balloons would fly apart. Together, however, they can withstand tensile and compressive loads with the degree of deformation under load depending on the magnitude of the load and the architecture and knots (crosslinks) of the string network and the number and degree of inflation of the balloons. A network containing a few floppy balloons will deform more than one stuffed full of highly inflated balloons. In the disc, the collagen network assumes the role of the string, while the role of the balloons is fulfilled by water drawn into the disc and held in it by aggrecan.

Little is known about how the collagen network organization affects the disc's mechanical properties. However, the lamellar arrangement of the collagen network in humans is by no means as simple as that represented in most schematic drawings of the disc (52) as the lamellae do not form perfect concentric rings. Many of the lamellae are incomplete and vary in thickness and they join or split (34); with aging they become more disorganized. The effect of these changes on the disc's mechanical properties is unknown. More is understood of the role of aggrecan. Aggrecan, on account of the highly sulfated glycosaminoglycan (GAG) chains, has a high swelling pressure that inflates the disc; the degree of inflation depends on the applied load and on the aggrecan content (57). A disc with a low aggrecan content will hold less water under any load than a normal disc (57).

The water content of the disc depends on the pressure applied to the disc by external loads and on aggrecan content (Fig. 2.1). Disc pressure arises more from muscular activity than from body weight and thus varies with posture and movement. In human lumbar discs, pressure is lowest when lying prone (at around 0.1 to 0.2 MPa) and increases five- to eightfold when standing or sitting (40). In order to maintain osmotic equilibrium fluid is expressed with increase in pressure but because of the disc's size and low hydraulic permeability, water loss is slow and equilibration takes many hours; thus the disc rarely achieves osmotic equilibrium. In humans, around 20% to 25% of the disc's water is expressed due to high loads imposed by muscle tensions during the day's activity, this is

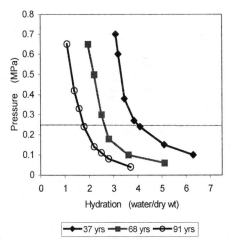
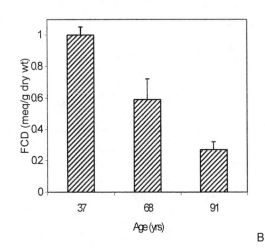

A   B

FIG. 2.1. A: Typical variation in disc swelling pressure with age. At a pressure of 0.25 MPa (three atmospheres) the hydration of the 37-year-old disc is around 4 g water per g dry weight, whereas that of the 91-year-old disc is around 1.8 g water per g dry weight. **B:** Aggrecan content, expressed as fixed charge density, of the same discs, showing the strong dependence of swelling pressure on fixed charge density. (Adapted from Urban JPG, McMullin JF. Swelling pressure of the intervertebral disc: influence of proteoglycan and collagen contents. *Biorheology* 1985;22:145–157, with permission.)

regained during the decrease in load under rest at night (3). This cyclic change in fluid content is thought to be responsible for the oscillating length of the spine (10), while increase of disc hydration under weightlessness can also account for the height gain experienced in space flight (6).

Solute Permeability: Normal Discs and Antibiotics

Aggrecan has another important role apart from regulating the disc's swelling pressure; it also governs movement of solutes through the disc. Aggrecan is negatively charged because of the presence of sulfated GAGs; positively charged molecules such as small cations are attracted into the tissue but negatively charged molecules are repelled to some extent (56). Aggrecan also confers on the disc a low effective "pore" size. Serum proteins, growth factor-binding protein complexes, and other large molecules are effectively excluded from the disc. Studies on antibiotic penetration into the disc have shown this to be important practically in treatment. Positively charged antibiotics such as gentamicin or tobramycin penetrate into the disc to a much greater extent than negatively charged penicillins or cephalosporins (53) and the charge on antibiotics should be considered when deciding on treatment of the intervertebral disc.

DISC CELLS

The disc also contains cells. Although these cells occupy only about 1% of tissue volume, their role is vital in maintaining the health of the disc (Fig. 2.2). The main function of the disc's cells is to synthesize and maintain an appropriate macromolecular composition. The disc cells produce proteoglycans and other molecules throughout life. They also produce proteases and their inhibitors (9,51). The disc remains healthy while the rate of macromolecular synthesis and breakdown are in balance. However, if the rate of breakdown increases over synthesis, the disc matrix ultimately begins to disintegrate (9,17). Disc degeneration thus results from failure of the disc's cells to produce, maintain, and repair the matrix.

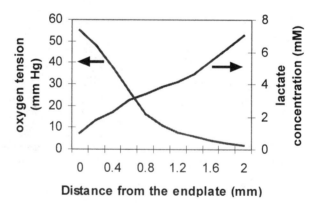

Distance from the endplate (mm)

FIG. 2.2. Schematic view of oxygen and lactate concentration gradients from the endplate toward the disc center in a dog. Oxygen tensions are highest at the disc–bone interface and decrease toward the center as oxygen is consumed by disc cells. Lactate concentrations are highest in the center as lactate is produced by disc cells and falls toward the disc–bone interface where it is removed by the blood supply. (Adapted from Holm S, Maroudas A, Urban JP, et al. Nutrition of the intervertebral disc: solute transport and metabolism. *Connect Tissue Res* 1981;8:101–119, with permission.)

Cell Types

The cell populations of the different regions of the intervertebral disc have different developmental origins. The annulus fibrosus develops embryologically from the mesenchyme while the nucleus pulposus develops from the notochord (59). Early in embryonic development, distinct differences in cellular organization and shape appear in the annulus with the cells of the outer annulus forming sheets of elongated cells orientated obliquely with respect to the axis. In contrast, the cells of the inner annulus remain rounded and chondrocyte-like, do not form distinct lamellae, and produce more matrix (19,48). The cell population of the nucleus varies with age and species. In the early embryo, the cells of the nucleus are notochordal and produce a highly hydrated translucent matrix whose matrix macromolecules differ in some respects from those of mature human discs (12,16) . In adulthood, the cell population varies with species. In some cases such as in rabbit, rat, pig, and nonchondrodystrophoid dogs, notochordal cells persist well into adult life, whereas in cattle, notochordal cells have virtually disappeared by birth (7). In humans, notochordal cells are present in infancy but disappear by 4 to 10 years of age (55,59) when they are replaced by chondrocyte-like cells with long cytoplasm-filled processes (14).

FACTORS INFLUENCING CELL METABOLISM

Effect of Nutrient Supply

Discs are the largest avascular tissues in the body. Cells in the center of an adult lumbar disc are 6 to 8 mm from the nearest blood supply. In order to function and remain viable, the cells require an adequate nutrient supply, and also an efficient means of removing products of metabolism such as lactate. Failure of nutrient supply can affect production of matrix and may even lead to cell death. It is thought to be one possible cause of disc degeneration (15).

Several different studies have indicated that a fall in blood supply or transport into the disc is associated with disc degeneration. In studies of postmortem spines, Kauppila and coworkers find that atherosclerosis of arteries supplies the disc and vertebral bodies correlate with disc degeneration (31). Smoking and vibration, both of which are associated with back pain, lead to decreased transport into the disc, probably through regulation of the peripheral blood supply to the disc (25). The endplates of degenerate and scoliotic discs are calcified, thus impeding nutrient transport into these discs (41).

The disc's metabolism is mainly through glycolysis. The disc produces lactic acid at high concentrations. Disc cells, however, use oxygen so the oxygen supply in the center of even a normal disc is very low (22). Loss of nutrient supply leads to a fall in pO_2, a rise in lactic acid concentration, and thus more acid pH in the disc's center (2,11,39) (Fig. 2.2).

The levels of metabolites have a marked affect on the production of extracellular matrix. Proteoglycan synthesis is maximal at pH 7.0 and 5% oxygen, where it is approximately 40% higher than under standard conditions of air and pH 7.4 (27,29,43) . However, if pH becomes more acidic or oxygen levels fall below 5% O_2, synthesis rates decrease rapidly. At pH 6.3, rates are less than 10% those at pH 7.2. Oxygen and pH however do not have such dramatic effects on production of agents involved in matrix breakdown; the activity of matrix metalloproteinases remains constant between pH 7.2 and pH 6.3. Thus under more acidic and hypoxic conditions the balance of cellular activity is tipped toward matrix degradation.

Effect of Mechanical Stress on Cellular Activity

The disc is subjected to varying mechanical forces at all times. Exposure to heavy mechanical stress over long periods is thought to lead to disc degeneration. It has been suggested that under normal conditions the disc is subjected to Wolff's law (i.e., that applied stress affects cellular activity and the disc remodels to build a matrix which minimizes the stress) (4); high levels of mechanical load are thought, however, to affect cellular activity adversely.

In Vivo *Effects of Load*

Little is known about how load affects cellular activity in normal life. In dogs whose exercise level was increased, there were indications that cell metabolism and proteoglycan and collagen synthesis increased in discs but the effects were not marked, even in dogs running up to 40 km per day (24,47). The evidence that abnormal loads can adversely affect disc cell metabolism is stronger. For instance, it has been long observed that spinal fusion has a deleterious effect on adjacent discs (46). *In vivo* tests that examine the effects of changes in the mechanical stress applied to the disc through spinal fusion (23), in bipedal mice (8,13,20), and after high continuous compressive loading (32) have all found deleterious changes in the disc matrix. In some *in vivo* cases the loading has produced wedged discs (37). These results all support the hypothesis that an abnormal mechanical load, applied to an otherwise healthy disc, can lead to disc degeneration, probably through changes in cellular activity rather than through matrix damage alone.

Cell Reaction to Mechanical Stress

Little is known about the effect of mechanical forces on disc cells in comparison to cells of other load-bearing tissues like bone or cartilage. However it is apparent that disc cells are very sensitive to mechanical signals. With every change in posture, the cells see changes in hydrostatic pressure, deformation, and matrix compaction and fluid expression (58). All these alterations to the environment of the cell may affect its metabolic responses as discussed below.

Hydrostatic Pressure

Hydrostatic pressure rises in the central regions of the disc when it is loaded with pressure level depending on posture and activity (36,38,60). Both isolated cells and explants have been exposed to hydrostatic pressures in the ranges seen physiologically. It has been shown that very short exposures (20 seconds) to a burst of pressure can affect cell metabolism over the following 2 hours, with physiologic pressures (0.2 to 3.0 MPa) stimulating synthesis while higher pressures repress it (28). Longer periods of physiologic pressure application inhibit production of agents involved in cartilage breakdown (18) and affect matrix turnover (26). Surprisingly, only nucleus and inner annulus cells are affected by pressure rise; outer annulus cells show no response to even high levels of pressure (28).

Static Compression and Change in Fluid Content

The disc undergoes a daily loss and regain of around 20% to 25% of its fluid content (3,45). Ohshima and colleagues (44) find that static loading has a strong influence on

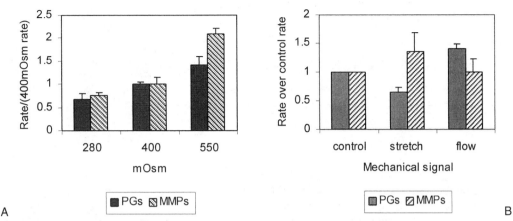

FIG. 2.3. The effect of mechanical signals on production of aggrecan (PGs) and on matrix metalloproteinase (MMP) activity (Bielby 2000, personal communication). **A:** The effect of fluid loss or regain in terms of osmolality. PG production and MMP activity both increase as fluid is expressed and osmolality increases. **B:** The effect of stretch and flow; stretch leads to a fall in PG production and an increase in MMP activity while flow increases PG production but has no effect on MMPs. Since the cells experience all these signals each time load is applied, the overall response is obviously complex and does not appear additive.

proteoglycan production, with synthesis maximal under normal physiologic hydration and falling if the disc swells under low loads, or if water is expressed under high loads (Fig. 2.3). The effect is shown to arise in part from changes in proteoglycan-induced osmotic pressure (30).

Stretch and Flow

Disc cells also appear to respond to deformation. Nucleus cells have been grown in monolayer on surfaces that are then "stretched" and the effect of such mechanical signals measured (35). Although the signals imposed are nonphysiologic as nucleus cells are unlikely to experience strains of the magnitudes tested and also do not attach to surfaces *in situ*, the cells respond strongly to tensile strain by increasing proliferation and collagen production; the response indicates the cells' potential to react even to mechanical signals not routinely encountered.

Overall Responses to Mechanical Stress

These *in vitro* tests have shown that disc cells are very responsive to mechanical signals such as pressure, compression, and stretch and that these signals lead to alterations in production of both proteoglycans and proteases (Fig. 2.3). However, the disc cells do not see these signals separately; during every application of load the signals are applied together at varying magnitudes and varying durations. Under normal conditions, the cell integrates these signals to produce a matrix appropriate for the load seen, but at present we understand little of this process. Change in customary mechanical stress could therefore potentially influence turnover of the matrix and ultimately disc composition and structure. (Scoliotic discs are an extreme example of the effects of mechanical stress on disc composition.) At present, however, it is difficult to relate these *in vitro* results to the disc's responses to load *in vivo*.

OTHER FACTORS INFLUENCING DISC CELL ACTIVITY

Disc cells also respond to and produce growth factors and cytokines such as interleukin-1 (1,33,49,54) . This aspect of disc cell behavior, though possibly very important, has not yet been thoroughly investigated.

CONCLUSIONS

An intact and well-organized extracellular matrix is vital for disc function. Appropriate cellular function is necessary to maintain this matrix throughout life. Very little is yet known about disc cells and the factors that regulate them. However, it is clear that ultimately disc degeneration arises from a failure of cellular activity. If we are to understand why the disc degenerates so early with possibly distressing consequences, we need to know how to protect these vital cells and how to influence them to produce and repair the disc matrix.

ACKNOWLEDGMENTS

This work was supported by the ARC (U0507).

REFERENCES

1. Ashton IK, Risley GL, Eisenstein SM. IL1-beta induces nitric-oxide production in intervertebral disc cells invitro. *J Orthop Rheumatol* 1995;8:151–154.
2. Bartels EM, Fairbank JCT, Winlove CP, et al. Oxygen and lactate concentrations measured in vivo in the intervertebral discs of scoliotic and back pain patients. *Spine* 1998;23:1–8.
3. Boos N, Wallin A, Gbedegbegnon T, et al. Quantitative MR imaging of lumbar intervertebral disks and vertebral bodies: influence of diurnal water content variations. *Radiology* 1993;188:351–354.
4. Brickley-Parsons D, Glimcher M. Is the chemistry of collagen in the intervertebral disc an expression of Wolff's law? A study of the human lumbar spine. *Spine* 1984;9:148–163.
5. Broom ND, Marra DL. New structural concepts of articular cartilage demonstrated with a physical model. *Connect Tissue Res* 1985;14:1–8.
6. Brown JW. Crew height measurement. The Apollo–Soyuz test project: medical report. *NASA* 1977;SP411.
7. Butler WF. Comparative anatomy and development of the mammalian disc. In: Ghosh P, ed. *The biology of the intervertebral disc*. Boca Raton: CRC Press, 1989:84–108.
8. Cassidy J, Yong-Hing M, Kirkaldy-Willis W, et al. A study of the effects of bipedalism and upright posture on the lumbosacral spine and paravertebral muscles of the Wistar rat. *Spine* 1988;13:301–308.
9. Crean JK, Roberts S, Jaffray DC, et al. Matrix metalloproteinases in the human intervertebral disc: role in disc degeneration and scoliosis. *Spine* 1997;22:2877–2884.
10. DePuky P. The physiological oscillation of the length of the body. *Acta Orthop Scand* 1935;6:338–348.
11. Diamant B, Karlsson J, Nachemson A. Correlation between lactate levels and pH in discs of patients with lumbar rhizopathies. *Experientia* 1968;24:1195–1196.
12. Domowicz M, Li H, Hennig A, et al. The biochemically and immunologically distinct CSPG of notochord is a product of the aggrecan gene. *Dev Biol* 1995;171:655–664.
13. Dong F, Dai K, Hou X. Changes of proteoglycans in lumbar intervertebral disc of bipedal rats with aging [in Chinese]. *Chung Hua I Hsueh Tsa Chih* 1995;75:352–383.
14. Errington RJ, Puustjarvi K, White IF, et al. Characterisation of cytoplasm-filled processes in cells of the intervertebral disc. *J Anat* 1998;192:369–378.
15. Eyre DR, Caterson B, Benya P, et al. The intervertebral disc. In: Gordon S, Frymoyer J, eds. *New perspectives on low back pain*. Philadelphia: American Institute of Orthopedic Surgery, 1991:147–209.
16. Gotz W, Kasper M, Miosge N, et al. Detection and distribution of the carbohydrate binding protein galectin-3 in human notochord, intervertebral disc and chordoma. *Differentiation* 1997;62:149–157.

17. Goupille P, Jayson MI, Valat JP, et al. Matrix metalloproteinases: the clue to intervertebral disc degeneration? *Spine* 1998;23:1612–1626.
18. Handa T, Ishihara H, Ohshima H, et al. Effects of hydrostatic pressure on matrix synthesis and matrix metallo-proteinase production in the human lumbar intervertebral disc. *Spine* 1997;22:1085–1091.
19. Hayes AJ, Benjamin M, Ralphs JR. Role of actin stress fibres in the development of the intervertebral disc: cytoskeletal control of extracellular matrix assembly. *Dev Dynamics* 1999;215:179–189.
20. Higuchi M, Abe K, Kaneda K. Changes in the nucleus pulposus of the intervertebral disc in bipedal mice. A light and electron microscopic study. *Clin Orthop* 1983;251–257.
21. Hirsch C, Schajowicz F. Studies on structural changes in the lumbar annulus fibrosus. *Acta Orthop Scand* 1952;22:184–231.
22. Holm S, Maroudas A, Urban JP, et al. Nutrition of the intervertebral disc: solute transport and metabolism. *Connect.Tissue Res* 1981;8:101–119.
23. Holm S, Nachemson A. Nutritional changes in the canine intervertebral disc after spinal fusion. *Clin Orthop* 1982;169:243–258.
24. Holm S, Nachemson A. Variation in the nutrition of the canine intervertebral disc induced by motion. *Spine* 1983;8:866–874.
25. Holm S, Nachemson A. Nutrition of the intervertebral disc: acute effects of cigarette smoking. An experimental animal study. *Ups J Med Sci* 1988;93:91–99.
26. Hutton WC, Elmer WA, Boden SD, et al. The effect of hydrostatic pressure on intervertebral disc metabolism. *Spine* 1999;24:1507–1515.
27. Ichimura K, Tsuji H, Matsui H, et al. Cell culture of the intervertebral disc of rats: factors influencing culture, proteoglycan, collagen, and deoxyribonucleic acid synthesis. *J Spinal Disord* 1991;4:428–436.
28. Ishihara H, McNally DS, Urban JG, et al. Effects of hydrostatic pressure on matrix synthesis in different regions of the intervertebral disk. *J Appl Physiol* 1996;80:839–846.
29. Ishihara H, Urban JP. Effects of low oxygen concentrations and metabolic inhibitors on proteoglycan and protein synthesis rates in the intervertebral disc. *J Orthop Res* 1999;17:829–835.
30. Ishihara H, Warensjo K, Roberts S, et al. Proteoglycan synthesis in the intervertebral disk nucleus: the role of extracellular osmolality. *Am J Physiol* 1997;272:C1499–C1506.
31. Kauppila LI, Penttila A, Karhunen PJ, et al. Lumbar disc degeneration and atherosclerosis of the abdominal aorta. *Spine* 1994;19:923–929.
32. Lotz JC, Colliou OK, Chin JR, et al. 1998 Volvo Award winner in biomechanical studies — Compression-induced degeneration of the intervertebral disc: an in vivo mouse model and finite-element study. *Spine* 1998;23:2493–2506.
33. Maeda S, Kokubun S. Changes with age in proteoglycan synthesis in cells cultured in vitro from the inner and outer rabbit annulus fibrosus. Responses to interleukin-1 and interleukin-1 receptor antagonist protein. *Spine* 2000;25:166–169.
34. Marchand F, Ahmed AM. Investigation of the laminate structure of lumbar disc annulus fibrosus. *Spine* 1990;15:402–410.
35. Matsumoto T, Kawakami M, Kuribayashi K, et al. Cyclic mechanical stretch stress increases the growth rate and collagen synthesis of nucleus pulposus cells in vitro. *Spine* 1999;24:315–319.
36. McNally DS. Biomechanics of the intervertebral disc—disc pressure measurements and significance. In: Aspden RM, Porter RW, eds. *Lumbar spine disorders: current concepts*. Singapore: World Scientific Publishing Co, 1995:42–50.
37. Mente PL, Aronsson DD, Stokes IA, et al. Mechanical modulation of growth for the correction of vertebral wedge deformities. *J Orthop Res* 1999;17:518–524.
38. Nachemson A. Lumbar intradiscal pressure. *Acta Orthop Scand* 1960[Suppl 43]:1–104.
39. Nachemson A. Intradiscal measurements of pH in patients with lumbar rhizopathies. *Acta Orthop Scand* 1969;40:23–42.
40. Nachemson A, Elfstrom G. Intravital dynamic pressure measurements in lumbar discs. A study of common movements, maneuvers and exercises. *Scand J Rehabil Med* 1970;2 [Suppl 1]:1–40.
41. Nachemson A, Lewin T, Maroudas A, et al. In vitro diffusion of dye through the end-plates and annulus fibrosus of human lumbar intervertebral discs. *Acta Orthop Scand* 1970;41:589–607.
42. Oegema TR. Biochemistry of the intervertebral disc. *Clin Sports Med* 1993;12:419–439.
43. Ohshima H, Urban JPG. Effect of lactate concentrations and pH on matrix synthesis rates in the intervertebral disc. *Spine* 1992;17:1079–1082.
44. Ohshima H, Urban JPG, Bergel DH. The effect of static load on matrix synthesis rates in the intervertebral disc measured in vitro by a new perfusion technique. *J Orthop Res* 1995;13:22–29.
45. Paajanen H, Lehto I, Alanen A, et al. Diurnal fluid changes of lumbar discs measured indirectly by magnetic resonance imaging. *J Orthop Res* 1994;12:509–514.
46. Penta M, Sandhu A, Fraser RD. Magnetic resonance imaging assessment of disc degeneration 10 years after anterior lumbar interbody fusion. *Spine* 1996;20:743–747.
47. Puustjarvi K, Lammi M, Kiviranta I, et al. Proteoglycan synthesis in canine intervertebral discs after long distance running training. *J Orthop Res* 1993;11:738–746.
48. Rufei A, Benjamin M, Ralphs JR. The development of fibrocartilage in the rat intervertebral disc. *Anat Embryol* 1995 (*in press*).

49. Shinmei M, Kikuchi T, Yamagishi M, et al. The role of interleukin-1 on proteoglycan metabolism of rabbit annulus fibrosus cells cultured in vitro. *Spine* 1988;13:1284–1290.

50. Szirmai JA. Structure of the intervertebral disc. In: Balazs EA, ed. *Chemistry and molecular biology of the intercellular matrix.* New York: Academic Press, 1970:1279–1308.

51. Sztrolovics R, Alini M, Roughley PJ, et al. Aggrecan degradation in human intervertebral disc and articular cartilage. *Biochem J* 1997;326:235–241.

52. Takeda T. Three-dimensional observations of collagen framework of human lumbar discs. *J Japan Orthop Assoc* 1975;49:45–57.

53. Thomas RdM, Batten JJ, Want S, et al. A new in-vitro model to investigate antibiotic penetration of the intervertebral disc. *J Bone Joint Surg* 1995;77-B:967–970.

54. Thompson JP, Oegema TR, Bradford DS. Stimulation of mature canine intervertebral disc by growth factors. *Spine* 1991;16:253–260.

55. Trout JJ, Buckwalter JA, Moore KC, et al. Ultrastructure of the human intervertebral disc. I. Changes in notochordal cells with age. *Tissue Cell* 1982;14:359–369.

56. Urban J, Maroudas A. Measurement of the fixed charge density and partition coefficients in the intervertebral disc. *BBA* 1992;586:166–178.

57. Urban JPG, McMullin JF. Swelling pressure of the intervertebral disc: influence of proteoglycan and collagen contents. *Biorheology* 1985;22:145–157.

58. Urban JG. The chondrocyte—a cell under pressure. *Br J Rheumatol* 1994;33:901–908.

59. Walmsley R. The development and growth of the intervertebral disc. *Edinburgh Med J* 1953;60:341–364.

60. Wilke HJ, Neef P, Caimi M, et al. New in vivo measurements of pressures in the intervertebral disc in daily life. *Spine* 1999;24:755–762.

3

Disc Herniation and Sciatica: The Basic Science Platform

Kjell Olmarker and Björn Rydevik

The lumbosacral nerve roots have been known to be intimately involved in disc herniation and sciatica for more than six decades (19). However, the basic pathophysiologic mechanisms are still not well understood. Over the last decade there has been an increasing interest in this topic. Recent research has been aimed at defining basic pathophysiologic events at the cellular or subcellular level responsible for the pathophysiology of sciatic pain. In this chapter, the current knowledge about these mechanisms will be discussed. The symptoms of sciatica may be divided into two main categories: pain and nerve dysfunction (26). The pain of sciatica is the typically radiating pain that may be related to a specific nerve root and commonly extends below the knee. Nerve dysfunction may be present in both motor and sensory modalities thus producing both motor weakness and sensory disturbances. One may assume that pain and nerve dysfunction are due to different pathophysiologic events, but because they usually coincide in sciatica, it is indicated that the pathophysiology of this disorder is very complex.

PATHOPHYSIOLOGY OF NERVE ROOT INVOLVEMENT

Two specific mechanisms for nerve root injury at the "tissue level" may be defined: (a) mechanical deformation of the nerve roots and (b) biologic or biochemical activity of the disc tissue with effects on the roots. The mechanical deformation theory is the oldest concept of nerve root injury induced by herniated disc tissue. This theory dates back partly to the beginning of the twentieth century when some clinical observations on injuries in the lumbosacral junction with subsequent leg pain were made, primarily to Mixter and Barr's early observations (3,11,26,37). The theory that biologic activity of the disc tissue may injure the nerve roots was just recently confirmed experimentally (24). These biologic mechanisms will be discussed here.

The clinical picture of sciatica with a characteristic distribution of pain and nerve dysfunction, but in the absence of herniated disc material both at x-ray examination and at surgery, has indicated that the mechanical component is not the only factor that may be responsible for sciatic pain. It has therefore been suggested that the disc tissue per se may have some injurious properties that may be of pathophysiologic significance (35). However, it has only been recently confirmed in an experimental setting that local, epidural application of autologous nucleus pulposus in the pig, with no mechanical deformation, induces significant changes in both structure and function of the adjacent nerve roots (24). This finding has opened up a new field of research. The knowledge gathered thus far is reviewed below.

Biologic Effects of Nucleus Pulposus

After placing autologous nucleus pulposus, obtained from a lumbar disc in a rabbit, onto the tibial nerve in a rabbit model, no changes in either nerve function or structure were observed (34). However, certain differences in microscopic anatomy and vascular permeability between peripheral nerves and nerve roots make the extrapolation from peripheral nerve experiments to spinal conditions difficult. McCarron and associates applied autologous nucleus pulposus from discs of dogs' tails in the epidural space of a dog (18). They observed an epidural inflammatory reaction that did not occur when saline was injected as control. The nerve tissue, however, was not assessed in this study.

Olmarker and colleagues recently presented a study demonstrating autologous nucleus pulposus may induce a reduction in nerve conduction velocity and light microscopic structural changes in a pig cauda equina model (Figs. 3.1, 3.2, and 3.3) (24). However, these axonal changes have a focal distribution and the quantity of injured axons is too low to be responsible for the significant neurophysiologic dysfunction observed. A follow-up study of areas of the nerve roots exposed to nucleus pulposus, and that appeared to be normal in the light microscope, revealed significant injuries of the Schwann cells with vacuolization and disintegration of the Schmidt-Lanterman incisures (28). The Schmidt-Lanterman incisures are essential for the normal exchange of ions between the axon and the surrounding tissues. An injury to this structure would therefore be likely to interfere with the normal impulse conduction properties of the axons. However, the distribution of changes is also too limited to fully explain the neurophysiologic dysfunction observed. For instance, a recent study that demonstrated freezing of the nucleus pulposus prevents the reduction in nerve conduction velocity also demonstrated these characteristic changes histologically in spite of normal nerve conduction (29). The potency of the nucleus pulposus, however, was further emphasized in an experiment using a dog model where it was

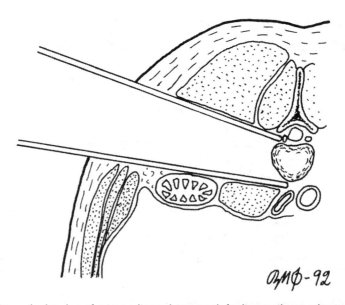

FIG. 3.1. Schematic drawing of retroperitoneal approach for harvesting nucleus pulposus from the L3-L4 intervertebral disc. (From Olmarker K, et al. Autologous nucleus pulposus induces neurophysiologic and histologic changes in porcine cauda equina nerve roots. *Spine* 1993; 18:11:1425–1432, with permission.)

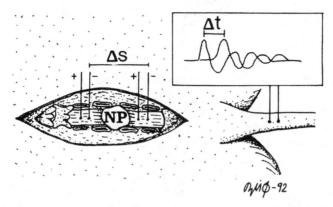

FIG. 3.2. Procedure for determination of nerve root conduction velocity. The cauda equina is stimulated cranial and caudal to the segment exposed to nucleus pulposus or control. The difference in distance (Δs) between these two stimulation sites is divided by the time difference (Δt) between the first peaks of the two recordings. (From Olmarker K, et al. Autologous nucleus pulposus induces neurophysiologic and histologic changes in porcine cauda equina nerve roots. *Spine* 1993;18:11:1425–1432, with permission.)

seen that a surgical incision of the annulus fibrosus, with minimal leakage of nucleus pulposus, was enough to induce significant changes in structure and function of the adjacent nerve root (13).

Since there is not a structural correlate to the functional changes, recent studies have assessed the potential effects of nucleus pulposus on the nerve root nutrition. It has thereby been seen that epidural application of autologous nucleus pulposus within 2 hours induces an intraneural edema (6) that within 3 hours leads to a reduction of the intraneural blood flow (6,7,31). Histologic changes of the nerve roots are present after 3 hours (5), and a subsequent reduction of the nerve conduction velocity will start between 3 to 24 hours after application (5,24).

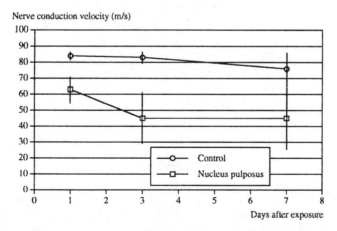

FIG. 3.3. Nerve conduction velocity for nerve roots exposed to retroperitoneal fat (control) and nucleus pulposus. Error bars indicate standard deviation. (From Olmarker K, et al. Autologous nucleus pulposus induces neurophysiologic and histologic changes in porcine cauda equina nerve roots. *Spine* 1993;18:11:1425–1432, with permission.)

From these initial experiments, it could therefore be concluded that nucleus pulposus has significant properties to injure the nerve roots after local application. However, the mechanisms for the nucleus pulposus-induced nerve root injury are not yet fully understood. There are indications in these studies that inflammatory reactions are present, at least epidurally. This initiated a study in which methylprednisolone, a potent antiinflammatory agent, was administered at different times intravenously after nucleus pulposus application (25). The results show clearly that the nucleus pulposus-induced reduction in nerve conduction velocity is eliminated if methylprednisolone is administered within 24 hours of application. If methylprednisolone is administered within 48 hours, the effect is not eliminated but is significantly lower than if no drug is used. This observation indicates that the negative effect does not occur immediately but will develop during the first 24 hours after application. However, if methylprednisolone is administered within 24 hours, there are still areas in the nerve roots demonstrating normal impulse conduction properties that have light microscopic axonal changes in the same magnitude as in the previous study (24). This further corroborates the impression that the structural nerve injury inducing nerve dysfunction may not be found at the light microscopic level but must be sought for at the subcellular level.

Although methylprednisolone may intervene with the pathophysiologic events of the nucleus pulposus-induced nerve root injury, it was not clear if this was due to the antiinflammatory properties of the methylprednisolone or some other property. To establish if the presence of autologous nucleus pulposus could initiate a leukotactic response from the surrounding tissues, a study was initiated to assess the potential inflammatogenic properties of the nucleus pulposus (27). Autologous nucleus pulposus and autologous retroperitoneal fat were placed in separate small perforated titanium-chambers and placed subcutaneously, together with a sham chamber, in a pig. Seven days later, the number of leukocytes was assessed for the chambers. The number of leukocytes was the same between the fat and the sham chambers. However, the chambers containing the nucleus pulposus had a number of leukocytes that exceeded the two others by 250%. Also, when injected locally in contact with the microvasculature of the hamster cheek pouch, nucleus pulposus induced an increase in permeability for macromolecules that was not present if the animals were simultaneously treated with indomethacin (27). In another experiment, autologous nucleus pulposus and muscle were placed in Gore-Tex tubes subcutaneously in rabbits (40). After 2 weeks, there was an accumulation of macrophages, T-helper cells, and T-suppressor cells in the tube with nucleus pulposus that persisted the full observation time of 4 weeks. Recent studies have confirmed that treatment of dogs subjected to disc incision with indomethacin reduces the effects on nerve conduction velocity (1). This further supports the impression that autologous nucleus pulposus may elicit inflammatory reactions when outside the intervertebral disc space.

Components of the Nucleus Pulposus

The nucleus pulposus mainly comprises proteoglycans, collagen, and cells (4,10). The observed effects as induced by the nucleus pulposus at local application should therefore probably be related to one or more of these components. The proteoglycans are the component that has gained the most attention and has been suggested to have a direct irritating effect on the nerve tissue (16,17,22). Neither the collagen nor the cells have previously been suggested to be of pathophysiologic importance. However, recent studies of the cells of the nucleus pulposus show that these cells are capable of producing metalloproteases such as collagenase or gelatinase, as well as interleukin-6 and prostaglandin E_2, and do so spontaneously in culture (12). Using the same pig model as described previously, the possible role of the nucleus pulposus cells for the nucleus pulposus-induced nerve injury has been assessed (29). In a blinded fashion, autologous nucleus pulposus was subjected to 24 hours of freezing at −20°C, digestion by hyaluronidase, or just a heating box at 37°C for 24 hours. The treated nucleus pulposus was reapplied after 24 hours and analyses were performed 7 days later. It was evident that in animals where the nucleus pulposus had been frozen, and the cells thus killed, there were no changes in nerve conduction velocity, whereas in the other two series, the results were similar to the previous study (24). It therefore seems reasonable to believe that the cells have been responsible in some way for inducing the nerve injury and that the structural molecules should be of less importance. This assumption is further supported by a recent study using the same model, which shows that application of cultured pig disc cells to the cauda equina reproduce the reduction in nerve conduction velocity (14). However, application of disc cell membranes also reproduce this reduction, indicating that the responsible substances probably are membrane-bound.

Substances like immunoglobulin G, hydrogen ions, and phospholipase A2 (PLA2) have previously been suggested to be responsible for the pathophysiologic reactions (9,21,23,32,36). However, tumor necrosis factor (TNF) is another substance found in disc cells, which exists both in the cytoplasm and also in a membrane-bound form, that can be intimately involved in the early pathophysiologic phases (30). TNF may induce both thrombus formation and increased vascular permeability (15,33), and seems to be closely related to neuropathic pain (20,39). Injected into nerve fascicles it produces histologic changes similar to those seen in nerve roots exposed to nucleus pulposus (38). Cyclosporin A, an immunosupressor that acts by interfering with TNF has been found to efficiently block the nucleus pulposus-induced reduction of nerve conduction velocity caused by incising lumbar discs in dogs (2,8). TNF will also initiate inflammatory reactions locally by stimulation and recruitment of inflammatory cells of the host. TNF thus seems to be one interesting candidate substance for the early phases of nucleus pulposus-induced nerve injury. However, one should be aware that pathophysiologic processes are complex events, with multiple interactions at molecular, cellular, and tissue levels, and that a considerable number of substances and mechanisms may be involved.

CONCLUSIONS

The pathophysiology of sciatica is a complex event with numerous substances and mechanisms acting at various levels. Recently, these mechanisms have attracted the attention of basic scientists, and thus a number of studies exploring these pathophysiologic events have been published. Disc-related cytokines, in particular TNF, have been suggested to be intimately involved in the pathophysiology of acute sciatica and clinical trials using selective inhibition of cytokines have been initiated. It is hoped that this may lead to a direct and efficient way to pharmacologically manage this very common and expensive spinal disorder.

ACKNOWLEDGMENTS

Based on research supported by the Swedish Research Council (#8685).

REFERENCES

1. Arai I, Mao GP, Otani K, et al. Indomethacin blocks nucleus pulposus-related effects in adjacent nerve roots. *Eur Spine J* (*in press*).
2. Arai I, Konno S, Otani K, et al. Cyclosporin A blocks the toxic effects of nucleus pulposus on spinal nerve roots. Submitted.
3. Bailey P, Casamajor L. Osteo-arthritis of the spine as a cause of compression of the spinal cord and its roots. With report of 5 cases. *J Nerv Ment Dis* 1911;38:588–609.
4. Bayliss MT, Johnstone B. Biochemistry of the intervertebral disc. In: Jayson MIV, ed. *The lumbar spine and back pain*. New York: Churchill Livingstone, 1992:111–131.
5. Byröd G, Olmarker K, Nordborg C, et al. Early effects of nucleus pulposus application on spinal nerve root morphology and function. *Eur Spine J* 1998;7:445–449.
6. Byröd G, Otani K, Brisby H, et al. Methylprednisolone reduces the early vascular permeability increase in spinal nerve roots induced by epidural nucleus pulposus application. J Orthop Res 2000 (*in press*).
7. Byröd G, Rydevik B, Johansson BR, et al. Transport of epidurally applied horseradish peroxidase to the endoneurial space of dorsal root ganglia. A light and electron microscopic study. *J Per Nerv Syst* 2000 (*in press*).
8. Dawson J, Hurtenbach U, MacKenzie A. Cyclosporin A inhibits the in vivo production of interleukin-1beta and tumor necrosis factor alpha, but not interleukin-6, by a T-cell-independent mechanism. *Cytokine* 1996;8(12): 882–888.
9. Diamant B, Karlsson J, Nachemson A. Correlation between lactate levels and pH in discs of patients with lumbar rhizopathies. *Experienta* 1968;24:1195–1196.
10. Eyre D, Benya P, Buckwalter J, et al. Basic science perspectives. In: Frymoyer JW, Gordon SL, eds. *Intervertebral disc. New perspectives on low back pain*. American Academy of Orthopaedic Surgeons Symposium, Airlie, VA 1988:149–207.
11. Goldthwait JE. The lumbo-sacral articulation. An explanation of many cases of "lumbago", "sciatica" and paraplegia. *Boston Med Surg J* 1911;164:365–372.
12. Kang JD, Georgescu HI, MacIntyre-Larkin L, et al. Herniated lumbar intervertebral discs spontaneously produce matrix metalloproteinases, nitric oxide, interleukin-6 and prostaglandin E2. *Spine* 1996 21:(3): 271–277.
13. Kayama S, Konno S, Olmarker K, et al. Incision of the annulus fibrosus induces nerve root morphologic, vascular and functional changes. *Spine* 1996;21:2539–2543.
14. Kayama S, Olmarker K, Larsson K, et al. Cultured, autologous nucleus pulposus cells induce structural and functional changes in spinal nerve roots. *Spine* 1998;23:20:2155–2158.
15. Koga S, Morris S, Ogawa S, et al. TNF modulates endothelial properties by decreasing cAMP. *Am J Physiol* 1995;268:(5pt1):C1104–1113.
16. Marshall LL, Trethewie ER. Chemical irritation of nerve-root in disc prolapse. *Lancet* 1973;2:320.
17. Marshall LL, Trethewie ER, Curtain CC. Chemical radiculitis. *Clin Orthop* 1977;129:61–67.
18. McCarron RF, Wimpee MW, Hudkins P, et al. The inflammatory effect of nucleus pulposus. A possible element in the pathogenesis of low-back pain. *Spine* 1987;12:8:760–764.
19. Mixter WJ, Barr JS. Rupture of the intervertebral disc with involvement of the spinal canal. *New Engl J Med* 1934;211:210–215.
20. Myers RR. The pathogenesis of neuropathic pain. *Reg Anaesth* 1995;20:173–184.
21. Naylor A. The biophysical and biochemical aspects of intervertebral disc herniation and degeneration. *Ann R Col Surg Engl* 1962;31:91–114.
22. Naylor A. Biochemical changes in human intervertebral disk degeneration and prolapse. *Orthop Clin N Am* 1971;2:2:343.
23. Nachemson A. Intradiscal measurements of pH in patients with lumbar rhizopathies. *Acta Orthop Scand* 1969; 40:23–42.
24. Olmarker K, Rydevik B, Nordborg C. Autologous nucleus pulposus induces neurophysiologic and histologic changes in porcine cauda equina nerve roots. *Spine* 1993;18:11:1425–1432.
25. Olmarker K, Byröd G, Cornefjord M, et al. Effects of methyl-prednisolone on nucleus pulposus-induced nerve root injury. *Spine* 1994;19:16:1803–1808.
26. Olmarker K, Hasue M. Classification and pathophysiology of spinal pain syndromes. In: JN Weinstein, B Rydevik, eds. *Essentials of the spine*. New York: Raven Press, 1995.
27. Olmarker K, Blomquist J, Strömberg J, et al. Inflammatogenic properties of nucleus pulposus. *Spine* 1995;20: 6,665–669.
28. Olmarker K, Rydevik B, Nordborg C. Ultrastructural changes in spinal nerve roots induced by autologous nucleus pulposus. *Spine* 1996;21:411–414.
29. Olmarker K, Brisby H, Yabuki S, et al. The effects of normal, frozen and hyaluronidase digested nucleus pulposus on nerve root structure and function. *Spine* 1997;24:471–475.
30. Olmarker K, Larsson K. TNFα and nucleus pulposus-induced nerve root injury. *Spine* 1998;23:2538–2544.
31. Otani K, Arai I, Mao GP, et al. Nucleus pulposus-induced nerve root injury: relationship between blood flow and nerve conduction velocity. *J Neurosurg* 1999;45(3):614–619.
32. Pennington JB, McCarron RF, Laros GS. Identification of IgG in the canine intervertebral disc. *Spine* 1988;13: 909–912.

33. Rowlinson-Busza G, Maraveyas A, Epenetos AA. Effects of tumor necrosis factor on the uptake of specific and control monoclonal antibodies in a human tumor xenograft model. *Br J Cancer* 1995;71:4:660–665.
34. Rydevik B, Brown MD, Ehira T, et al. Effects of graded compression and nucleus pulposus on nerve tissue: an experimental study in rabbits. *Acta Orthop Scand* 1983;54:670–671.
35. Rydevik B, Brown MD, Lundborg G. Pathoanatomy and pathophysiology of nerve root compression. *Spine* 1984;9:7–15.
36. Saal JS, Franson RC, Dobrow R, et al. High levels of inflammatory phospholipase A2 activity in lumbar disc herniations. *Spine* 1990;15:674–678.
37. Sachs B, Fraenkel J. Progressive anchylotic rigidity of the spine. *J Nerve Ment Dis* 1900;27:1–15.
38. Selmaj KW, Raine CS. Tumor necrosis factor mediates myelin and oligodendrocyte damage in vitro. *Ann Neurol* 1988;23(4):339–346.
39. Sorkin LS, Xiao WH, Wagner R, et al. TNF-alpha applied to the sciatic nerve trunk elicits background firing in nociceptive primary afferents fibers. 8th World Congress for Pain, August 1996. *IASP abstracts.* Vancouver: IASP Press, 1996:354.
40. Takino T, Takahashi K, Miyazaki T, et al. Immunoreactivity of nucleus pulposus. Trans. International Society for the Study of the Lumbar Spine; Helsinki, Finland, 1995:107.

SECTION 2

Pathology

4

Schmorl's Nodes: Are They Herniations?

J. Assheuer

SCHMORL'S FINDINGS

In 1926, at the annual meeting of the Deutsche Orthopädische Gesellschaft at Cologne, Schmorl described displacement of nucleus material through the cartilaginous plate and bony endplate (34). The lesions seem to start with hemispheric bulging of the endplates in the second decade of growth or even in childhood (Fig. 4.1). The bulging occurs mainly in a restricted area opposite the nucleus and by this appearance it is different from the concave shape of the osteoporotic vertebra. The force that causes the cartilaginous plate to bulge is the turgor of the nucleus. If the pressure of the nucleus becomes higher than the retaining strength of the cartilaginous plate, fissures appear in the plate through which the nucleus material is pressed into the spongious bone (Fig. 4.2). This may happen even by minor additional load to the spine if the bony endplate is weak enough.

Weak points are the former location of the chorda, former vessel channels and ossification gaps, or disturbances of the endochondral growth. The affected levels are in the lower thoracic and upper lumbar spine.

Bulging and displacement of nucleus material may be present in one, but mostly in several subsequent segments. The upper endplate is more often affected than the lower.

In older persons degenerative processes may lead to weakness of the cartilaginous plate with fissures into which nucleus material will be pressed, leading to further weakness of the endplate (Fig. 4.3). Additional load may provoke fractures, opening the spongious space for displacement of nucleus material into it. Fractures of the endplates may also occur in osteoporotic situations or in every disease which effects the stability of the endplate.

The displaced nucleus material seems to undergo different modifications. The progress of displacement may be stopped by reaction of the surrounding spongious bone forming a sclerotic shield. This is the case mainly for the protruded nucleus. The displaced nucleus material induces atrophy of the trabeculae, forming holes. From the walls cartilaginous growth starts forming a node—the "Knorpelknoten"—replacing the nucleus material (Fig. 4.4). This replacement is often incomplete and fibers of the disc remain, passing from the disc into the node. Secondary to the development of the node, vascularization and fibrosation of the disc may occur. If the repair by the cartilaginous transformation or the sclerotic shield is insufficient, the displacement may progress. At the moment when peripheral cartilaginous growth starts, Schmorl thought that the expression "discus herniation or nucleus herniation" could be adopted as it was used first by Geipel.

In 1920, Scheuermann described a kyphotic malformation in adolescents which was different from kyphosis due to infection, mainly tuberculosis, or to degenerative diseases in older patients (33). This malformation develops around puberty and affects mainly the segments Th6 to Th11. It is characterized radiographically by one or more wedge-shaped

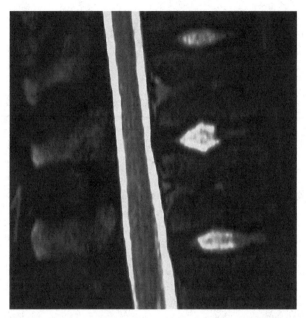

FIG. 4.1. STIR 1900/135, sagittal. Hemispheric bulging of the nucleus at the level Th 11/12 (short time Jayension recovery).

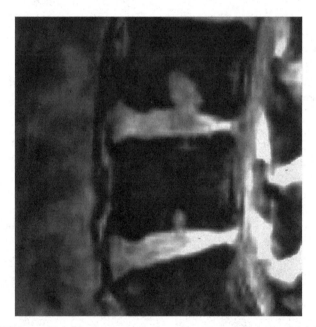

FIG. 4.2. GE 500/10, sagittal. Displacements of nuclear material into the L3-L4 vertebrae (gradient echo).

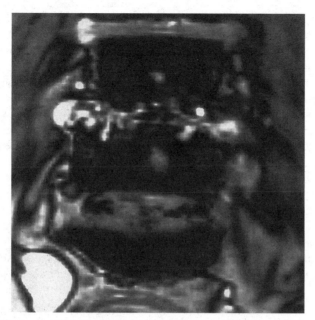

FIG. 4.3. GE 500/10, coronal after i.v. application of gadolinium diethylenetriamine. Multiple enhancing lesions of the endplates in severe osteochondrosis of L4-L5.

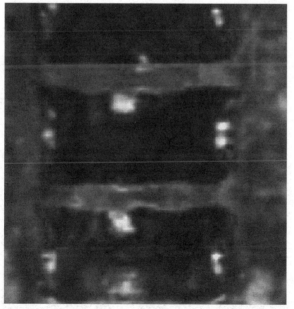

FIG. 4.4. GE 500/10 coronal after i.v. application of gadolinium diethylenetriamine. Two enhancing Schmorl's nodes in the L1 and L2 vertebrae.

vertebrae, irregular endplates, and irregularity of the epiphyseal ring. Scheuermann suggested that the disease is caused by disturbances of growth plate between the epiphyseal ring and the vertebra body, and that the disease is equivalent to osteochondrosis dissecans of the hip as described by Perthes and Calvé.

In 1930, Schmorl published pathoanatomic studies on juvenile kyphosis (35). He rejected the hypothesis that necrosis of the epiphyseal ring leads to kyphosis. Kyphosis is induced by changes of the disc forming protrusions toward the endplates. Through clefts in the cartilaginous plate—preformed or formed by fissures due to overstress—nucleus and annulus material is pressed into the spongious bone. This may happen more ventrally in the thoracic–lumbar region because the nucleus extends more anteriorly in the teenagers and load is greater anteriorly due to the physiologic kyphosis. When material is lost, the disc becomes deformed. Endochondral bone growth is enhanced at those regions where the disc is narrowed (Edgren-Vaino sign). The disc is sloped at the sides where the cartilaginous plate is destroyed by the disc displacement and it is delayed at the ventral border of the vertebrae by increased pressure.

In his last paper published in 1932, Schmorl pointed out that the separation of the epiphyseal ring of the lower lumbar spine and the first sacral vertebra from the vertebral body—radiologically a limbus vertebra—is more often due to herniation of annulus material passing through the junction zone of the epiphyseal ring and the cartilaginous plate than to fracture (36) (Fig. 4.5). In the same paper he underlined the importance of annulus herniations for the development of spondylosis deformans. Again, as in all previous papers, Schmorl made a sharp distinction between herniation of disc material and cartilaginous nodes. He was very cautious with regard to the clinical relevance of intravertebral herniation of disc material.

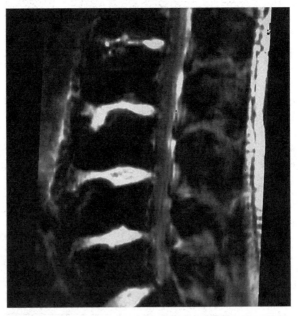

FIG. 4.5. GE 500/10 sagittal. Displacement of disc material between the junction zone of the endplate and the apophyseal ring.

WEAK POINTS OF THE ENDPLATES

Until recently Schmorl's concept of displacement of disc material has been widely accepted. There are different opinions on what are the weak points of the endplates: ossification gaps, former chorda—through passing, residual channels of former cartilaginous vessels. Coventry and colleagues describe the ossification gaps and the obliterated channels as only factors predisposing to nuclear protrusion (10). Aufdermaur finds no evidence that these structures—chorda, vessels, ossification gaps—are weak points of the endplate (3). He describes translucent areas of varying size with partial or total absence of collagen fibers in the cartilaginous endplate. Roberts and associates find fewer proteoglycans in the disc and endplates at the side of Schmorl's nodes (30). Tanaka and Kimula suppose that in older individuals the impaired function of the degenerated disc in absorbing static and dynamic stress together with thinning of the subcortical trabeculae lead to multiple endplate fractures without disc prolapse necessarily occurring (45). Hansson and coworkers find the weakness of the cancellous bone principally responsible for the formation of those Schmorl's nodes that are asymmetric to the nucleus and mushroom-shaped (14,15). Chandraraj and colleagues favor regressed blood vessel channels as weak points for later disc herniation (8). Prescher proposes the thinner cartilage plate in the center due to the former chorda as the reason for the disc herniation (28).

That additional stress is needed for vertebral disc herniation, as Schmorl pointed out, is a common belief. It is confirmed by Fahey and associates for posteriorly situated lesions (12) and by Swärd and colleagues and Henales and coworkers for anteriorly situated lesions (17,41,43).

THE CONCEPT OF SCHEUERMANN'S DISEASE

There is more discussion on Schmorl's theory on Scheuermann's disease. His concept of intravertebral disc prolapse as the starting point of juvenile kyphosis is supported by Resnick and Niwayama and McFadden and Taylor (29,24).

The main objections to Schmorl's theory on Scheuermann's disease are cited in the literature by Aufdermaur (4–6). The cartilaginous endplates with reduced numbers of irregularly arranged collagen fibers may decrease the mechanical stability of the endplates, resulting in their identification and dislocation. It may further induce changes in the pressure distribution within the vertebral bodies with resulting disturbances of growth. Prolapses of disc material through gaps in the endplates are thought to be secondary to loss of mechanical strength in the described areas. Alexander underlines the importance of stress to the growth plate (2). In his opinion the radiologic smooth node is to be regarded as a traumatic growth arrest of Schmorl's "nuclear expansion," and the irregular node—the true node—is due to endplate fracture without any antecedent cartilage defect. The fracture is due to failure, under dynamic load, and the irregular ossification in Scheuermann's disease represents spondylodystrophy due to excessive static load, which is consistent with the findings of Aufdermaur. The distribution of disc pressure in different positions and different load is extensively examined by Nachemson (26).

DEFINITIONS OF SCHEUERMANN'S DISEASE

Nodes are not always associated with kyphosis, and kyphosis may occur without nodes. Sörensen defines Scheuermann's kyphosis as "a kyphosis including at least 3 adjacent vertebrae with wedging of 5 degrees or over" (38). This criterion was adopted by Blumenthal and coworkers in classification of lumbar Scheuermann's disease as type I and the presence of anterior Schmorl's node disc space narrowing and vertebral end-plate irregularities of only one or two vertebrae as type II (7). On the other hand, Stoddard and Osborn, using the expression "spinal osteochondrosis" as equivalent to Scheuermann's disease, find that at least three of the following radiologic features should be present for diagnosis: (a) increased anteroposterior diameter of vertebral bodies; (b) wedge-shaped vertebral bodies; (c) irregular-shaped and narrowed disc spaces; (d) kyphosis or loss of lordosis; (e) Schmorl's nodes; (f) a flattened area on the superior surface in the region of the epiphyseal ring anteriorly; and/or (g) a detached epiphyseal ring anteriorly (40). Lemire's radiographic criteria for Scheuermann's disease are: (a) irregular vertebral endplates; (b) thoracic kyphosis greater than 45 degrees; (c) narrowing of intervertebral disc spaces; and (d) one or more wedged vertebrae greater than 5 degrees. Schmorl's nodes seem to be associated for unknown reasons (21).

In clinical practice the differences Schmorl made between bulging disc, cartilaginous node, and displacement of disc material have disappeared, and the term Schmorl's node is used for nearly all impressions of the endplates with exception of balloon disc (46).

PREVALENCE OF SCHMORL'S NODES

The prevalence of displacement of disc material into the vertebra varies widely in the findings from investigator to investigator. Differences in the selected material being studied and in technique account for the great range of the reported prevalence (Table 4.1).

Differences in the reported prevalence are mainly due to the method chosen for investigation. Obviously, plain radiograph will not detect all nodes as translucent areas due to superposition of other tissues, or they will be only detected when sclerosis around the herniation occurs. Discography will better detect defects of the endplate but cannot be employed for all thoracic and lumbar segments (22,47,49). Magnetic resonance (MR) imaging seems to be more sensitive in detecting nodes *in vivo* (13,16,17,27,39,42,48). But all *in vivo* imaging modalities are inferior to cadaveric studies, for they are macroscopic examinations.

DEFINITION OF SCHMORL'S NODE

A great difficulty arises from the lack of clear definition of nodes in the *in vivo* imaging modalities. Most commonly the criterion "impression of the endplate with a sclerotic shell" is used (19,25,41). Alexander gives the radiologic definition of a localized, incongruous depression of the endplate 3 mm or more in diameter (2). The same definition is given by Stäbler and associates for MR examination (39). Wagner and others cite mar-

TABLE 4.1. *Prevalence of displacement of discus material into the vertebra*

Type of Study
Cadaveric: Schmorl (1929) (34) 38%; Coventry, et al. (1945) (10) 64%; Malmivaara, et al. (1987) (22) 79%; Yasuma, et al. (1988) (50) 46%
Skeletal: Saluja, et al. (1986) (31) 56%
Cadaveric and x-ray: Coventry, et al. (1945) (10) 3.6%; Hansson (1983) (14) 66.6%
X-ray: Schmorl and Junghanns (1959) (37) 13.5%; Hurxthal (1966) (18) 15%; Stoddard and Osborn (1979) (40) 14%; Tsuji, et al. (1985) (46) 3.6%; Yasuma, et al. (1988) (50) 5.6%
Magnetic resonance imaging: Heithoff, et al. (1994) (16) 20%; Hamanishi, et al. (1994) (13) 17%

row edema or disc signal in an endplate defect as characteristic for acute endplate disc extrusions (48).

CLINICAL RELEVANCE OF SCHMORL'S NODE

The clinical relevance of intravertebral herniation of disc material and formation of subsequent cartilaginous nodes have been widely discussed since the first description by Schmorl. He was very cautious in his determinations, taking into account that he was a pathologic anatomist who received poor clinical information. Schmorl did not consider the lesions to be responsible for major clinical symptoms. However, he pointed out that displacement of disc material would necessarily induce disc degeneration with derangement of the motional segment. Krämer has denied the clinical importance of Schmorl's nodes (20). Hamanishi and coworkers believe Schmorl's nodes are associated with low back pain in younger patients (13). Stäbler and colleagues find correlation of enhancing Schmorl's node in MR examination with localized symptoms (39). Wagner and others refer to symptomatic acute nodes and endplate fractures (48). In athletes, Swärd and colleagues find significant correlation between nonapophyseal Schmorl's nodes and low back pain, but nodes were found to be more anteriorly in these individuals than in controls (41). Nodes were also found more often in athletes with low back pain by Aggrawal and associates; however, these athletes also presented other pathologies of the lumbar spine (1). On discography, thoracic discs with prominent Schmorl's nodes may be intensely painful (49).

BACK PAIN AND SCHEUERMANN'S DISEASE

Back pain is more often associated with Scheuermann's disease with or without Schmorl's node. Sörensen notes pain in 39% of high kyphosis cases, 50% in long kyphosis cases, and 78% in low kyphosis cases (38). Blumenthal and colleagues report on six patients with lumbar Scheuermann's disease with anterior Schmorl's nodes suffering from back pain, whereas, only one of six with classic Scheuermann's disease had pain. One patient suffering from back pain had classic and lumbar Scheuermann's disease. Four of seven patients with lumbar Scheuermann's disease were athletes or had a traumatic incident (7). In the study by Paajanen and associates, 21 young patients with low back pain had Scheuermann's disease with a rate of disc degeneration five times higher than in the control group (27).

In examining five children with lumbar disc herniation or protrusion, Cleveland and Delong observed additional Scheuermann's disease in two, one had two adjacent midthoracic discs with Schmorl's nodes, and one had narrowing of thoracic discs. From this observation they suggested a unitary concept of childhood lumbar disc disease with only different vectors of the mechanical stress to presumably degenerated discs (9). For the same reasons and as a result of examination of 120 patients with lumbar disc degeneration and associated Scheuermann's disease, Heithoff and others propose the term "juvenile discogenic disease" (16). Similar findings in young patients are reported by Swischuk and coworkers, who suggest grouping Schmorl's node, Scheuermann's disease, limbus vertebra, and disc degeneration together into one category (44).

The underlying reason for early disc degeneration, Scheuermann's disease, and Schmorl's node may be a genetic one as most investigators suppose and as supported by Hurxthal's study of identical twins (18).

With regard to the foregoing review of literature, the answer to the question: "Schmorl's nodes: are they herniations?" is twofold.

1. *In vivo* detection of local impressions of the endplates can be called Schmorl's nodes subsuming displacement of disc material and formation of cartilaginous nodes. They are expressions of weakness of the disc–vertebra junction.
2. In the strict sense of meaning I give the answer I have received from a well-known pathologist: Schmorl's nodes are not herniations, but I would not mind saying they are.

REFERENCES

1. Aggrawal ND, Kaur R, Kumar S, et al. A study of changes in the spine in weight lifters and other athletes. *Br J Sports Med* 1979;13:58–61.
2. Alexander CJ. Scheuermann's disease: A traumatic spondylodystrophy? *Skeletal Radiol* 1977;1:209–221.
3. Aufdermaur M. Zur pathogenese der Scheuermannschen krankheit. *Dtsch Med Wschr* 1964;2:73–76.
4. Aufdermaur M. Zur pathologischen anatomie der Scheuermannschen krankheit. *Schweizerische Med Wschr* 1965;8:264–268.
5. Aufdermaur M. Die Scheuermannschen adoleszentenkyphose. *Orthopäde* 1973;2:153–161.
6. Aufdermaur M. Juvenile kyphosis (Scheuermann's disease): radiography, histology, and pathogenesis. *Clin Orthop Rel Res* 1979;154:166–174.
7. Blumenthal SL, Roach J, Herring JA. Lumbar Scheuermann's; a clinical series and classification. *Spine* 1987;9: 929–932.
8. Chandraraj S, Briggs CA, Opeskin K. Disc herniations in the young and end-plate vascularity. *Clin Anat* 1998;11:171–176.
9. Cleveland RH, Delong GR. The relationship of juvenile lumbar disc disease and Scheuermann's disease. *Pediatr Radiol* 1981;10:161–164.
10. Coventry MB, Ghormley R, Kernohan JW. The intervertebral disc: its microscopic anatomy and pathology. Part II. *J Bone Joint Surg* 1945;2:233–247.
11. Coventry MB, Ghormley R, Kernohan JW. The intervertebral disc: its microscopic anatomy and pathology. Part III. *J Bone Joint Surg* 1945;3:460–474.
12. Fahey V, Opeskin K, Silberstein M, et al. The pathogenesis of Schmorl's nodes in relation to acute trauma. *Spine* 1998;21:2272–2275.
13. Hamanishi C, Kawabata T, Yosii T, et al. Schmorl's nodes on magnetic resonance imaging; their incidence and clinical relevance. *Spine* 1994;4:450–453.
14. Hansson T, Roos B. The amount of bone mineral and Schmorl's nodes in lumbar vertebrae. *Spine* 1983;3: 266–271.
15. Hansson TH, Keller TS, Spengler DM. Mechanical behavior of the human lumbar spine. II. Fatigue strength during dynamic compressive loading. *J Orthop Res* 1987;5: 479–487.
16. Heithoff KB, Gundry CR, Burton Ch, et al. Juvenile discogenic disease. *Spine* 1994;3:335–340.
17. Henales V, Hervás JA, Lopez P, et al. Intervertebral disc herniations (limbus vertebrae) in pediatric patients: report of 15 cases. *Pediatr Radiol* 1993;23:680–610.
18. Hurxthal LM. Schmorl's nodes in identical twins. *Lahey Clin Found Bull* 1966;3:89–92.
19. Köhler, Zimmer. *Grenzen der normalen und anfänge des pathologischen. Röntgenbildes des skeletts.* Stuttgart: Thieme Verlag, 1994.
20. Krämer J. *Bandscheibenbedingte erkrankungen.* Stuttgart: Thieme Verlag, 1994.
21. Lemire JJ, Mierau DR, Crawford CM, et al. Case reports: Scheuermann's juvenile kyphosis. *J Manipulative Physiologic Therapeutics* 1996;3:195–201.
22. Malmivaara A, Videman T, Kuosma E, et al. Plain radiographic, discographic, and direct observations of Schmorl's nodes in the thoracolumbar junctional region of the cadaveric spine. *Spine* 1987;5:453–457.
23. Facet joint orientation, facet and costovertebral joint osteoarthrosis, disc degeneration, vertebral body osteophytosis, and Schmorl's nodes in the thoracolumbar junctional region of cadaveric spines. *Spine* 1987;5:458–463.
24. McFadden KD, Taylor JR. End-plate lesions of the lumbar spine. *Spine* 1989;5:867–869.
25. Müller W. Das röntgenologische bild und die klinische bedeutung der sogenannten knorpelknötchen. *Beitr Zur Klin Chir* 1928;145:191.
26. Nachemson A. Lumbar intradiscal pressure. *Acta Orthop Scand* 1932;43:371–377.
27. Paajanen H, Alanen A, Erkintalo M, et al. Disc degeneration in Scheuermann disease. *Skeletal Radiol* 1989;18: 523–526.
28. Prescher A. Anatomy and pathology of the aging spine. *Eur J Radiol* 1998;27:181–195.
29. Resnick D, Niwayama G. Intravertebral disk herniations: cartilaginous (Schmorl's) nodes. *Diagnostic Radiol* 1978;126:57–65.
30. Roberts S, Menage J, Urban JPG. Biochemical and structural properties of the cartilage end-plate and its relation to the intervertebral disc. *Spine* 1989;2:166–174.
31. Saluja G, Fitzpatrick K, Cross MB, et al. Schmorl's nodes (intravertebral herniations of intervertebral disc tissue) in two historic British populations. *J Anat* 1986;145:87–96.

32. Deleted in proof.
33. Scheuermann H. Kyphosis dorsalis juvenilis. *Zeit Orthopäd Chir* 1920;20:306–317.
34. Schmorl G. Über Knorpelknštchen an den wirbelbandscheiben. *Fortschritte a.d.Gebiete d. Röntgenstrahlen* 1929;20, 266–279.
35. Schmorl, G. Die pathogenese der juvenilen kyhose. *Fortschritte a.d. Gebiete d.Röntgenstrahlen* 1930;41: 359–383.
36. Schmorl G. Über verlagerung von bandscheibengewebe und ihre folgen. *Anat Klin Chir* 1932;241–276.
37. Schmorl G, Junghanns H. *The human spine in health and disease: anatomicopathologic studies.* New York: Grune & Stratton, Inc, 1959.
38. Sörensen KH. *Scheuermann's juvenile kyphosis.* Copenhagen: Munksgaard 1964.
39. Stäbler A, Bellan M, Weiss M, et al. MR imaging of enhancing intraosseous disk herniation (Schmorl's nodes). *AJR* 1997;168: 933–938.
40. Stoddard A, Osborn JF. Scheuermann's disease or spinal osteochondrosis. *J Bone Joint Surg* 1979;1:56–58.
41. Swúrd L, Hellstrom M, Jacobsson B, et al. Back pain and radiologic changes in the thoraco-lumbar spine of athletes. *Spine* 1990;2:124–129.
42. Swärd L, Hellstrorm M, Jacobsson B, et al. Acute injury of the vertebral ring apophysis and intervertebral disc in adolescent gymnasts. *Spine* 1990;2: 144–148.
43. Swärd L. The thoracolumbar spine in young elite athletes. *Sports Med* 1992;13:357–364.
44. Swischuk LE, John SD, Allbery S. Disk degenerative disease in childhood: Scheuermann's disease, Schmorl's nodes, and the limbus vertebra: MRI findings in 12 patients. *Pediatr Radiol* 1998;28:334–338.
45. Takana Y, Kimula Y. Terminal plate fracture in vertebrae of the aged. *Virchows Arch Path Anat Histol* 1976; 371:351–362.
46. Tsuji H, Yoshioka T, Sainoh H. Developmental balloon disc of the lumbar spine in healthy subjects. *Spine* 1985; 10:907–911.
47. Videman T, Nurminen M, Troup JDG. Lumbar spinal pathology in cadaveric material in relation to history of back pain, occupation, and physical loading. *Spine* 1990;8:728–740.
48. Wagner AL, Murtagh FR, Arrington JA, et al. Relationship of Schmorl's nodes to vertebral body endplate fractures and acute endplate disk extrusions. *AJNR* 2000;21: 276–281.
49. Wood KB, Schellhas KP, Garvey TA, et al. Thoracic discography in healthy individuals. *Spine* 1999;24: 1548–1555.
50. Yasuma T, Saito S, Kihara, K. Schmorl's nodes: correlation of x-rays and histological findings in postmortem specimens. *Acta Pathol Jpn* 1988;38:723–733.

5

Intervertebral Disc Herniation in Children

Federico Balagué and André J. Kaelin

In his recent review of the topic, Kling characterized disc herniation in children as "infrequent and different in its presentation" compared with their adult counterparts (24). Bartolozzi and colleagues even consider disc herniation "quite exceptional" before puberty (3).

One of the problems one has to face in a literature review is the lack of agreement concerning the age limits of childhood. To resolve this problem we have searched for a definition that could be generally accepted.

According to the World Health Organization (WHO) definition, adolescence spans the years between 10 and 19 (54). Therefore, when possible in this chapter we will focus on subjects younger than 10 years of age. This definition is much more restrictive than that used by other authors (24) but it seems justified because another chapter in this book focuses on the same pathology in adolescents.

Adolescence is characterized by several physiologic and psychologic modifications that occur sequentially during this period of life with individual differences (29,49,52). At 10 years of age a majority of children cannot be considered adolescents, and because of this we do include discussion of children older than 10 years in this chapter.

The term disc herniation is generally used for posterior or lateral herniations into the spinal canal or the intervertebral foramina. This will be the main focus of this chapter. However, intracorporeal and anterior herniations exist (9) and we will summarize some relevant information about these lesions.

From a historical standpoint, the first case of disc herniation in a child cited in the reviewed literature was that of a 12-year-old published by Wahren in 1945 (55). However, if we take into account subjects below the age of 10 years, the first reported cases were published in 1968 according to a review of the literature by Bartolozzi and colleagues (3).

EPIDEMIOLOGY

Accurate figures of prevalence and/or incidence of disc herniation among children within the general population are missing (24), with the exception of a survey conducted in Japan. This survey included 20,257 students between the ages of 10 and 12 and revealed an incidence of surgically treated juvenile disc herniation of 1.69 per 100,000 persons per year (32).

Most of the epidemiologic data currently available concern reported series of surgically treated patients. In these specific settings, children and adolescents considered together represent around 1% of subjects undergoing surgery (24,27,30). In his review, Shillito finds figures of frequency of herniated disc under 15 years of age ranging from 0.05% (among patients of all ages) to 42% in the age-limited group at the Hospital for Sick Children in Toronto (44). Similar figures were found in a review limited to the Italian literature (3).

Patients younger than 19 years represented 15.4% of all the patients treated surgically during a period of 26 years (26). Moreover, figures ranging from 7.8% to 22.3% have been found in Japan (26). Incidence is much lower among children chronologically defined according to the WHO. A review of the literature by Bussière and coworkers includes 248 cases of individuals up to 18 years of age. Among those, only three (1.2%) were children under 10 years of age (6). Ishihara and colleagues reviewed a group of 378 patients less than 16 years of age who were surgically treated for lumbar disc herniation between 1982 and 1989. Only two of these patients (0.5%) were less than 10 years of age (both were 9-year-old girls) (23). In a recent article Papagelopoulos and associates report on 72 subjects 16 years of age or younger at the time of surgery. This cohort represented approximately 3% of all the adolescents less than 17 years of age evaluated at their institution because of lower back or lower limb pain. Children and adolescents considered together represented 0.4% of all patients who underwent lumbar discectomy during the same period ($N = 16,586$) (35).

In the same article the Papagelopoulos team reviewed the literature and found ten studies (341 subjects) in which the clinical results of surgery in children and adolescents were reported. The lowest limit in age range was 10 years in one study, 9 years in another, and 8 years in two other series (35). No single case among their own ($N = 72$) was younger than 11 years at the time of surgery (35). Nelson and colleagues compared three age groups, and found the youngest subjects among these groups to be 9 years of age (33). In Ishihara and coworkers' series of surgically treated subjects ($N = 11$), the youngest cases were three girls who were, respectively, 9, 9, and 11 years of age (23). In a cohort of 101 surgically treated cases reported by Savini and colleagues, the youngest subjects were 13-years old (42).

Among the studies included in Table 5.1, subjects 10 years of age or less represented 7.7% of the children and adolescent group. The youngest case of disc herniation confirmed at surgery we are aware of was that of a 27-month-old child (37).

Previously, we reviewed the statistics of the Department of Neurosurgery of the University Hospital of Lausanne (Switzerland) concerning 4,102 patients surgically treated for disc herniation during a period of 15 years (1). We found that 1.2% of the patients were younger than 20 years of age. The youngest subject was a girl who was 10 years, 11

TABLE 5.1. *Overall percentage of children and their gender distribution in review of literature*

Reference	Less than 10 years: more than 10 years (N[a])	Girls	Boys
Da Silva, et al. (1977) (10)	4:12	2	2
Ishihara, et al. (1997) (23)	2:9	2	0
Zamani and MacEwan (1982) (58)	4:19	NR	NR
Liquois	2:8	1	1
Gennuso	3:87	NR	NR0
Kurihara and Kataoka (1980) (26)	2:68	2	0
Bartolozzi[b], et al. (1989) (3)	2:?	2	0
Shillito (1996) (44)	1:19	0	1
Kaelin	1:4	1	0
Overall:	19:226 ~1:12	71.4%	28.6%

NR, not reported.

[a]The upper limit of age varies from one study to another between 15 and 19 years of age.

[b]The two cases reported by Bartolozzi, et al. are not included in the comparisons with other age groups as this author did not provide epidemiologic data.

months of age at the time of surgery. This is in agreement with a series reviewed by Russ-wurm and associates in which the two youngest patients were 10-years old (39).

In the last 15 years, five children were treated surgically for lumbar disc herniation in the Pediatric Orthopedic Unit. These five patients were all girls. One was 10-years old and the other four were adolescents. Two girls also had dysplastic spondylolisthesis at the L4-L5 level.

Other data can be found in retrospective studies focused specifically on young patients who did not undergo surgery. Da Silva and colleagues report on 16 patients younger than 16 years treated either conservatively or surgically. Their youngest patients were two boys who were 8- and 9-years old, respectively, and two girls, both of whom were 10 years and 10 months of age when their symptoms began (10). Similarly, Zamani and MacEwen's comparison of surgically ($N = 13$) and conservatively ($N = 10$) treated patients, shows only three subjects in the surgically treated group (8, 9, and 10 years, respectively) and one in the conservative group (10 years) who were within the age limits used in this chapter (58).

Some data have been published in Finland with repeated magnetic resonance imaging (MRI) studies performed in small groups of subjects not drawn from surgical series (i.e., athletes and healthy controls [25]; random samples of schoolchildren [14,40,41,48], etc.) In a study by Kujala and colleagues 43 girls (27 athletes and 16 nonathletes) whose mean age was below 12 years, underwent MRI studies at baseline and at 3-year follow-up. At baseline, disc protrusion or prolapse was found in one athlete and one nonathlete; at follow-up disc protrusion or prolapse was evident in five athletes and two nonathletes (25). In studies of schoolchildren no disc protrusion was found by MRI among 15-year-old subjects who did not complain of lower back pain (LBP) (14,40,41), except in one case reported by Tertti and others (48). Curiously, this article seems to concern the same population of schoolchildren as the previous references. However, the prevalence of signs of disc degeneration is much more common than protrusion even among asymptomatic adolescents (14,40,41,48).

Within the limits of the small number of subjects examined, these studies suggest that disc protrusions or herniations are uncommon among asymptomatic children.

The prevalence of disc prolapse through the endplates (Schmorl's nodes) has been described in a MRI study of 506 patients between the ages of 1 and 82 years performed in Japan. Eleven subjects between the ages of 1 and 9 years underwent MRI examinations for different neurologic disorders other than suspicions of lumbar lesion. None of these subjects had Schmorl's nodes (19). The authors state that this type of nuclear prolapse seems unlikely in children due to the thickness of the cartilaginous endplate (19).

In another radiologic study, Heithoff and associates focused on the association of degenerative disc disease (lower lumbar region) and thoracolumbar signs of Scheuer-mann's disease (20). Only one child (7 years of age) with these two types of lesions was identified in this study among 1,419 patients examined by MRI (20).

According to a recent review, it is not clear from the literature whether or not the frequency of disc herniation is significantly higher among girls or boys (24). Russwurm and colleagues (39) find a slight predominance of girls, particularly in younger patients but the figures are not significant. Bartolozzi and coworkers (3) find that there is a significant predominance of females before the age of 16 years, while males predominate over 16 years.

Among the studies summarized in Table 5.1, girls accounted for 69% of all subjects under 10 years of age, even with all authors not reporting on patients' gender.

The most commonly cited risk factors leading to disc herniation are trauma, congenital spine malformations, and family predisposition (12,24). Nutritional factors have been cited by Revuelta and coworkers (37).

Trauma, either significant traumatic events or repetitive cumulative trauma, has been reported to be a potential risk factor in disc herniations. A clear history of trauma preceding the onset of pain is related to half of the patients (24). Epstein and associates state that in young people, disc herniation "represents more of a fracture with a hinge-like displacement of fibrocartilage..." (12). In recent reviews different types of separate bone fragments are described under the label "rim fractures" (4) or slipped vertebral apophysis (24). The youngest reported case of apophyseal fracture was in a 9-year-old boy (24).

Disc herniations have been classified by Takata and colleagues into three types (46); a fourth type was later described by Epstein and coworkers (13).

Other authors stated that limbus vertebra, Schmorl's hernia, and Scheuermann's disease have an identical pathogenesis (21).

In their discussion, Kurihara and Kataoka suggest that Japanese people probably have a smaller spinal canal than Caucasians. Thus with the same incidence of herniated disc, sciatica might be much more frequent among the Japanese. This could explain the high epidemiologic figures found in the Japanese literature (26). Another fact highlighted by these authors is the etiologic role of repeated trauma (26). However, the fact that the incidence among Japanese males is two to three times higher than among females (26) does not support their first hypothesis, as Japanese males are generally bigger than their female counterparts.

According to Kling's review of literature, congenital anomalies have been observed in 30% of young patients with lumbar disc herniation. The most common of these are transitional vertebrae and spina bifida occulta, however absent lamina, congenital narrowed lumbar spinal canal, and spondylolisthesis have also been described (24). In Kurihara and Kataoka's study, congenital anomalies were observed in 33% (23/70) of patients with lumbar disc herniation (26).

Cases of familial clustering for lumbar disc herniation have been described among adults (36,38,43,45) as well as teenagers (18,34).

Family predisposition for disc herniation in young subjects has also been specifically studied by different authors (32,53). In a very impressive project, Matsui and colleagues studied the incidence of lumbar disc herniation among the siblings and relatives of 40 patients 18 years of age or younger who underwent surgery for lumbar disc herniation. This group of 111 subjects and 120 age- and sex-matched patients with normal spines (controls) were evaluated by standardized questionnaire about history of sciatica or specific surgery. Those suspected of having disc herniation were physically examined and underwent MRI in order to evaluate the prevalence of disc herniation. In addition, a survey was conducted among 75,237 students from elementary school age through high school age to define the expected values in general populations. Comparing these data, it appears that the incidence of lumbar disc herniation among individuals 18 years of age or younger show a family clustering. In the conclusions of these studies, the authors highlight the fact that family clustering is not synonymous with genetic factors (32). The relative risk of disc herniation among first-degree relatives of patients was been found to be 5 and 5.61 in the two studies (32,53).

In a study performed at the Mayo clinic, young patients who were surgically treated were approximately 2% taller than control subjects matched for age and gender (35). The differences in weight were not significant (35).

SPECIFIC SYMPTOMS AND SIGNS

Disc herniation is a difficult diagnosis among these age groups (8,12,24,37,44). For this reason the duration of symptoms before diagnosis ranges from several months to 1 year (24).

Kling reports his personal observation that young patients generally tend to "grin and bear" the pain as long as they can function to some extent. Thus direct questioning is necessary to make the diagnosis (24). The apparent good tolerance to pain has been attributed to "the lack of the emotional component of pain" present in adults (31).

Review articles state that the main signs and symptoms of disc herniation are mechanical back pain and positive straight leg raising (SLR) test, while other neurologic symptoms and findings are uncommon (24,50). Disabling pain together with the paucity of neurologic findings often leads clinicians to suspect a psychologic origin (12). According to Shillito, the absence of sciatica is the main difficulty in diagnosis of a herniated disc in pediatric patients (44). A high prevalence of hamstring tightness among young patients with disc herniation has been described (47). Overall, the main signs and symptoms reported in the literature are summarized in Table 5.2.

TABLE 5.2. *Most frequently reported signs and symptoms of disc herniation in young patients*

Author/year	N[a] (children)	Pain	Neurologic symptoms	SLR	Neurology (deficit)	Other signs
Papagelopoulos, et al. (1998) (35)	72	LBP + sciatica: 90% Sciatica only: 10%	Weakness: 4%	89%	Weakness: 47% Reflex: 32% Sensory: 6%	Muscle spasm: 56% Scoliosis: 40%
Russwurm, et al. (1978) (39)	37 (2)	LBP ± sciatica: 43% Sciatica only: 21.6%		100%	Weakness: 29% Reflex: 10% Sensory: 21%	Muscle spasm: 100% Scoliosis: 51%
Ishihara, et al. (1997) (23)	11 (2)	LBP ± sciatica: 82% Sciatica only: 18%		100% contralateral SLR: 64%	Slight weakness and sensory deficit: 55%	Tight hamstrings: 91%
Da Silva, et al. (1977) (10)	16 (4)	LBP ± sciatica: 62.5% Lower limb: 37.5%	Paresthesia: 6.25%	100% Reflex: 44%	Weakness: 19% Postural faults decreased mobility: 100% Sensory: 25%	Muscle spasm: 31%
Gennuso (1992)	90 (3)	LBP ± sciatica: 100%		Specific values not reported	Weakness: 28% Reflex: 16% Sensory: 9%	Acquired scoliosis ± decreased mobility ± SLR: 100%
Zamani and MacEwan[b] (1982) (58)	23 (4)	LBP ± sciatica: 100%		100%	Weakness: 2/4 Reflex: 2/4 Sensory: 1/4	Functional scoliosis: 3/4 Muscle spasm: 100%
Kurihara and Kataoka (1980) (26)	70 (2)	Sciatica: 100% LBP: 78%	Bowel/urine disturbance: 1%	97%	Weakness: 86% Reflex: 4% Sensory: 83%	[c]lord: 90% Scoliosis: 56% [c]L mobility: 100% Muscle spasm: 87%
Shillito (1996) (44)	20 (1)	Never sciatica: 20% LBP or kyphoscoliosis: 80%		100%		Pain on back motion: 100%

LBP, lower back pain; SLR, straight leg raising test.
[a]These series include children and adolescents. Individual patient's data were only reported by Zamani and MacEwan. Therefore it is impossible to report exclusively on children's signs and symptoms.
[b]The neurologic data concern exclusively the few children included in this study.
[c]Means decreased or reduced.

Kurihara and Kataoka highlight the fact that scoliosis and paravertebral muscle spasm "are evident even under general anesthesia and tend to persist for a long time after surgery" (26). Progressive scoliosis with vertebral rotation reversible after disc herniation surgery has been reported in a 10-year-old girl (17). Bartolozzi and colleagues report two girls aged 9 and 10 years who presented with decreased lumbar lordosis and marked rigidity and antalgic scoliosis were much more prominent features than lumbar and sciatic pain (3). A case report describes a 7-year-old boy complaining of LBP and presenting with a scoliosis due to an L1 intravertebral herniation of a calcified disc (57).

In a 27-month-old boy, to our knowledge the youngest described case, the symptoms noticed by the mother were "irritability, low-back pain, and difficulty in walking" (37). Lumbar muscle spasm, positive SLR test, and right leg monoparesis were found at the physical examination (37).

Our review of literature shows rather large differences between the clinical findings reported in the published studies both in terms of symptoms and clinical findings. It is difficult to know whether or not biases due to geographic factors, origin of the studies, methodologic factors, and so forth can explain these different results.

The symptoms presented by patients with slipped vertebral apophysis are "similar to those observed with soft disc herniation" (24).

To further illustrate this topic, we summarize a case treated by one of the authors (A.K.) at the University Hospital of Geneva.

Case Report

An 11-year-old girl who was very active in gymnastics (15 hours per week) complained after a workout session of acute lumbar pain radiating to the lower limbs. The clinical evaluation showed important spasm of the lumbar paravertebral muscles, a positive SLR test at 30 degrees, with hamstring tightness and Achilles tendon reflexes decreased on both sides but no significant sensory or motor deficit. Standard radiographs revealed a dysplastic spondylolisthesis L4-L5 with a posterior calcification. Both MRI and computed tomography (CT) scan showed a large disc herniation with a fracture of the posterior vertebral rim leading to a narrowed canal that was functionally relevant (Figs. 5.1 and 5.2). Therapy consisted of decompression, combined with curettage of the disc, and a posterior intercorporeal graft combined with posterior instrumented fusion of L4-L5.

The outcome was excellent both in terms of pain and function. Leisure time sports activities were possible 6 months after surgery.

DIFFERENTIAL DIAGNOSIS

The differential diagnosis of disc herniation in this age group includes tumor, infection, inflammatory diseases, or spondylolisthesis (8). In pediatric populations, this problem was specifically addressed in a recent paper (7). In this study, malignancies were finally diagnosed in 29 children (mean age 8 years at onset of symptoms) referred to two pediatric rheumatology centers. Back pain as a principle presenting feature was reported in nine patients whose referring diagnoses were "discitis" (three cases), spondyloarthropathy (one case), and juvenile rheumatoid arthritis (JRA) (five cases). The authors highlight that "back pain is not a usual presenting feature of any chronic childhood arthritis...." This statement includes ankylosing spondylitis and other spondyloarthropathies, where back pain usually develops late in the course of the disease. The

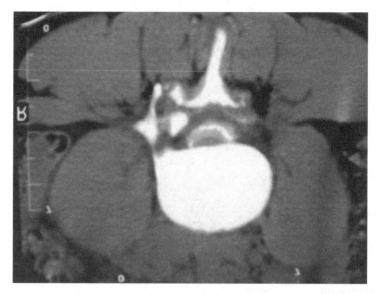

FIG. 5.1. The computed tomography shows a large L4-L5 disc herniation with posterior calcification in an 11-year-old girl.

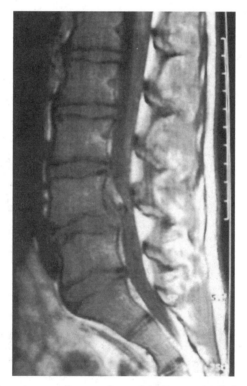

FIG. 5.2. This magnetic resonance image shows L4-L5 spondylolisthesis combined with disc herniation in an 11-year-old girl.

same authors cite some "atypical" features as well (e.g., night sweats, focal neurologic abnormalities, and bruising) (7).

In another pediatric rheumatology series, underlying neoplasia was found in ten out of 1,254 patients complaining of musculoskeletal symptoms. However, LBP was an uncommon complaint. Moreover, nocturnal pain and sweats, fever, and weight loss alerted the physician (51).

Martinez-Lage and colleagues report on two groups of pediatric patients whose main complaints were LBP and/or sciatica; 17 of the subjects were diagnosed with disc herniation while 16 were suffering from neoplasms of the lower thoracic and lumbosacral region. The main differences between these two groups were:

1. Age. Mean age at diagnosis was 14.5 years in the lumbar disc herniation and 6.8 years in the spinal neoplasm group ($P = 0.018$). No patient in the disc herniation group was younger than 11 years.
2. Clinical signs. Motor deficit (8/16 versus 1/17) and impaired reflexes (11/16 versus 4/17) were significantly more frequent among children with neoplasms (31).
3. Standard radiographs were considered especially useful in the diagnosis of spinal masses (31).

Some patients can present with atypical symptoms such as the recently reported case of a 6-year-old boy complaining of abdominal pain and progressive difficulty in walking to the point of refusing to walk. His final diagnosis was anterior disc protrusion attributed to a discitis and treated as such even though blood cultures grew no organism (56). In another case, a 19-month-old girl presented with irritability, progressive scoliosis, reluctance to walk and finally, inability to stand due to an aseptic inflammation of the intervertebral disc space L3-L4 (28). The empiric approach to the management of patients with negative cultures is stressed by the authors (28).

Intracorporeal herniations are "almost always asymptomatic," but anterior herniations have been confused with fractures or discitis. In the latter, some blood tests could be helpful to differentiate between the two diagnoses (15).

RADIOGRAPHIC EVALUATION

Plain radiographs are considered "an integral part of the examination of an adolescent with LBP" (24). The evaluation begins with standing anteroposterior and lateral radiographs when a slipped vertebral apophysis is suspected (24). Plain radiographs show the avulsed fragment in approximately four out of ten patients (30). Structural anomalies such as spina bifida occulta and sacralization of L5 or lumbarization of S1 have been reported to occur in one-third of adolescents with disc herniation (24). Mild nonstructural scoliosis and loss of lumbar lordosis are common findings (24).

In our experience, a narrowed intervertebral disc space does not always harbor pathology, and one has to rule out hypotheses like developmental disc anomalies (2). Disc space narrowing is considered "rare" by Kling (24). In a recent study performed in adults using quantitative volumetric MRI, it appears that the loss of the volume of the herniated nucleus pulposus does not cause a significant decrease in the intervertebral space width (22).

Modern imaging techniques (CT/MRI) either plain or with a contrast agent have reduced the need for myelography (24). When the latter is performed, it should be done with CT scanning to identify avulsed cartilage and bone from apophyseal fractures (24).

There are some disadvantages of MRI. First, bone and cartilage cannot be visualized very well, which means slipped vertebral apophysis may not be recognized. Because the examination is done in the supine position and not in a standing one or in physiologic lordosis, interpretation of the room available for the nerve roots should be done cautiously (24). Finally, abnormal signal on MRI has also been reported in asymptomatic schoolchildren (14,16,40,41,48).

TREATMENT

According to Kling, "treatment is aggressive whether it is nonoperative or surgical" (24). A course of conservative treatment should be offered to all patients except those with progressive neurologic deficits (24). However, the program of nonoperative treatment proposed by this author (complete bed rest with or without traction for 2 to 4 weeks, utilization of corsets for 3 months, etc.) is very different from those used with adult patients. Moreover, it is unclear if these recommendations are supported by the results of clinical trials or just based on the author's personal ideas (24).

In Kurihara and Kataoka's series, 40% of their 70 subjects improved with conservative management, but symptoms recurred when these individuals returned to their usual activity level and all the patients eventually underwent surgery. Sciatica disappeared or decreased within the first 24 hours in all the subjects (26). All patients with neurologic signs required surgery; the long-term results of conservative methods were not positive and recurrences for pain and neurologic signs were frequent.

In one of the cases by Bartolozzi and coworkers, it is clearly stated that conservative management failed (3).

Intensive conservative management failed in all patients in the cohort described by Epstein and others (12). The results of surgery were rated as "excellent" in 18 of 25 (72%) cases but the authors did not define what they considered an "excellent" result. Moreover, they did not report the duration of follow-up or state who performed the follow-up evaluation or how it was done (12).

Isolated cases of excellent response to conservative treatment for herniated discs have been reported (34). Yaniv and associates report one patient who, at 30 months following diagnosis, had an excellent outcome both radiologically and clinically after a short treatment with a nonsteroidal antiinflammatory drug (57). Bartolozzi and coworkers state that conservative management must be attempted although this approach is less effective in children than in adults. These authors do not subscribe to the proposal made by other authors that intersomatic fusion has to be performed in association with discectomy (3).

Classic disc herniation could be treated by the usual technique of discectomy without fusion. In case of epiphyseal plate slipping, vertebral rim fracture or spondylolisthesis at the same level, fusion has to be considered by different methods: intracorporeal bone graft, anterior fusion, and posterior segmental instrumentation. A grossly unstable level after discectomy must be fused.

OUTCOME

We have not found any study on disc herniation limited to the definition of "children" we are using here. Therefore it is very difficult to gather information about long-term outcome. Instead we have decided to present some data concerning the published cases of younger patients.

According to Epstein and colleagues, the results following discectomy are "uniformly good" (12). However, this statement is difficult to accept today because from a methodologic point, most of the reviewed articles do not fulfill the current standards (e.g., standardized evaluation, validated tools, independent observer, and at least 2 years follow-up).

After a minimum follow-up of 5 years postsurgery, Kurihara and Kataoka evaluated 26 of their initial 70 patients. At this time 17 subjects were totally asymptomatic while five (19%) patients reported LBP, three (12%) reported weakness of the leg, and three (12%) reported numbness of the leg (26). After long-term follow-up (up to 20 years) the results of surgical procedures has been considered successful in 88% of cases by Shillito (44).

A case reported by Callahan and colleagues remained symptom-free for 2 years (8).

At 7-year follow-up, the child discussed previously who had been operated on at 27 months was asymptomatic (37).

At 1 and 3 years, respectively, the two girls treated surgically by Bartolozzi and coworkers were asymptomatic (3).

The results recently reported by Luukkonen and associates after a mean follow-up time of 6.2 years (range: 3.5 to 9.1 years) seem less optimistic. Among 12 patients under 15 years of age at the time of the surgical procedure, only five (42%) were totally asymptomatic at follow-up, while 58% reported both pain and disability. However, none of the patients underwent a second surgery or physiotherapy by the time of follow-up (27). It should be noted that the short-term outcome was rated as good or excellent in all patients, which indicates that at 6 months none of the subjects reported any disability, four of them had minor pain occasionally, and one also reported occasional lumbar stiffness (27). According to their review of literature, these authors conclude that their results appear somewhat less favorable than those in two pediatric series published several years earlier (in 1980 and 1982, respectively) (27).

Durham and colleagues report on a cohort of 29 patients who underwent surgery for lumbar disc herniation and were reevaluated after a mean follow-up of 8.5 years (range: 4 months to 30.5 years). It should be noted that the rate of subsequent surgery was 24% and that the authors could not identify any predictor of the need for subsequent surgery or of poor outcome (11). The authors conclude that surgical treatment in the pediatric population "does not appear to lead to chronic complaints of back pain and it does not appear to have a negative impact on overall health or quality of life" (11).

Bradbury and coworkers compared outcome in two groups of adolescents treated by surgery or chymopapain, respectively 7.2 years and 8.5 years earlier. These authors conclude that "long-term results of surgery are no better than the results of first-line chymopapain treatment with surgery being reserved for the failures" (5).

CONCLUSION

Intervertebral disc herniation in children under 10 years of age has a very low occurrence. No specific epidemiologic paper was found in the literature. Low back pain and hamstring contracture are the main symptoms. MR studies are the best imaging technique when radiographs cannot explain the cause of pain. In case of progressive neurologic deficit, surgical treatment is always indicated. Otherwise orthopedic, physical therapy, and antiinflammatory treatment should be tried first. In case of treatment resistance or recurrence of pain, surgery has to be considered. Association of fusion depends on the presence of local instability or morphologic changes.

Outcome is difficult to analyze from the literature but general results seem to be better for children than for adults.

REFERENCES

1. Balagué F, Nordin M. Back pain in children and teenagers. *Baillière's Clin Rheumatol* 1992;6:575–593.
2. Balagué F, Sadry F. Narrowed intervertebral discs in a teenager: should these be considered pathologic? *J Clin Rheumatol* 1995;1:253–255.
3. Bartolozzi P, Lombardini G, Floris G. Herniated lumbar disc in the child: a description of two cases. *Ital J Orthop Traumatol* 1989;15:115–120.
4. Beggs I, Addison J. Posterior vertebral rim fractures [Review]. *Br J Radiol* 1998;71:567–572.
5. Bradbury N, Wilson L, Mulholland R. Adolescent disc protrusions. A long-term follow-up of surgery compared to chymopapain. *Spine* 1996;21:372–377.
6. Bussière JL, Leblanc B, Lopitaux R, et al. Sciatiques par hernie discale de l'enfant. *Rev Rhum Mal Osteoartic* 1981;48:543–548.
7. Cabral DA, Tucker LB. Malignancies in children who initially present with rheumatic complaints. *J Pediatr* 1999;134:53–57.
8. Callahan DJ, Pack LL, Bream RC, et al. Intervertebral disc impingement syndrome in a child. Report of a case and suggested pathology. *Spine* 1986;11:402–404.
9. Chandraraj S, Briggs CA, Opeskin K. Disc herniations in the young and end-plate vascularity. *Clin Anat* 1998; 11:171–176.
10. Da Silva V, Beyeler F, Mumenthaler M, et al. Die lumbale diskushernie im kindesalter anhand von 16 eigenen beobachtungen. *Therapeutische Umschau* 1977;34:405–408.
11. Durham SR, Sun PP, Sutton LN. Surgically treated lumbar disc disease in the pediatric population: an outcome study. *J Neurosurg (Spine 1)* 2000;92:1–6.
12. Epstein JA, Epstein NE, Marc J, et al. Lumbar intervertebral disc herniation in teenage children: recognition and management of associated anomalies. *Spine* 1984;9:427–432.
13. Epstein N, Epstein J, Mauri T. Treatment of fractures of the vertebral limbus and spinal stenosis in five adolescents and five young adults. *Neurosurgery* 1989;24:595–604.
14. Erkintalo MO, Salminen JJ, Alanen AM, et al. Development of degenerative changes in the lumbar intervertebral disc: results of a prospective MR imaging study in adolescents with and without low back pain. *Radiology* 1995;196:529–533.
15. Fitzer PM. Anterior herniation of the nucleus pulposus: radiologic and clinical features. *South Med J* 1985; 78:1296–1300.
16. Gibson M, Szypryt E, Buckly J, et al. Magnetic resonance imaging of adolescent disc herniations. *J Bone Joint Surg (Br)* 1987;69–B:699–703.
17. Grass JP, Dockendorff IB, Soto VA, et al. Progressive scoliosis with vertebral rotation after lumbar intervertebral disc herniation in a 10-year-old girl. *Spine* 1993;18:336–338.
18. Gunzburg R, Fraser R, Fraser GA. Lumbar intervertebral disc prolapse in teenage twins. *J Bone Joint Surg (Br)* 1990;72–B:914–916.
19. Hamanishi C, Kawabata T, Yosii T, et al. Schmorl's nodes on magnetic resonance imaging. Their incidence and clinical relevance. *Spine* 1994;19:450–453.
20. Heithoff KB, Gundry CR, Burton CV, et al. Juvenile discogenic disease. *Spine* 1994;19:335–340.
21. Henales V, Hervas JA, Lopez P, et al. Intervertebral disc herniations (limbus vertebrae) in pediatric patients: report of 15 cases. *Pediatr Radiol* 1993;23:608–610.
22. Holodny A, Kisza P, Contractor S, et al. Does a herniated nucleus pulposus contribute significantly to a decrease in height of the intervertebral disc? Quantitative volumetric MRI. *Neuroradiol* 2000;42(6):451–454.
23. Ishihara H, Matsui H, Hirano N, et al. Lumbar intervertebral disc herniation in children less than 16 years of age. long-term follow-up study of surgically managed cases. *Spine* 1997;22:2044–2049.
24. Kling TF. Herniated nucleus pulposus and slipped vertebral apophysis. In: Weinstein SL, ed. *The pediatric spine. principles and practice.* New York: Raven Press, 1994:603–618.
25. Kujala UM, Taimela S, Erkintalo M, et al. Low-back pain in adolescent athletes. *Med Sci Sports Exerc* 1996; 28:165–170.
26. Kurihara A, Kataoka O. Lumbar disc herniation in children and adolescents. A review of 70 operated cases and their minimum 5-year follow-up studies. *Spine* 1980;5:443–451.
27. Luukkonen M, Partanen K, Vapalahti M. Lumbar disc herniations in children: a long-term clinical and magnetic resonance imaging follow-up study. *Br J Neurosurg* 1997;11:280–285.
28. Maliner LI, Johnson DL. Intervertebral disc space inflammation in children. *Childs Nerv Syst* 1997;13:101–103.
29. Marcelli D. L'adolescence: une épreuve psychique particulière. In: Michaud PA, Deschamps JP, Frappier JY, et al. eds. *La santé des adolescents. Approches, soins, prévention.* Lausanne: Payot, 1997:44–54.
30. Martinez-Lage J, Poza M, Arcas P. Avulsed lumbar vertebral rim plate in an adolescent: trauma or malformation? *Childs Nerv Syst* 1998;14:131–134.
31. Martinez-Lage JF, Robledo AM, Lopez F, et al. Disc protrusion in the child—particular features and comparison with neoplasms. *Childs Nerv Syst* 1997;13:201–207.
32. Matsui H, Terahata N, Tsuji H, et al. Familial predisposition and clustering for juvenile lumbar disc herniation. *Spine* 1992;7:1323–1328.
33. Nelson CL, Janecki CJ, Gildenberg PL, et al. Disc protrusions in the young. *Clin Orthop* 1972;88:142–150.

34. Obukhov SK, Hankenson L, Manka M, et al. Multilevel lumbar disc herniation in 12-year-old twins. *Childs Nerv Syst* 1996;12:169–171.
35. Papagelopoulos PJ, Shaughnessy WJ, Ebersold MJ, et al. Long-term outcome of lumbar discectomy in children and adolescents sixteen years of age or younger. *J Bone Joint Surg [Am]* 1998;80A:689–698.
36. Postacchini F, Lami R, Pugliese O. Familial predisposition to discogenic low-back pain. an epidemiologic and immunogenetic study. *Spine* 1988;13:1403–1406.
37. Revuelta R, De Juambelz PP, Fernandez B, et al. Lumbar disc herniation in a 27-month-old child. Case report. *J Neurosurg (Spine)* 2000;92:98–100.
38. Richardson JK, Chung T, Schultz JS, et al. A familial predisposition toward lumbar disc injury. *Spine* 1997;22: 1487–1493.
39. Russwurm H, Bjerkreim I, Ronglan E. Lumbar intervertebral disc herniation in the young. *Acta Orthop Scand* 1978;49:158–163.
40. Salminen JJ, Erkintalo (Tertti) M, Laine M, et al. Low back pain in the young. a prospective three-year follow-up study of subjects with and without low back pain. *Spine* 1995;20:2101–2108.
41. Salminen JJ, Erkintalo MO, Pentti J, et al. Recurrent low back pain and early disc degeneration in the young. *Spine* 1999;24:1316–1321.
42. Savini R, Martucci E, Nardi S, et al. The herniated lumbar intervertebral disc in children and adolescents. Long-term follow-up of 101 cases treated by surgery. *Ital J Orthop Traumatol* 1991;17:505–511.
43. Scapinelli R. Lumbar disc herniation in eight siblings with a positive family history for disc disease. *Acta Orthop Belg* 1993;59:371–376.
44. Shillito J. Pediatric lumbar disc surgery: 20 patients under 15 years of age. *Surg Neurol* 1996;46:14–18.
45. Simmons ED, Guntupalli M, Kowalski JM, et al. Familial predisposition for degenerative disc disease. *Spine* 1996;21:1527–1529.
46. Takata K, Inoue S, Takahashi K, et al. Fracture of the posterior margin of a lumbar vertebral body. *J Bone Joint Surg (Am)* 1988;70:589–594.
47. Takata K,Takahashi K. Hamstring tightness and sciatica in young patients with disc herniation. *J Bone Joint Surg (Br)* 1994;76–B:220–224.
48. Tertti M, Salminen J, Paajanen H, et al. Low-back pain and disc degeneration in children: a case-control MR imaging study. *Radiology* 1991;180:503–507.
49. Theintz G. Le développement pubertaire normal. In: Michaud PA, Deschamps JP, Frappier JY, eds. *La santé des adolescents. Approches, soins, prévention.* Lausanne: Payot, 1997:25–43.
50. Thompson GH. Back pain in children. *J Bone Joint Surg (Am)* 1993;75A:928–938.
51. Trapani S, Grisolia F, Simonini G, et al. Incidence of occult cancer in children presenting with musculoskeletal symptoms: a 10-year survey in a pediatric rheumatology unit. *Semin Arthritis Rheum* 2000;29:348–359.
52. Tursz A, Cook J. Les adolescents dans une société en transition. In: Michaud PA, Deschamps JP, Frappier JY, eds. *La santé des adolescents. Approches, soins, prévention.* Lausanne: Payot, 1997:11–13.
53. Varlotta GP, Brown MD, Kelsey JL, et al. Familial predisposition for herniation of a lumbar disc in patients who are less than twenty-one years old. *J Bone Joint Surg* 1991;73–A:124–128.
54. World Health Organization. *The health of young people: a challenge and a promise.* Geneva: 1993.
55. Wahren H. Herniated nucleus pulposus in a child of twelve years. *Acta Orthop Scand* 1945;16:40–42.
56. Wong-Chung JK, Naseeb SA, Kaneker SG, et al. Anterior disc protrusion as a cause for abdominal symptoms in childhood discitis. A case report. *Spine* 1999;24:918–920.
57. Yaniv M, Bar-Ziv J, Wientroub S. Herniation of calcified intervertebral disc in a lumbar vertebral body presenting as acute scoliosis in a child. A case report and literature review. *J Pediatr Orthop* 1999;8:306–307.
58. Zamani MH, MacEwen GD. Herniation of the lumbar disc in children and adolescents. *J Pediatr Orthop* 1982;2:528–533.

6

Intervertebral Disc Herniation in Adolescents

Dietrich Schlenzka

Lumbar intervertebral disc herniation in adolescents is rare. In operative series reported in the literature, the number of patients under the age of 19 varies between 1% and 15%. A history of trauma is often expressed as an etiologic factor in young patients. Congenital anomalies as well as genetic factors have also been mentioned. The gender distribution is equal between boys and girls. Diagnosis is often delayed in this age group. Symptoms may be intermittent and differ from typical sciatica in adults. Final diagnosis is based on magnetic resonance imaging. Primary treatment is nonoperative if no progressive neurologic signs are present. Surgery should be considered if there is no satisfactory relief of symptoms after nonoperative measures. Surgical treatment follows the rules of adult disc excision. Results of disc excision in young patients are very satisfactory in short-term as well as in long-term follow-up studies.

Lumbar disc herniation, a common problem in the adult population, is rare in children and adolescents. The exact incidence of disc herniations in growing individuals is not known. The only reports on this are based on surgical series. Giroux and Leclercq (6) report that 1% of patients undergoing surgery for lumbar disc herniation were between 13 and 18 years of age and 4% were between 13 and 21 years of age. According to Epstein and Lavine (5), the incidence among surgically treated patients is 1.8%. However, Kurihara and Kataoka (9) report a frequency as high as 15% for patients undergoing surgery for disc herniation under the age of 19 years. A history of trauma is often expressed as an etiologic factor in young patients (2,18). The underlying condition seems to be early disc degeneration, which was described in the 1990s in several magnetic resonance (MR) studies in symptomatic as well as asymptomatic children and adolescents (13,15). Also congenital anomalies (4) and genetic factors (7,17) have been mentioned. The gender distribution is equal between girls and boys.

The possibility of the occurrence of disc herniations at a young age is not very well known. Besides, the clinical picture of lumbar disc herniation in young people differs considerably from the typical sciatica in the adult age group. Due to that, diagnosis is often delayed. The leading symptoms in young patients are a stiff spine, secondary scoliosis, low back pain increasing during activities, and hamstring tightness. Leg pain may be absent or if present, it is usually mild. In some patients symptoms are intermittent. Some youngsters are totally pain-free, but they exhibit a stiff and unbalanced spine as well as a limp due to the inability to tilt the pelvis in the normal way during the gait cycle. Positive neurologic findings are very rare in this age group.

Plain anteroposterior and lateral radiographs of the lumbar spine taken in standing position very often show a secondary scoliosis without vertebral rotation. In some cases they may reveal lumbosacral anomalies or mild disc space narrowing. MR imaging is presently the diagnostic procedure of choice. Computed tomography (CT) imaging, which is superior in visualizing bony structures, may be helpful in special cases (e.g., fractures of the ring apophysis). In assessing MR or CT images one should bear in mind that those are taken with the patient in horizontal position when the spine is unloaded. Thus, bulging discs or protrusions, typical findings in the young population, may appear much smaller or even disappear. In such cases compression CT as described by Willén and colleagues (19) may be indicated for further clarification. Laboratory investigations show normal results in children and adolescents with disc herniation. Electroneuromyography (ENMG) is usually normal, too.

Primary treatment of lumbar disc herniation in children and adolescents is nonoperative, as long as there is no progressive neurologic deficit. A short period of bed rest and analgesic drugs may be helpful in acute cases. Physical activities should be restricted. Application of massage, local heat, ultrasound and/or diadynamic currents, and traction are recommended. Cast or brace treatment may also prove beneficial. No reliable data on the effectiveness of nonoperative measures are available, nor is there any evidence-based knowledge indicating which of the above-mentioned treatment modalities should be preferred.

Immediate surgical treatment is indicated in extremely rare cases with a progressive neurologic deficit. In other cases, surgery should be considered if symptoms do restrict activities of daily living too much despite a sufficient period of intensive nonsurgical measures. The surgical technique follows the rules for adult disc excision. The surgery is performed under general anaesthesia with the patient in a kneeling position. Identification of the level requiring surgery using image intensifier is mandatory. A minimal invasive approach using proper illumination and magnification should be preferred. The intraoperative findings in this age group are somewhat different from the adult. Sequestrated fragments are very rare. Usually a disc protrusion consisting of soft elastic disc material is found. Due to the positioning of the patient intraoperatively, the size of the protrusion is sometimes surprisingly small and the nerve root appears to be free. In those cases, confirmation of the disc level by fluoroscopy is recommended before opening the disc. In patients with congenitally short pedicles, the nerve root may be impinged between the articular process and the bulging disc. In such a case, some resection of the articular process may be necessary in addition to the disc excision. After decompression of the nerve root and exact hemostasis, a free fat graft from the subcutaneous layer is placed onto the dura to diminish scar formation. Patients are mobilized the day after the surgery without external support. They should undergo an intensive muscle rehabilitation program before resuming sports activities.

The primary results after disc excision in young patients are usually good in the vast majority of patients (1,6,8,11,12). Back and leg pain often resolve immediately. Posture changes, secondary scoliosis, and hamstring tightness may persist for some time after surgery, especially in cases with a prolonged preoperative history. The availability of long-term follow-up studies demonstrating favorable results in the majority of young patients are limited (3,14,16).

We studied 18 patients, 9 boys and 9 girls, between the ages of age 11 to 17 years at surgery, with a mean follow-up time of 10.5 (5 to 22) years (10). On preoperative myelograms no signs of a congenitally narrow spinal canal were found. Five of the patients were operated on at the presacral level, and 13 were operated on at the L4-L5 level. Follow-up investigation was performed by an independent observer and included interview, Oswestry disability score, pain drawing, physical examination, and standing anteroposterior and lateral lumbar spine radiographs. MR images were taken in 10 patients at follow-up. At follow-up, the clinical result was good in all patients. The mean Oswestry score was 3.5 (0 to 10). There was no statistical correlation between age at surgery or length of follow-up and clinical result. On plain radiographs, disc height at the surgical level was 50% to 100% as compared to the third lumbar disc. No correlation could be established between disc height at follow-up and age at surgery or length of follow-up. MR images, taken at follow-up from 10 patients, 15 years of age or younger at the time of surgery, revealed signs of disc degeneration (dehydration) in the two lowermost lumbar discs in all but two cases. Three patients also showed disc degeneration in the third lumbar disc. These findings seem to support the assumption that an early degenerative process may play a role in the etiology of juvenile disc herniation.

Good patient outcome after long-term follow-up speaks for the policy of surgical treatment in young patients with lumbar disc herniation if the diagnosis is clear and a reasonable period of nonsurgical treatment and observation does not lead to a satisfactory result.

REFERENCES

1. Borgesen SE, Vang PS. Herniation of the lumbar intervertebral disc in children and adolescents. *Acta Orthop Scand* 1974;45:540–549.
2. Bradford D, Garcia A. Herniations of the lumbar intervertebral disc in children and adolescents. A review of 30 surgically treated cases. *JAMA* 1969;210:2045–2051.
3. DeOrio JK, Bianco AJ. Lumbar disc excision in children and adolescents. *J Bone Joint Surg* 1982; 64–A:991–996.
4. Epstein JA, Epstein NE, Marc J, et al. Lumbar intervertebral disc herniation in teenage children: recognition and management of associated anomalies. *Spine* 1984;9:427–432.
5. Epstein JA, Lavine LS. Herniated lumbar intervertebral discs in children and adolescents. *J Neurosurg* 1964;21:1070–1075.
6. Giroux J-C, Leclercq TA. Lumbar disc excision in the second decade. *Spine* 1982;7:168–170.
7. Gunzburg R, Fraser RD, Fraser GA. Lumbar intervertebral disc prolapse in teenage twins. *J Bone Joint Surg* 1990;72–B:914–916.
8. Korkala O, Poussa M, Merikanto J, et al. Juvenile lumbar disc herniation. *Proc Orthop Hosp Invalid Found* 1986;1:21–22.
9. Kurihara A, Kataoka O. Lumbar disc herniation in children and adolescents. A review of 70 operated cases and their minimum 5-year follow-up studies. *Spine* 1980;5:443–551.
10. Poussa M, Schlenzka D, Mäenpää S, et al. Disc herniation in the lumbar spine during growth: long-term results of operative treatment in 18 patients. *Eur Spine J* 1997;6:390–392.
11. Rugtveit A. Juvenile lumbar disc herniations. *Acta Orthop Scand* 1966;37:348–356.
12. Russwurm H, Bjerkreim I, Ronglan E. Lumbar intervertebral disc herniation in the young. *Acta Orthop Scand* 1978;49:158–163.
13. Salminen JJ, Erkintalo MO, Pentti, J, et al. Recurrent low back pain and early disc degeneration in the young. *Spine* 1999;24:1316–1321.
14. Savini R, Martucci E, Nardi S, et al. The herniated lumbar intervertebral disc in children and adolescents. Long-term follow-up of 101 cases treated by surgery. *Ital J Orthop Traumatol* 1991;17:505–511.
15. Schlenzka D, Seitsalo S, Poussa M, et al. Premature disc degeneration: source of pain in isthmic spondylolis-thesis in adolescents? *J Pediatr Orthop* (Part B) 1993;1:153–157.
16. Silvers HR, Lewis PJ, Clabeaus DE, et al. Lumbar disc excisions in patients under the age of 21 years. *Spine* 1994;19:2387–2392.
17. Varlotta GP, Brown MD, Kelsey JL, et al. Familial predisposition for herniation of a lumbar disc in patients who are less than twenty-one years old. *J Bone Joint Surg* 1991;73–A:124–128.
18. Wahren H. Herniated nucleus pulposus in a child of twelve years. *Acta Orthop Scand* 1946;16:40–42.
19. Willén J, Danielson B, Gaulitz A, et al. Dynamic effects on the lumbar spinal canal. Axially loaded CT–myelography and MRI in patients with sciatica and/or neurogenic claudication. *Spine* 1997;24:2968–2976.

7

Physiologic Aging of the Intervertebral Disc and Herniation in the Adult

Gunnar B. J. Andersson

The term lumbar disc disease is used variably by health professionals involved in the care of back patients to include the full spectrum of degenerative disc disorders or to be limited to the specific entity of disc herniation. When discussing the natural history, diagnosis, and treatment, it is in the area of disc herniations where most of our knowledge exists. This chapter reviews the natural history, evaluation, and treatment of disc herniation while briefly discussing the process of disc degeneration, which, as will become obvious, almost always is present before a herniation occurs.

Disc degeneration is defined by changes in the biochemical and structural components of the disc. This development, which occurs in all individuals as part of the normal aging process, can be diagnosed early using magnetic resonance imaging (MRI) scans, and only much later with radiographs. It is not a painful process as such, but weakens the disc mechanically and changes the relationship between different components of the motion segment. As part of the degenerative process, the disc loses some of its height (narrows) and bulges. Further, fissures (cracks) occur in its substance through which disc material can herniate. Disc bulge and disc herniation are different entities. A bulge is an expansion of disc material beyond its normal border as is a herniation. The difference is that the bulge is circumferential rather than discrete or local. The main reasons for circumferential bulges are that the disc is healthy and subject to compressive load or that it is degenerated (or aged) and disc material has been displaced as part of the reduction in disc height. In both cases, symptoms are not caused by the bulge as such, but large bulges can cause spinal stenosis and impinge on neural tissue.

A localized bulge in the annulus is often referred to as a protrusion. Here disc material is displaced through one or more cracks in the annulus and therefore, a true herniation is present. This protrusion may or may not cause symptoms, depending on its effect on neural tissue. When the annular fibers are completely disrupted and penetrated by disc material, but the disc material still remains in contact with the material inside the disc, we refer to it as an extrusion. Sequestration occurs when there is a truly free fragment that is separated from the annulus and can migrate (16).

DISC DEGENERATION

We do not know in detail how disc degeneration starts. There are probably a number of different initiating events at a biological and biomechanical level that can cause similar pathology. The nucleus, which at birth is gelatinous and well separated from the annulus, begins to change its consistency by the third decade, and by the fifth decade it is dry and fibrotic, merging into the annulus (22). At the same time there is a gradual loss of cells and formation of nuclear clefts. Once formed, these clefts tend to propagate posteriorly and posterolaterally, extending into and sometimes penetrating the annulus. Annular changes accompany the nuclear changes. Over time, annular clefts, often called tears, develop. These are initially mostly concentric (circumferential), separating the annular lamellae, and occasionally progressing to radial tears penetrating the annular fiber rings. The radiating tears, which most commonly develop posterolaterally, typically occur in the fourth and fifth decades. They are most often found in the lower lumbar discs, and are the tears through which disc material herniates.

As the discs degenerate, they narrow and osteophytes develop from the merging of the vertebral bodies. Further, the facet joint surfaces lose their congruency and as a result degenerative changes of the apophyseal joints develop (facet osteoarthritis), contributing to the development of degenerative spinal stenosis (12).

Biochemical changes accompany the morphologic changes. With aging there is gradual change in collagen from type II to type I and III, while the total collagen content remains unchanged (8). There is also an age-related decrease in the amount of enzymatically mediated collagen crosslinks and an increase in nonenzymatically mediated crosslinks which may contribute to mechanical weakening (15). The proteoglycan content in the nucleus pulposus decreases with age, and the size of the aggrecan molecules decreases. This reduces the amount of hydration in the disc because of a loss of osmotic power (21). The end result of the biochemical changes is decrease in the proteoglycan to collagen ratio of the disc, which is most pronounced in the nucleus and changes its load-carrying functions.

Disc degeneration has been studied epidemiologically using radiographs, autopsy material, and MRI techniques (2). By age 50, disc degeneration is present in all spines at autopsy. Radiographs document significant degenerative changes in most spines by the fourth decade. More recently MRI studies, which are more sensitive, show degenerative changes as early as in teenaged individuals, becoming increasingly common with aging. Male discs appear to degenerate earlier and to a greater degree than female discs. Disc degeneration is more severe and starts earlier at L4 and L5 levels, and is least often present at L1 and L2 levels.

Disc degeneration has been classified on MRI into five grades (20). This grading method, shown in Table 7.1, does have good inter- and intraobserver reliability, but its

TABLE 7.1. *Thompson's classification for disc degeneration*

Grade	Nucleus	Annulus	Endplate	Vertebral body
I	Bulging gel	Discrete fibrous lamellae	Hyaline, uniformly thick	Margins rounded
II	White fibrous tissue	Mucinous material peripherally	Thickness irregular between lamellae	Margins pointed
III	Consolidated fibrous tissue	Extensive mucinous infiltration; loss of annular–nuclear demarcation	Focal defects in cartilage	Early chondrophytes or osteophytes at margins
IV	Horizontal clefts parallell to endplate	Focal disruptions	Fibrocartilage extending from subchondral bone; irregularity and focal sclerosis in subchondral bone	
V	Clefts extend through nucleus and annulus		Diffuse sclerosis	Osteophytes greater than 2 mm

clinical importance must still be established. Other MRI findings related to disc degeneration have also been classified. Modic describes signal changes in the vertebral bodies adjacent to the endplates of degenerated discs (14). Type I changes have a decreased signal intensity on T1 and increased intensity on T2 images. Anatomically, there is fissuring of the endplates and vascularized fibrous tissue within the adjacent marrow in these cases. Type II changes have increased intensity on T1 images and an isointense signal on T2 images. In these cases there is also endplate disruption, but at this point there is yellow marrow replacement in the adjacent vertebral body. Finally, Type III changes show decreased signal intensity on both T1 and T2 images. In these cases there is bony sclerosis on radiographs, and absence of marrow adjacent to the endplate histologically. Type I and II changes can be confused with discitis, resulting in unnecessary treatment.

THE NATURAL HISTORY OF DISC HERNIATION

Most of our knowledge to date concerns the symptomatic lumbar disc herniations, but it is well documented that a large number of herniations occur without the presence of symptoms. In addition to anterior herniations, MRI scans of healthy (asymptomatic) individuals reveal the presence of posterior or posterolateral herniations in 21% to 40%, and of disc bulges in up to 79% (5,11,24). These studies confirm similar prevalences previously observed using myelography and computed tomography (CT) scans (10). Both asymptomatic and symptomatic herniations are most common at the L5 and L4 levels, while herniations at L1 and L2 levels are quite rare (9,19). This parallels the distribution of disc degeneration. The fact that both disc herniation and degeneration occur at an earlier age at L5 than at L4, and earlier at L4 than at L3, is further epidemiologic evidence of the relationship between degeneration and herniation.

The natural history of asymptomatic lumbar disc herniations and the natural history of untreated symptomatic herniations are unknown. Most clinicians recall the often quoted study by Weber (23) when natural history is discussed. This study, however, is not really a study of the natural history. Weber's control group underwent considerable clinical intervention (a 2-week hospital stay) and before randomization patients were excluded if they had severe clinical symptoms. Indeed 25% of patients underwent surgery rather than were randomized. What Weber's study showed was that patients with herniations affecting L5 and S1, who did not initially improve or deteriorated, had similar results at 4 and 10 years whether they underwent surgery or not. At 1 year the results were clearly in favor of surgery (90% good versus 60% good), and a significant number of conservatively treated patients (17 patients or 26%) transferred to surgery during this year. Still 60% of patients who were randomized to nonsurgical care improved without a surgical intervention. This is powerful information for patients who for one reason or another are not candidates for surgery. Saal and Saal (17) report a 90% good or excellent outcome for patients with lumbar disc herniations, who receive epidural corticosteroid injections and undertake active exercise treatment. Interestingly, the result was unaffected by the size of the herniation and the presence of neurologic deficits. Extrusions appear to have the best prognosis, and only three of 15 patients with extruded fragments required surgery. Saal and coworkers (18) also report on a smaller group of patients in which 46% had a 75% to 100% resorption of their herniation, and 36% had a 50% to 75% decrease in size. This MRI study also revealed that the largest extrusions were those that had the greatest degree of resorption (16). Although not known in detail, this may be due to the fact that the barrier to vascular invasion and breakdown is broken when the herniation extrudes or sequestrates permitting resorption. Thus, the presence of a large herniation is not in and of itself a surgical indication; it is the patient's pain that is the primary determinant.

Clinically, it is the patient's pain that first improves with treatment. Only later do neurologic deficits normalize. Although the timing of improvement varies, the greatest chance for improvement occurs within the first 6 to 12 weeks of treatment. Neurologic dysfunction is not a surgical indication as such. Most agree, however, that a progressive loss of motor function is a reason for surgical intervention. While patients with a motor loss that is mild to moderate typically regain function over a 3- to 6-month period, it is not uncommon for patients with a severe loss of motor function (grade III and below) to have a slow and only partial recovery. Importantly, in the evaluation of results and recurrences, a lost tendon reflex will rarely return. Weber reports that after 10 years about one-third of patients had some degree of sensory loss, which typically did not influence function (23).

The natural history of a cauda equina syndrome is also not known in detail. There is agreement that once the diagnosis is made delay in surgical treatment should be avoided, but it is uncertain whether or not this is critical to the end result (13). In a metaanalysis, Ahn and colleagues (1) found no difference in result comparing interventions within 24 hours to those within 24 to 48 hours. Improved outcomes occurred, however, in patients treated within 48 hours compared to those treated after 48 hours.

EVALUATION

The clinical symptoms and signs of disc herniations provide the basis on which the diagnosis is made. The typical patient will have a history of back pain which, often suddenly, is accompanied by a "sharp, burning, stabbing, electrical" pain radiating down the back or lateral aspect of one leg reaching below the knee and often to the foot (4). The pain distribution is radicular (dermatomal) and sometimes affects more than one dermatome. Radicular pain, as described above, is a symptom with high sensitivity (0.98) and good specificity (0.88) (6). Numbness, paresthesias (pins and needles), and weakness may be present in these patients, but the sensitivity and specificity are low.

The physical findings almost always include a positive root tension sign (straight leg raise, Lasègue's test, etc.). The raising of a leg will normally move the L4, L5, and S1 nerve roots 1 to 4 mm. A herniated disc can prevent this motion causing radicular pain when the leg is lifted. The reverse straight leg raising test or femoral stretch test causes tension of the L2, L3, and L4 nerve roots. Root tension tests are sensitive (0.80) but unspecific (0.40). The sensitivity decreases with advancing age. Crossed straight leg raising (well leg-raising), on the other hand, is a test with low sensitivity (0.25) and high specificity (0.90). Neurologic tests are important to assess which root is affected. Table 7.2 lists the main neurologic levels (L4-S1). Knee reflexes typically represent L4 function, while S1 function is represented by the ankle reflexes. Minor asymmetry may be due

TABLE 7.2. *Neurologic level diagnosis for herniated lumbar discs*

Disc	Root	Reflex	Muscles	Sensation
L3-L4	L4	Patellar	Anterior tibialis	Medial leg/foot
L4-L5	L5	None	Exterior hall. long	Lateral leg/dorsum foot
L5-S1	S1	Achilles	Peroneus long/brev	Lateral foot

to poor relaxation. To be valid the reflex should show marked asymmetry on repeated testing. A previous herniation will make the reflex test difficult to evaluate, as does advancing age which often causes the reflexes to diminish. The most important motor strength test involves the extensor hallucis longus (L5 innervated), but other muscle strength tests may be helpful as well. A significant cross-innervation exists which can result in misinterpretation (Table 7.3). Sensory changes (sharp pin, light touch, vibrating fork) should be dermatomal rather than diffuse. Most neurologic tests have only moderate sensitivity and specificity.

Because history and physical examination have low diagnostic accuracy by themselves, confirmatory tests are necessary for a definitive diagnosis. While myelograms and CT scans were often used in the past, they have become almost completely replaced by MRI (10). Myelography is currently used mainly in patients where contraindications to MRI exist, or where metallic constructs produce artifacts on a CT or MRI study. And, when used, it is almost always followed by a CT (CT–myelography). Severe deformity is another indication for myelography because the planes of MR images can be difficult to interpret. The advantages of the MRI over CT are that an MRI produces no ionizing radiation, allows multiplanar images with high spatial and contrast resolution, and provides a comprehensive overview of the entire lumbar spine including the conus medullaris. A high quality MRI provides information about the precise location of a herniation, allows classification as to the type of herniation, and informs about the anatomic effect of a herniation on the neural tissues. An open MRI is less informative than a closed, but may still provide sufficient information for decisions on treatment. Although the precise timing of an imaging study varies, depending on the clinical reality and need for the treatment decisions, it is usually not necessary to order one during the initial 4 to 6 weeks after the onset of pain.

Neurophysiologic tests are mainly of use when there is a discrepancy between the clinical findings and the imaging results. Routine use should be discouraged because of the low overall sensitivity and specificity and the excellent available imaging which, together with the clinical symptoms and signs, provides sufficient information. Still, neurodiagnostics are helpful to exclude peripheral nerve damage, to objectively verify muscle weakness, and sometimes for medicolegal reasons (7).

TABLE 7.3. *Segmental innervation of the lower limb musculature*

Joints and muscle groups	Cord segments						
	L2	L3	L4	L5	S1	S2	S3
Knee							
Extensors	O	X	X				
Flexors			O	X	X	O	O
Ankle							
Extensors (dorsiflexors)			X	X	O		
Flexors (plantar flexors)				O	X	X	
Pretalar–subtalar joint							
Invertors			X	X	O		
Evertors				X	X	O	
Toes							
Extensors				X	X	O	
Flexors					X	X	O
Intrinsic foot muscles					X	O	

O, secondary cord segment; X, principal cord segment.

TREATMENT

More detailed information on treatment is available in later chapters of this book. The following is intended as a brief summary.

There is only a minor difference in the initial care of a patient with a disc herniation and one with acute low back pain. The prognosis in disc hernia patients is for a slower recovery and a more frequent need for surgery thus justifying a more aggressive approach. Bed rest and medication are the most frequent early interventions. If used, bed rest should be short (no more than one to two days). Analgesics are almost always indicated and, if pain is severe, narcotics may be used for 3–5 days. Nonsteroidal antiinflammatory drugs (NSAIDs) are indicated in these patients, when tolerated, since there is good evidence of the inflammatory effect of nuclear material, and inflammation plays a major role in the response of nerve roots to compression and traction. For the same reasons the use of Medrol dose packs (oral corticosteroids), epidural steroid injections, and nerve root blocks are advocated. There is no high quality clinical study available on the usefulness of oral steroids in patients with disc herniations. Steroid injections (epidurally and as root blocks) have been studied but with conflicting results (16). As an isolated treatment, modality steroid injections are probably not particularly helpful, but symptomatic relief may allow the patient to be more physically active. Manipulation, braces and corsets, transcutaneous nerve stimulation, and tricyclic medication have no documented effect.

Overall it appears that appropriate pain management, good information to the patient, emphasis on functional return, and time allow for a resolution of symptoms over a 6- to 12-week period in most patients. Passive care should be avoided.

Surgical treatment becomes an option in patients with cauda equina syndrome, progressive neurologic deficit, or persistent symptoms not responding to nonsurgical care. For reasons mentioned earlier, there is rarely an indication to perform surgery during the first 6 to 12 weeks since so many patients recover. The most common surgical procedure is the open discectomy, with or without the use of a microscope. Chemonucleolysis, percutaneous discectomies, and arthroscopic discectomies are procedures that, in some hands and in selected patient groups, can produce good results but overall produce less predictable results than the open discectomy (3).

CONCLUSIONS

Degenerative changes of the lumbar discs occur as a natural part of the aging process. Disc degeneration, while not painful in itself, sets the stage for the development of disc herniations, spinal instability, and spinal stenosis.

The natural history of disc herniation is not known in detail. Generally it is favorable with resolution of symptoms over 6 to 12 weeks in the majority of patients.

The diagnosis of a disc herniation should never be made using history and physical examination alone. Imaging, mainly MRI, is necessary to confirm the clinical suspicion because the clinical assessment has low accuracy. In addition, good imaging provides information on location, allows classification, and can determine the influence of the herniation on neural tissue. A positive imaging study without appropriate clinical symptoms is not very useful either since herniations occur in many individuals without clinical symptoms.

Nonoperative treatment includes a short period of rest, analgesics, and antiinflammatory medication. Epidural steroid injections or root blocks are controversial, but appear to be helpful in some patients, particularly when combined with an aggressive physical therapy program. Good information to the patient, symptomatic treatment, and emphasis on functional return allow for symptom resolution over a 6- to 12-week period in most patients.

For patients in whom nonsurgical treatment is unsuccessful, treatment alternatives include chemonucleolysis, percutaneous discectomy, arthroscopic discectomy, and open discectomy (microdiscectomy or similar). The open discectomy is the gold standard with good to excellent results in over 90% of cases.

REFERENCES

1. Ahn UM, Ahn NU, Buchowski JM, et al. Cauda equina syndrome secondary to lumbar disc herniation: meta analysis of surgical outcomes. Paper #222 presented at: The 66th Annual Meeting of the American Academy of Orthopedic Surgeons; 1999; Anaheim, CA.
2. Andersson GBJ. The epidemiology of spinal disorders, In: Frymoyer JW, ed. The adult spine: principles and practice, 2nd ed. Philadelphia: Lippincott-Raven Publishers, 1997:93–141.
3. Andersson GBJ, Brown MD, Dvorak J, et al. Consensus summary on the diagnosis and treatment of lumbar disc herniation. *Spine* 1996;21:75S–78S.
4. Andersson GBJ, Deyo RA. History and physical examination in patients with herniated lumbar discs. *Spine* 1996;21:10S–18S.
5. Boden SD, Davis DO, Dina TS, et al. Abnormal magnetic resonance scans of the lumbar spine in asymptomatic subjects. *J Bone Joint Surg (Am)* 1990;72:403–408.
6. Deyo RA, Rainville J, Kent DL. What can history and physical examination tell us about low back pain? *JAMA* 1992;268:760–765.
7. Dvorak J. Neurophysiologic tests in diagnosis of nerve root compression caused by disc herniation. *Spine* 1996;21:39S–44S.
8. Eyre D, Benya P, Buckwalter J, et al. The intervertebral disc: basic science perspectives. In: Frymoyer J, Gordon S, eds. *New perspectives on low back pain*. Park Ridge, IL: American Academy of Orthopedic Surgeons; 1993: 391–412.
9. Heliovaara M. *Epidemiology of sciatica and herniated lumbar intervertebral disc* [Thesis]. Helsinki: The Research Institute for Social Security, 1988:1–147.
10. Herzog RJ. The radiologic assessment for a lumbar disc herniation. *Spine* 1996;21:19S–38S.
11. Jensen MC, Brant-Zawedzki MN, Obuchowski N, et al. Magnetic resonance imaging of the lumbar spine in people without back pain. *N Engl J Med* 1994;331:69–73.
12. Kirkaldy-Willis WH. The three phases of the spectrum of degenerative disease. In: Kirkaldy-Willis WH, Burton CV, eds. *Managing low back pain*. New York: Churchill Livingstone, 1992:105–119.
13. Kostuick JP, Harrington I, Alexander D, et al. Cauda equina syndrome and lumbar disc herniation. *J Bone Joint Surg (Am)* 1986;68:386–391.
14. Modic MT, Skimberg PM, Ross JS, et al. Degenerative disc disease: assessment of changes in the vertebral bone marrow with MR imaging. *Radiology* 1988;166:193–199.
15. Pokharna HK, Phillips FM. Collagen crosslinks in human lumbar intervertebral disc aging. *Spine* 1998;23: 1645–1648.
16. Saal JA. Natural history and nonoperative treatment of lumbar disc herniation. *Spine* 1996;21:2S–9S.
17. Saal JA, Saal JS. Nonoperative treatment of herniated intervertebral disc with radiculopathy. *Spine* 1989;14: 431–437.
18. Saal JA, Saal, JS, Herzog RJ. The natural history of lumbar intervertebral disc extrusions treated non-operatively. *Spine* 1990;15:683–686.
19. Spangfort EV. The lumbar disc herniation. *Acta Orthop Scand* 1972[Suppl 142]:1–95.
20. Thompson JP, Pearce RH, Schechter MT, et al. Preliminary evaluation of a scheme for grading the gross morphology of the human intervertebral disc. *Spine* 1990;15:411–415.
21. Urban JP, McMullin JF. Swelling pressure of the lumbar intervertebral discs: influence of age, spinal level, composition, and degeneration. *Spine* 1988;13:179–187.
22. Vernon-Roberts B, Pirie CJ. Degenerative changes in the intervertebral discs and their sequelae. *Rheum Rehabil* 1997;16:13–21.
23. Weber H. Lumbar disc herniation: a controlled, prospective study with ten years of observation. *Spine* 1983; 8:131–140.
24. Weishaupt D, Zanetti M, Hodler J, et al. MR imaging of the lumbar spine: prevalence of intervertebral disc extrusion and sequestration, nerve root compression, endplate abnormalities, and osteoarthritis of the facet joints in asymptomatic volunteers. *Radiology* 1988;209:661–666.

8

Aging and Degeneration: Cause and Effect of Intervertebral Disc Damage?

Keita Ito, Max Aebi, and Mauro Alini

Low back pain is the most common cause of disability in individuals between 20 and 50 years old and it can have enormous socioeconomic consequences (1). Although evidence for an indisputable link between clinical symptoms and intervertebral disc (IVD) degeneration remains elusive, disorders of the IVD have been some of the most widely supported and intensely investigated mechanisms for low back pain (2). While the majority of those affected will not require prolonged medical care or absence from work, about one-third will require more extensive care involving hospitalization. The direct costs of low back pain, as analyzed in 1990 by Frymoyer and Cats-Baril (3), have been estimated to exceed $24 billion. The indirect costs related to lost productivity have been estimated to exceed $27 billion.

Aging and degeneration of the disc may be considered different processes, with degeneration having a more deleterious influence on its structure and function. Their frequent coexistence, however, causes difficulty distinguishing these processes. Mechanisms that may contribute to the age-related and/or degenerative changes of the disc include reduction in nutrient supply, diminished cell viability, loss of notochordal cells, cell senescence, and cell apoptosis, which lead to biochemical alterations in the composition and structure of the extracellular matrix. In addition, disc tissue alterations are also associated with or aggravated by mechanical factors as well as being influenced by genetic factors.

ALTERATIONS IN DISC COMPOSITION AND STRUCTURE WITH AGING

Intervertebral discs are characterized by their abundant extracellular matrix and low cell density, coupled with an absence of blood vessels, lymphatics, and nerves in all but the most peripheral annulus layers. In many respects, this absence leaves the disc prone to degeneration because the cells have a large matrix to maintain without nociceptive feedback to limit and detect damage and no source of repair through the vasculature.

Intervertebral discs are not uniform in composition, but consist of two distinct regions. The outer annulus fibrosus is fibrocartilage and contains concentric lamellae rich in collagen, whereas the inner nucleus pulposus is a less structured gelatinous substance rich in proteoglycans. Degeneration and age-related changes in both the biochemical composition and structure of each component of the IVD have been widely reported (4–8). As discs degenerate, the nucleus pulposus becomes more consolidated and fibrous and is less clearly demarcated from the annulus fibrosus. Focal defects appear in the cartilage endplate, and there is a decrease in the number of layers of the annulus with an increase in thickness and interbundle spacing (9). Degeneration causes decreased hydration especially in the nucleus (4). Water in the nucleus pulposus drops from about 90% of the tissue wet weight in the infant to less than 70% in older adults (4,10). In the annulus fibrosus, the water content remains relatively constant with age, accounting for approximately 60% to 70% of the tissue wet weight (4,10).

At least seven distinct collagen types have been identified in the IVD, types I, II, III, V, VI, IX, and XI. The annulus fibrosus of the IVD has been reported to contain all these collagen types, whereas the nucleus pulposus contains only collagen types I, II, VI, and IX (11–16). In addition, type X collagen has recently been shown to be present in discs with histomorphologic alterations consistent with disc degeneration (17,18). Type I and II collagens constitute about 80% of the collagens in the IVD (4,11). They are distributed radially in opposing concentration gradients, with type II composing the major part of the nucleus pulposus and type I being the major constituent of the annulus fibrosus (4,19). Type I and type II collagens are particularly important to the integrity of the disc because they form the fibrous framework of the tissue. Although the other collagen types identified in the disc account for a smaller proportion of the total collagen, they may make a very significant contribution to the overall function of the tissue. Collagen represents about 15% to 20% of the nucleus and 65% to 70% of the annulus dry weight (4,11,20,21).

The trend is reversed for proteoglycans, which represent approximately 50% of the dry weight in the nucleus, and drop to 10% to 20% in the annulus (4,11,20,21). The ability of disc tissue to resist compressive forces is largely due to its high content of the proteoglycan aggrecan. Many aggrecan molecules can bind to a single hyaluronate chain, producing large proteoglycan aggregates (22–24). Versican at the mRNA level, another proteoglycan with the ability to form aggregates with hyaluronate, has been shown to be present within the IVD (25). In addition to aggregating proteoglycans, these tissues also contain proteoglycans that do not have the ability to interact specifically with hyaluronate. Such distinct molecules that have been definitively identified include decorin and biglycan (26,27), and it has been recently shown that fibromodulin and lumican, which also belong to the expanding family of leucine-rich repeat protein, are present in the human IVD (28).

Aging and degeneration are accompanied by a marked decrease in proteoglycan content in the nucleus and significant alterations in proteoglycan structure (4,6,29). The collagen content remains relatively constant in the nucleus with aging and degeneration, whereas a decrease is observed in the annulus (4). In addition, a change in the distribution of collagen types I and II has been reported (4,8,30,31).

Noncollagenous proteins represent up to 45% of the dry weight of the nucleus pulposus and 25% of the annulus fibrosus in a human disc (32). Several of the identifiable noncollagenous proteins include fibronectin, thrombospondin, and elastin. However, their significance and their possible changes with degeneration are presently unknown (53).

The process of disc degeneration involves the destruction of structural proteins, including collagens and proteoglycans within the extracellular matrix. It is generally agreed that proteinases play a major role in this process. The primary proteinases thought to be involved in the direct destruction of the cartilage tissue are the matrix metalloproteinases (MMPs), particularly stromelysin and collagenase (33–35). There are three collagenases: the interstitial enzyme produced by connective tissue cells (MMP-1), that produced by PMN leukocytes (MMP-8), and the recently cloned MMP-13 (36). Three forms of stromelysin have also been described: the original form (MMP-3), stromelysin-2 (MMP-10) and, more recently, stromelysin-3 (MMP-11). Stromelysin (MMP-3) has received particular attention because of its action on a wide range of connective tissue matrix components, including aggrecan and type IX collagen (37–39). Furthermore, it is able to activate procollagenase by proteolytic cleavage (40). Once activated, collagenase can degrade type I and type II collagens by cleavage in the helical domains, thus making these collagens susceptible to further enzymatic degradation. In addition, it has been shown that aggrecan cleavage products at the metalloproteinase and aggrecanase sites are present in the IVD tissue, suggesting that these enzymes are also present in this tissue (41). Indeed, these results indicate that the two enzyme systems act independently of each other and exhibit differences in the degree to which they contribute to aggrecan degradation in the different regions of the disc (41). Unlike most other connective tissue cell types little is known about the ability of disc cells to produce the different metalloproteinases. The only proteinase extracted directly from IVD appears to be a serine proteinase rather than a metalloproteinase, and it has properties similar to plasmin (42,43). However, human disc in organ culture has been shown to synthesize stromelysin, which can become activated within the matrix (44). MMP-2 and MMP-9 have also been shown to be present at higher levels in degenerated human discs, suggesting a key role for these metalloproteinases in disc degeneration (45).

MECHANISMS THAT CONTRIBUTE TO AGE-RELATED DEGENERATIVE ALTERATIONS

Notochordal Cells

The vertebral column develops in the embryonic mesoderm at about 4 weeks gestational age in humans (46). The vertebral bodies mature under the combined influence of the notochord and neuronal tube. The disc grows initially in an environment that contains few blood vessels and is surrounded by a perichondral layer, the future longitudinal vertebral ligaments. Between the vertebrae, the notochord expands, as local aggregations of cells (the notochordal cells) within a proteoglycan matrix, forming the gelatinous center of the IVD, the nucleus pulposus. The nucleus is later surrounded by the circularly arranged fibers of the annulus fibrosus, which are derived from the perichordal mesenchyme. The rapid increase in notochordal nucleus pulposus volume in fetuses occurs at the expense of the inner annulus region. At this point, the cells populating the nucleus pulposus are a mixture of notochordal and chondrocyte-like cells, while the rest of the IVD contains fibroblast-like cells. However, at the junction with the notochordal sheath, the cells of the inner annulus are closer in shape to the chondrocyte-like cells found within the nucleus. The exact role and interaction of notochordal cells with the other disc cells is unknown. However, a recent study suggests an important function of notochordal cells in stimulating proteoglycan synthesis by nucleus pulposus cells (48). This synergy may be of importance in maintaining a normal nondegenerated disc. Interestingly, notochordal cells disappear from the human disc as well as in chondrodystrophoid dogs, cattle, and sheep during early life, whereas in other animals (i.e., nonchondrodystrophoid dogs, cats, pigs, mice, rats, and rabbits) notochordal cells persist into adulthood (47). Remarkably, animals that preserve notochordal cells into later life do not have degenerated discs, or if they do, it is to a much lesser degree. Thus, the loss of notochordal cells may be seen as the first step toward aging of the disc.

Nutrition and Fluid Flow

It has been proposed that insufficient nutrition may cause degradation of nucleus pulposus material properties and hence its load-bearing properties, leading to damage of other spinal structures (i.e., disc collapse or herniation). This is appealing not only because of the tenuous nutritional supply of the disc but also because of evidence showing its restriction.

The adult human disc is the largest avascular structure in the body. In adult discs, some cells may be as much as 6 to 8 mm from the nearest blood supply, which resides in the osseous endplate of the adjacent vertebral bodies. Similar to the articulating ends of long bones, the vertebral endplate is covered by a thin layer of hyaline cartilage, the cartilaginous endplate. However, unlike long bones, the deep calcified layer and the underlying subchondral bone is penetrated by marrow contact channels (MCCs) through which capillary buds emerge. These capillary buds connect the trabecular spaces to the cartilaginous endplate, but do not penetrate into it (49). In addition to the endplate, there is also a vascular network in the outer annulus. The relative importance of these two sources of nutrition has been investigated using hydrogen washout, (50) fluorescent dyes, (51) and radiologic techniques (52). All of these studies supported the general consensus that the central region of the endplate is the predominant route of transport for metabolic processes of the disc.

The actual complex transport mechanisms of disc nutrition and metabolism have also been studied. For small solutes, it has been shown in isolated functional spine units that diffusion is the predominant molecular transport mechanism from the endplate to the nucleus, (53), and that it is sufficient for transport rates consistent with the metabolic needs of the disc (51). These conclusions were also supported by in vivo studies in anesthetized dogs showing transport by molecular diffusion. (54,55). In addition to steric considerations, there are also electric charge considerations. Because the extracellular matrix of cartilaginous endplate and nucleus consist of highly concentrated proteoglycans, these tissues have a high negative charge density. Thus, positively charged solutes may exchange freely with the nuclear matrix and uncharged solutes may cross the endplate relatively easily, but negatively charged solutes may have difficulty travelling through the endplate and nuclear matrix (55).

It has also been suggested that convective solute transport may play a role in nourishing the disc. Biomechanically, the nucleus pulposus is a poroelastic material, a mixture of solid and fluid. Because of its poroelastic nature, fluid flow is inextricably coupled to the deformation of the tissue such as the diurnal change in disc volume, which has been reported to be as high as 20% (56,57). Hence, there is a cyclic flow of fluid, exudation, and imbibition, accompanying loss in disc height during loading of the spine over the course of a day and return of this height with unloading during overnight rest. This fluid exchange with the nucleus occurs through the endplates similar to the exchange of nutrition and metabolites. During compressive creep of canine spinal motion segments, fluid was observed to exude out of the endplates but not from the annulus (58). More recently, fresh lumbar SMS without ligaments from adult White New Zealand rabbits was allowed to swell immersed in normal saline with a Procion red stain (59). Histologic examination of the fluorescent dye penetration showed that in all specimens, the stain penetrated from the trabecular spaces, through the MCCs and cartilage endplate, into the nucleus pulposus (Fig. 8.1), but did not penetrate the annulus (Fig. 8.2). This spatial correlation of fluid flow and nutritional source suggests that fluid flow may aid the transport of solutes in the disc by convection. In vivo studies with radioactive tracers in exercised versus anesthetized dogs show only moderately deeper penetration of the tracer in more active dogs. However, it must be kept in mind that the greatest fluid exchange volume occurs over a diurnal cycle. Furthermore, since the fluid flow is cyclic, the assistance of fluid flow would be combined convection and diffusion (i.e., convective mixing). Hence for small solutes, diffusion may still predominate, but transport of larger solutes such as proteins may be significantly facilitated by the bulk flow of fluid (53,60).

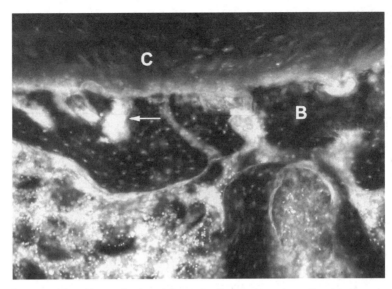

FIG. 8.1. Cross-section of vertebral endplate of spinal segment swollen in normal saline with fluorescent dye. Subchondral bone (*B*); cartilage (*C*); marrow contact channel (*arrow*).

Nevertheless, whether diffusion alone or in combination with convection is the transport mechanism for nutrients and metabolites in the disc, the predominant route remains through the endplates. Interestingly, endplate blood vessels have been observed to diminish after the age of 20 years when the first signs of disc degeneration are evident (61). Also reduced permeability of endplates is generally seen in association with disc degeneration and age-related changes (49,62). Both of these changes may be due to calcifica-

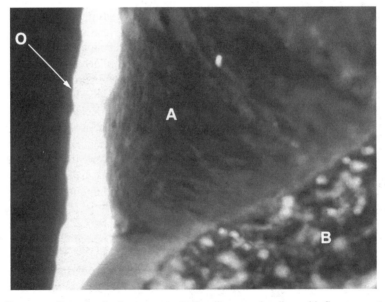

FIG. 8.2. Cross-section of spinal segment swollen in normal saline with fluorescent dye. Subchondral bone (*B*); exterior edge of annulus fibrosis (*O*).

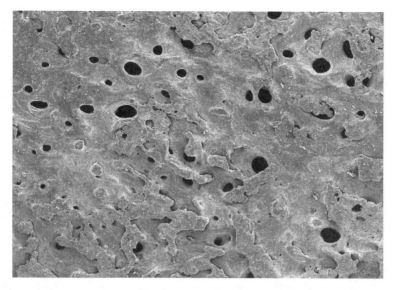

FIG. 8.3. Typical scanning electron micrograph of an emaciated human osseous endplate surface from a younger donor.

tion of the endplates and occlusion of the MCCs observed with disease and age (63–65). These changes can be clearly illustrated by emacerated endplates examined with scanning electron microscopy. Figures 8.3 and 8.4 produced in pilot experiments on lumbar endplates harvested from young and older human donors clearly show that the marrow contact channels are patent in a younger endplate, whereas in an older endplate, the increased mineral deposition has occluded the channels (66).

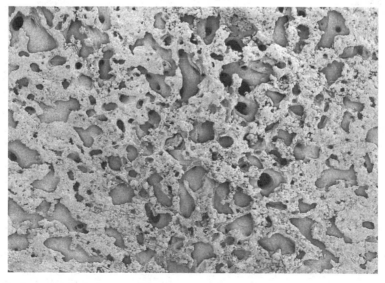

FIG. 8.4. Typical scanning electron micrograph of an emaciated human osseous endplate surface from an older donor.

With a decrease in the number and caliber of the channel openings in the endplate, exchange of solutes from the capillary buds would be diminished and diffusion would be inhibited. Finite element analyses of the fluid flow through the channels have also showed that both the exuding and imbibing resistances decrease with occlusion and that the resistances become similar (66). These changes in the fluid flow with occlusion would cause the volume of fluid exchanged over a diurnal cycle to decrease and a net loss in fluid exchanged over each diurnal cycle to occur. With the decreased bulk flow, convective transport may be hindered and loss of fluid would result in disc dehydration. Even without the aid of fluid flow, occlusion of the channels would diminish diffusion from and to the capillary buds. Hence, with decreased nutrient and metabolite transport, it is believed that the cells are unable to maintain the matrix necessary for the normal function of the disc, resulting in degeneration. These predictions are both consistent with disc dehydration (4) and decreasing proteoglycan content observed in degenerated discs (4,67).

Cell Metabolism

The lack of an appropriate nutritional supply will subsequently affect cell metabolism and cell viability. *In vivo* metabolic studies have mainly examined $^{35}SO_4{}^{2-}$ incorporation into newly synthesized proteoglycans at different time points after injection of radiolabeled materials (68–73). Among these studies, two analyzed changes in proteoglycan synthesis with aging and one explored the effect of strenuous running exercise on proteoglycan synthesis (71–73). These studies showed that with aging and degeneration a new proteoglycan population was synthesized which was of larger average hydrodynamic size and richer in keratan sulfate (72). Excessive running induced alterations in the disc proteoglycans in the most strained area of the dog's spine (upper thoracic) (73).

Metabolic studies also support the idea that many disc proteoglycans may be synthesized as large aggrecan molecules, which are subsequently subjected to proteolysis in the matrix (68,74). This has now been confirmed by a human study, using anti-neoepitope antibodies specific for the amino–terminal degradation products generated by cleavage within the interglobular domain at the metalloproteinase and aggrecanase sites (41). Recently, it has been reported that biosynthetic changes also contribute to the age-related increase in the heterogeneity of human disc proteoglycans (75), and that a progressive decrease in aggrecan synthesis in human lumbar IVDs occurs with aging (4). Thus the reduction in aggrecan content observed with age within the disc may be the result of the observed drop in the synthetic activity of the disc cells, or increased degradative capacity of these cells. In addition, the disc contains link proteins, which stabilize the interaction between aggrecan molecules and hyaluronate chains (76). However, the disc link proteins show increased proteolytic modification compared to those extracted from cartilage, and their abundance drops considerably with age (77). There is also evidence that disc link proteins may have a lower capacity to stabilize proteoglycan aggregates than their cartilage counterparts (78). Such properties of disc link protein may play a role in the loss of proteoglycan and in its ability to aggregate, as observed in an experimental model of disc degeneration (79), and may also be related to the observed loss in human disc proteoglycan that precedes tissue degeneration (80).

Only a recent study has investigated changes in collagen synthesis rate with aging and degeneration. In this study, it was demonstrated that type II collagen degradation of the human lumbar IVD was increased with aging and degeneration (4). In addition, the authors also showed that synthesis for type II collagen was strongly suppressed with aging, while that for type I collagen increased, presumably resulting in the fibrotic appearance of degenerated disc tissue. In addition, this reversal suggested independent regulatory mechanisms in the synthesis of these two collagens during aging and degeneration.

Few *in vitro* experiments have been performed to study alterations of the metabolic activity of disc cells. Explant cultures maintained at *in vivo* hydration levels using poly-ethylene glycol (PEG) (81,82) or in a free swelling environment (83), and alginate bead cultures (84) have been used to measure changes in the proteoglycan synthesis rates with aging. The results of these works show that the age-related decline in proteoglycan biosynthesis observed in human disc tissue *in vivo* is also reflected in these culture systems (4). Not only was there a decline in proteoglycan synthesis with age, but the number of viable cells isolated from the adult tissue was also dramatically reduced compared to fetal or calf tissues, suggesting a decline in the number of viable cells present within the disc tissue with aging (84). This diminished cell density with aging and degeneration occurs most probably by programmed cell death, as has been reported in recent studies (85). Cell apoptosis has been also shown to increase with excessive mechanical load (86).

Mechanical Loading

Mechanical factors are often associated with disc diseases and low back pain. The development of lumbar disc rupture is reported to be associated with activities including frequent bending and twisting as well as heavy physical work (87). In general, pathology of the spine and back is often considered to be associated with or aggravated by mechanical factors. Mechanical studies of the motion segment have been performed to assess the structural response to a variety of loading modes, such as compression, flexion/extension, lateral bending, shear, and torsion (88–108). These studies document some fundamental mechanical characteristics of the motion segment, such as viscoelasticity, nonlinear behaviors, and sensitivity to environmental factors (temperature and humidity). The overall results of these studies give evidence that torque and rotation applied to the disc are related to deformation of the annulus, while compressive forces are more related to disc bulging. Furthermore, studies of motion segments with aging or degenerated discs report increased deformability, decreased nucleus pressure, reduced stiffness and fatigue strength, altered failure properties, and changes in the viscoelastic effects of the motion segment compared to motion segments with nondegenerated IVDs (89,94,96,98,101, 109–111). These studies provide evidence that changes in disc extracellular matrix composition (with aging or degeneration) alter the mechanical properties of the disc.

The influence of mechanical factors, however, is not so clear. Only recently has there been confirmation of a link between disc degeneration, mechanical loading, and low back pain (112). Even so, the causal relationship between mechanical loading and changes in matrix composition are poorly understood. Specifically, gross structural failures are noted to be associated with tissue composition changes, but did an unobserved mechanical change stimulate cellular-mediated degeneration leading to the end stage or did biochemical changes of the matrix degrade mechanical function by itself? Both are reasonable conclusions.

In addressing the former, investigations have exhibited some possible mechanisms. Severe (113,114) or repetitive loading (115,116) in normal discs has been shown to produce disc prolapse and radial fissures. Also biological degeneration of the disc was induced following scalpel-induced damage to the annulus fibrosus (117,118). However, what about mechanical loading causing disc degeneration without a noted prior injury? Fatigue damage to endplates has been simulated with normal range of loading (119). A method was then developed whereby similar minor damage to endplates could be created such that SMS height was reduced by only 1% (120). During subsequent moderate repetitive loading, the nucleus became decompressed with significantly lower pressures and increased stress concentrations were observed within the annulus as compared to the same SMS prior to endplate damage. Also the magnitude of these changes was more significant with older motion segments (121). Finally, these pressure changes created by minor mechanical damage of the endplates were consistent with those that inhibit cell metabolism (122,123).

On the other hand, recent studies have investigated the direct effect of mechanical loading on disc cell metabolism and matrix biochemistry both *in vitro* and *in vivo*. An increase in the glycosaminoglycan content was observed in rat tail discs loaded at approximately 0.15 MPa above physiologic loading with Ilizarov-type apparatus compared with content of those at the control levels (124). This result was not anticipated in light of stud-

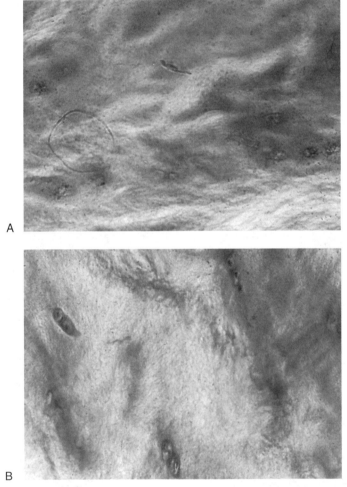

FIG. 8.5. Localization of type II collagen mRNA in histologic sections of bovine nucleus pulposus region by *in situ* hybridization using a 180-base pair probe. An entire functional spine unit was loaded for 2 hours at either (**A**) 150 N (physiological load); or (**B**) 700 N (excessive load). A clear hybridization signal for type II collagen mRNA was observed in the control disc (**A**) while in the disc with the excessive load for an extended period of time, no signal was detected (**B**).

ies on spine and cartilage, in which results showed decreased proteoglycan synthesis or content with increased static compression, hydrostatic pressure, or immobilization (125–127). However, results in studies *in vitro* using human and bovine tail discs indicate that the response to load is not monotonic (122,123,128). This bimodal response has also been found for articular cartilage and is partially attributed to decreased interstitial pH or transient changes in the mechanical environment of the cells with compressive deformations (129,130). Taken together these studies clearly indicate that at high compressive forces catabolic effect and cell apoptosis occur (Fig. 8.5), whereas at more physiologic compressions cell anabolic activities are favored. In addition, it should also be noted that the presence of notochordal cells in rats, mice, and other animals may enable discs in these species to respond to their mechanical environment in a different manner, or at different stress magnitudes than human discs (48).

CONCLUSIONS

The first change that IVDs undergo is the loss of notochordal cells. This is complete by the age of 10 in humans. The role and importance of these cells is not yet well known. Recent evidence indicates a possible function for these cells in stimulating the synthesis of extracellular matrix proteins by nucleus pulposus cells (48). Interestingly, a tenfold decrease in the synthesis of aggrecan and collagen types I and II has been shown to occur by the age of 15 in humans (4). Is this striking diminished cell activity a consequence of the notochordal cells lost? If so, it may be concluded that the aging process starts in humans by the age of 10, which is not a very promising situation for many of us.

However, not all of us will experience back pain in our lives, although, all of us will lose notochordal cells approximately at the same age. So, what are the other concomitant factors that may induce disc degeneration? Lack of an appropriate nutritional supply and excessive loading may accelerate disc degeneration, in addition to genetic predispositions. Thus, studies related to solute transport and cellular response to mechanical load will be fundamental to improving our knowledge of intervertebral disc aging and degeneration.

REFERENCES

1. Andersson GB. *Acta Orthop Scand Suppl* 1998;281:28–31.
2. Nachemson AL. *Clin Orthop Relat Res* 1985;200:266–278.
3. Frymoyer JW, Cats-Baril WL. *Orthop Clin North Am* 1991;22:263–271.
4. Antoniou J, Steffan T, Nelson F, et al. *J Clin Invest* 1996;98(4):996–1003.
5. Cole TC, Ghosh P, Taylor TKF. *Biochim Biophys Acta* 1986;880:209–219.
6. Lyons G, Eisenstein S, Sweet M. *Biochim Biophys Acta* 1981;673:443–453.
7. Miller J, Schmatz C, Schultz A. *Spine* 1988;13:173–178.
8. Pearce R. In: Buckwalter JA, Goldberg VM, Woo SLY, eds. *Musculoskeletal soft-tissue aging. Impact on mobility*. Rosemont, IL: American Academy of Orthopaedic Surgeons, 1993:363–379.
9. Marchand F, Ahmed A. *Spine* 1990;15:402–410.
10. Gower WE, Pedrini V. *J Bone Joint Surg* 1969;51A:1154–1162.
11. Eyre DR. Collagens of the disc. In: Ghosh P, ed. *The biology of the intervertebral disc*. Vol 1. Boca Raton, FL: CRC Press, 1988:171–188.
12. Adam M, Deyl Z. *Ann Rheum Dis* 1984;43:258–263.
13. Ayad S, Abedin MZ, Weiss JB, et al. *FEBS Lett* 1982;139:300–304.
14. Ayad S, Abedin MZ, Grundy SM, et al. *FEBS Lett* 1981;123:195–199.
15. Ayad S, Weiss JB. Biochemistry of the intervertebral disc. In: Jayson MIV, ed. *The lumbar spine and back pain*, 3rd ed, London: Pitmann Publishers, 1986:100–137.
16. Wu JJ, Eyre D, Slayter HS. *Biochem J* 1987;248:373–381
17. Boos N, Nerlich AG, Wiest I, von der Mark K, et al. *Histochem. Cell Biol* 1997;108:471–480.
18. Aigner T, Greskotter K, Fairbank JCT, et al. *Calcif Tissue Int* 1998;63:262–268.
19. Eyre DR, Muir H. *Biochim Biophys Acta* 1977;492:29–42.

20. Eyre DR, Benya P, Buckwalter J, et al. The intervertebral disc. Part B: Basic sciences perspectives. In: Frymoyer JW, Gordon SL, eds. *New perspectives on low back pain.* Park Ridge, IL: American Academy of Orthopaedic Surgeons, 1989:147–207.
21. Eyre DR. Biochemistry of the intervertebral disc. *Int Rev Connect Tissue Res* 1979;8:227.
22. Hascall VC. *J Supramolec Struc* 1977;7:101–120.
23. Heinegård D, Axelsson I. *J Biol Chem* 1977;252:1971–1979.
24. Nilsson B, DeLuca S, Lohmander S, et al. *J Biol Chem* 1982;257:10920–10927.
25. Dours-Zimmermann MT, Zimmermann DR. *J Biol Chem* 1994;269:32992–32998.
26. Roughley PJ, White RJ, Magny M-C, et al. *Biochem J* 1993;295:321–426.
27. Johnstone B, Markopoulos M, Neame P, et al. *Biochem J* 1993;292:661–666.
28. Sztrolovics R, Alini M, Mort JS, et al. *Spine* 1999;24:1765–1771.
29. Buckwalter JA. *Spine* 1995;20:1307–1314.
30. Brickley-Parsons D, Gilmcher M. *Spine* 1984;9:148–163.
31. Pearce RH, Grimmer BJ, Adams ME. *J Orthop Res* 1987;5:198–205.
32. Melrose J, Ghosh P. The noncollagenous proteins of the intervertebral disc. In: Ghosh P, ed. *The biology of the intervertebral disc.* Vol. 2. Boca Raton, FL: CRC Press, 1988:190–237.
33. Poole AR. Enzymatic degradation: cartilage destruction. In: Brandt KD, ed. *Cartilage changes in osteoarthritis.* Indiana University School of Medicine, Ciba-Geigy Co. 1990:63–72.
34. Mort JS, Dodge GR, Roughley PJ, et al. *Matrix* 1991;13:95–102.
35. Nguyen W, Murphy G, Roughley PJ, et al. *Biochem J* 1989;259:61–67.
36. Freije JM, Diez-Itza I, Balbin M, et al. *J Biol Chem* 1994;269:16766–16773.
37. Chin JR, Murphy G, Werb Z. *J Biol Chem* 1985;260:12367–12376.
38. Okada Y, Nagase H, Harris ED. *J Biol Chem* 1986;261:14245–14255.
39. Okada Y, Konomi H, Yada T, et al. *FEBS Letts* 1989;244:473–476.
40. Murphy G, Cockett MI, Stephens PE, et al. *Biochem J* 1987;248:265–268.
41. Sztrolovics R, Alini M, Mort JS, et al. *Biochem J* 1997;326:235–241.
42. Melrose J, Ghosh P, Taylor TKF. *Biochim Biophys Acta* 1987;923:483–495.
43. Cole TC, Melrose J, Ghosh P. *Biochim Biophys Acta* 1989;990:254–262.
44. Liu J, Roughley PJ, Mort JS. *J Orthop Res* 1991;9:568–575.
45. Crean JK, Roberts S, Jaffray DC, et al. *Spine* 1997;15:2877–2884.
46. Humzah MD, Soames RW. *Anat Rec* 1988;220:337–356.
47. Taylot JR, Twomey LT. The development of the human intervertebral disc. In: Ghosh P, ed. *The biology of the intervertebral disc.* Vol 1. Boca Raton, FL: CRC Press, 1988:40–82.
48. Aguiar DJ, Johnson SL, Oegema TR. *Exp Cell Res* 1999;246:129–137.
49. Nachemson A, Lewin T, Maroudas A, et al. *Acta Orthop Scand* 1970;41:589–607.
50. Ogata K, Whiteside LA. *Spine* 1981;6:211–216.
51. Holm S, Maroudas A, Urban JP, et al. *Connect Tissue Res* 1981;8:101–119.
52. Crock HV, Goldwasser M. *Spine* 1984;9:702–706.
53. Maroudas A, Stockwell RA, Nachemson A, et al. *J Anat* 1975;120:113–130.
54. Urban JP, Holm S, Maroudas A, et al. *Clin Orthop* 1977;122:587–593.
55. Urban JP, Holm S, Maroudas A. *Biorheology* 1978;15:203–221.
56. Botsford DJ, Esses SI, Ogilvie-Harris DJ. *Spine* 1994;19:935–940.
57. Malko JA, Hutton WC, Fajman WA. *Spine* 1999;24:1015–1022.
58. Cassidy JJ, Hiltner A, Baer E. *Connect Tissue Res* 1989;23:75–88.
59. Ayotte D, Tepic S, Ito K. *J Bone Joint Surg (Br)* 1999;81[Suppl]:67.
60. Tomlinson N, Maroudas A. *J Bone Joint Surg (Br)* 1980;62:251–259.
61. Putschar W. Comparative disc pathology. *Lab Invest* 1959;8:1259–1263.
62. Brown MD, Tsaltas TT. *Spine* 1976;1:240–244.
63. Bernick S, Cailliet R. *Spine* 1982;7:97–102.
64. Roberts S, Menage J, Eisenstein SM. *J Orthop Res* 1993;11:747–757.
65. Roberts S, Urban JP, Evans H, et al. *Spine* 1996;21:415–420.
66. Ayotte D, Tepic S, Perren SM. *J Biomech Eng* 2000;122:587–593.
67. Adams P, Eyre DR, Muir H. *Rheumatol Rehabil* 1977;16:22–29.
68. Cole TC, Burkhardt D, Frost L, et al. *Biochim Biophys Acta* 1985;839:127–138.
69. Lohmander S, Automopoulus CA, Frieberg S. *Biochim Biophys Acta* 1973;304:430–448.
70. Venn G, Mason RM. *Biochem J* 1983;215:217–225.
71. Venn G, Mason RM. *Biochem J* 1986;234:475–479.
72. Cole TC, Ghosh P, Taylor TKF. *Biochim Biophys Acta* 1986;880:209–219.
73. Puustjarvi K, Lammi M, Helminen H, et al. *Connect Tissue Res* 1994;30:225–240.
74. Oegema TR, Bradford DS, Cooper KM. *J Biol Chem* 1979;254:10579–1058.
75. Johnstone B, Bayliss MT. *Spine* 1996;20(6):674–684.
76. Donohue PJ, Jahnke MR, Blaha JD, et al. *Biochem J* 1988;251:739–747.
77. Pearce RH, Mathieson J, Mort JS, et al. *J Orthop Res* 1989;7:861–867.
78. Tengblad A, Pearce RH, Grimmer BJ. *Biochem J* 1984;222:85–92.
79. Lipson SJ, Muir H. *Arthritis Rheum* 1981;24:12–21.

80. Pearce RH, Grimmer BJ, Adams, ME. *J Orthop Res* 1987;5:198–205.
81. Bayliss T, Johnstone B, O'Brien JP. *Spine* 1988;13(9):972–981.
82. Bayliss MT, Urban JPG, Johnstone B, et al. *J Orthop Res* 1986;4:10–17.
83. Thompson JP, Oegema TR, Bradford DS. *Spine* 1991;16:253–260.
84. Heathfield TF, Goudsouzian NM, Aebi M, et al. *Trans Orthop Res Soc* 1998;22:149.
85. Gruber HE, Hanley EN. *Spine* 1998;23(7):751–757.
86. Lotz JC, Chin SR. *Spine* 2000;25(12):1477–1483.
87. Frymoyer J. *Epidemiology*. Park Ridge, IL: American Academy of Orthopedic Surgeons, 1989:19–34.
88. Adams M, Hutton W. *Spine* 1981;6:241–248.
89. Andersson G, Schultz A. *J Biomech* 1979;12:453–458.
90. Brinckmann P, Frobin W, Hierholzer E, et al. *Spine* 1983;8:851–856.
91. Brown T, Hanson R, Yorra A. *J Bone Joint Surg* 1957;39A:1135–40.
92. Goel V, Nishiyama K, Weinstein J, et al. *Spine* 1986;11:1008–1012.
93. Hickey D, Hukins D. *Spine* 1980;5:106–116.
94. Hirsch C, Nachemson A. *Acta Orthop Scand* 1954;23:254.
95. Kahmann R, Buttermann G, Lewis J, et al. *Spine* 1990;15:971–978.
96. Kazarian L. *Orthop Clin North Am* 1975;6:3–18.
97. Keller T, Holm S, Hansson T, et al. *Spine* 1990;15:751–761.
98. Keller T, Spengler D, Hansson T. *J Orthop Res* 1987;5:467–478.
99. Krag M, Wilder D, Pope M. *Spine* 1987;12:1001–1007.
100. McNally D, Adams M. *Spine* 1992;17:66–73.
101. Myers B, McElhaney J, Doherty B. *J Biomech* 1991;9:811–817.
102. Nachemson A, Schultz A, Berkson M. *Spine* 1979;4:1–8.
103. Panjabi M, Krag M, Chung T. *Spine* 1984;9:707–713.
104. Reuber M, Schultz A, Denis F, et al. *J Biomech Eng* 1982;104:187–192.
105. Rolander S, Blair W. *Orthop Clin North Am* 1975;6:75–81.
106. Seroussi R, Krag M, Muller D, et al. *J Orthop Res* 1989;7:122–131.
107. Stokes I. *J Orthop Res* 1987;5:348–355.
108. Virgin W. *J Bone Joint Surg* 1951;33B:607–611.
109. Koeller W, Muehlhaus S, Meier W, et al. *J Biomech* 1986;19:807–816.
110. Krag M, Pflaster D, Johnson C, et al. *Trans Orthop Res Soc* 1993;18:207.
111. Panjabi M, Brown M, Lindahl S, et al. *Spine* 1988;13:913–917.
112. Videman T, Nurminen M, Troup JD. *Spine* 1990;15:728–740.
113. Adams MA, Hutton WC. *Spine* 1982;7:184–191.
114. McNally DS, Shackleford IM, Goodship AE, et al. *Spine* 1996;21:2580–2587.
115. Adams MA, Hutton WC. *Spine* 1985;10:524–531.
116. Shirazi-Adl A. *Spine* 1989;14:96–103.
117. Osti OL, Vernon-Roberts B, Fraser RD. *Spine* 1991;15:762–767.
118. Pfeiffer M, Griss P, Franke P, et al. *Eur Spine J* 1994;3:8–16.
119. Hansson TH, Keller TS, Spengler DM. *J Orthop Res* 1987;5:479–487.
120. Adams MA, McNally DS, Wagstaff J, et al. *Eur Spine J* 1993;1:214–221.
121. Adams MA, Freeman BJ, Morrison HP, et al. *Spine* 2000;25:1625–1636.
122. Handa T, Ishihara H, Ohshima H, et al. *Spine* 1997;22:1085–1091.
123. Ishihara H, McNally DS, Urban JPG, et al. *J Appl Physiol* 1996;80:839–846.
124. Iatridis JC, Mente PL, Stokes IAF, et al. *Spine* 1999;24:996–1002.
125. Hutton WC, Toribatake Y, Elmer WA, et al. *Spine* 1998;23: 2524–2537.
126. Hall AC, Urban JPG, Gehl KA. *J Orthop Res* 1991;9:1–10.
127. Kiviranta I, Jurvelin J, Tammi M, et al. *Arthritis Rheum* 1987;30:801–809.
128. Ohshima H, Urban JPG, Bergel DH. *J Orthop Res* 1995;13:22–29.
129. Bachrach NM, Valhmu WB, Stazzone E, et al. *J Biomech* 1995;28:1561–1569.
130. Gray ML, Pizzanelli AM, Grodzinsky AL, et al. *J Orthop Res* 1988;6:777–792.

9

The Natural History
of Lumbar Disc Herniation

Michel Benoist

The majority of patients suffering from a radiculopathy caused by a herniated nucleus pulposus heal spontaneously without surgery or chemonucleolysis. The clinical course of the radiculopathy varies as well as the efficacy of conservative treatment. In some patients the symptoms decline after a week or two; in others the pain may continue for many months or years. Despite an abundance of literature there is still a controversy concerning the treatment of radiculopathies related to ruptured lumbar intervertebral discs. Obviously, knowledge of the natural history of disc herniation and of the mechanisms leading to the changes in the extruded disc tissue would be of great help in planning the therapeutic procedure. The purpose of this chapter is to review the reliable data concerning the clinical and pathomorphologic evolution and the biological mechanisms associated with the morphologic changes in disc herniation.

CLINICAL EVOLUTION

Very few studies concern the natural evolution of the clinical symptoms of disc herniation, as most patients undergo some kind of medical treatment. Hakelius (10) reviewed the course of the acute sciatica syndrome with conservative treatment in 38 patients with a disc herniation on myelography, who did not undergo surgery. Treatment consisted only of bed rest and bracing. Appreciation of the evolution of symptoms was made according to patient's subjective assessment and to the period of official sick registration. As shown in Table 9.1, 35 out of the 38 patients (92%) were free of symptoms after 6 months, but 11 of them were still registered as sick. Weber (22) analyzed a group of 126 patients with uncertain indication for surgical treatment. Their therapy was determined randomly, which permitted comparison between the results of surgical and conservative treatment. Sixty-six patients were randomized in the conservative group. All had a positive myelography and were treated by rest, bracing, and paracetamol. Tables 9.2 and 9.3 show the assessments of results in the conservatively treated patients after 1 and 4 years. After one year 60% ($N = 40$) of patients had good or fair results, 17 had undergone surgery, and nine were still incapacitated by back pain and sciatica. After 4 years, five of the 49 patients remaining in the original group who did not undergo surgery were still suffering from sciatica. At that follow-up time the difference with the randomized surgical group was no longer significant. Only minor changes took place during the last 6 years of observation.

In a multicenter prospective study, Weber and colleagues (23) analyzed 208 patients with obvious symptoms and signs of lumbar radiculopathy probably due to a disc herniation. All patients were examined within 14 days of onset. A concomitant double-

TABLE 9.1. *Evolution of sciatica in nonoperated patients (n = 38) with positive myelography*

	10–30 days	2 months	3 months	6 months
Free of symptoms	58%	60%	75%	88%

(From Hakelius A. Prognosis in sciatica: a clinical follow-up of surgical and nonsurgical treatment. *Acta Orthop Scand* [Suppl]:1970; 129, with permission.)

blind investigation of the effect of the nonsteroidal antiinflammatory drug piroxicam was performed. Results were assessed at 2 and 4 weeks using a visual analog scale and Roland's functional tests. In addition, questionnaires were sent at 3 and 12 months. During the first month, significant decrease of pain (VAS mean score 54 to 19) was observed in 70% of the patients; 60% returned to work. After one year, 30% still complained of back pain and/or sciatica and 20% had not returned to work. Four patients had undergone surgery. The piroxicam-treated group had the same results as the placebo control group.

In a randomized double-blind study Fraser (7) analyzed 60 patients with a disc herniation documented by myelography. Thirty underwent a chymopapain chemonucleolysis and 30 received a placebo. At 6 weeks, 37% of the placebo group had a good outcome, which increased to almost 60% at 6 months. By 2 years 40% of patients had undergone surgery (6).

In spite of the paucity of information, results of these studies and personal experience suggest that natural evolution of the clinical symptoms can be summarized as follows: in the first 2 months there is a marked decrease of back and leg pain in approximately 60% of patients. At 1 year, 20% to 30% are still complaining of back and /or leg pain. The decision to perform surgery is usually made within the first year.

PATHOMORPHOLOGIC EVOLUTION

In recent years numerous studies have shown that a disc herniation may decrease in size and even disappear spontaneously. No report on this subject could be found before the advent of computed tomography (CT). In order to evaluate the frequency and time frame of regression of disc herniation in patients recovering with a conservative treatment, a computer literature search was performed. As the clinical course of a symptomatic lumbar disc herniation is generally unpredictable, it would be very helpful to document the predictive parameters of regression. The literature data are analyzed here in chronological order.

Teplick (21) was the first to report on 11 patients in whom there was unequivocal regression or disappearance of a herniated lumbar disc on follow-up CT study, with a clinical improvement accompanying the morphologic changes.

TABLE 9.2. *66 patients conservatively treated with positive myelography (assessment at 1 year)*

Good and fair	40	
Poor and bad	9	} 40%
Operated	17	
Total:	66	

(From Weber H. Lumbar disc herniation. A controlled prospective study with 10 years of observation. *Spine* 1983; 18:1433–1438, with permission.)

TABLE 9.3. *66 patients conservatively treated with positive myelography (assessment at 4 years)*

Good and fair	44		
Poor and bad	5	}	33%
Operated	17		
Total:	66		

(From Weber H. Lumbar disc herniation. A controlled prospective study with ten years of observation. *Spine* 1983:8:131–140, with permission.)

In 1990, Saal and associates (19) reported on 12 patients treated nonsurgically. After a successful treatment the patients underwent follow-up magnetic resonance imaging (MRI) scans which revealed 46% had 75% to 100% resorption, 36% had 50% to 75% decrease in size, and 11% had 0 to 50% diminution. The mean interval between the two scans was 25 months. Total resorption was more often observed in the largest herniations. Clinical improvement and morphologic changes did not necessarily follow the same time course.

In 1992, several authors reported similar findings. Bozzao and coworkers (2) reported on a series of 69 patients with disc herniations of various locations and sizes found on MRI. The mean interval between diagnosis and follow-up scans was 11 months. Reduction of more than 70% was observed in 48% of patients; reduction of 30% to 70% in was observed in 15% of patients. No change or increase was observed in 29% and 8%, respectively, of the remaining patients. There was no significant correlation between the location of the herniations and the reduction of the herniations. In contrast, the high rate of resorption (over 70%) was observed in the large and medium herniations.

Delauche-Cavallier and colleagues (4) have successfully and conservatively treated 21 patients with a lumbar disc herniation observed on CT scan. A subsequent CT was performed with a mean interval of 6 months. Disappearance or major decrease of herniation was observed in 10 patients, moderate diminution was evident in four, and no change was seen in the remaining patients in spite of the disappearance of the clinical symptoms. Maigne and others (17) followed the course of 48 patients who had a second scan 1 to 40 months after the first imaging. A decrease in the size by 75% or more was observed in 64% of patients, with a diminution from 50% to 75% in 17%, and from 25% to 50% in 19%. Tables 9.4 and 9.5 respectively summarize the comparison between a first CT scan and a follow-up one, and the evolution according to the size of

TABLE 9.4. *Comparison CT1–CT2*

	No. of cases
Group 1 (decrease less than 25%)	9
Group 2 (decrease from 50% to 75%)	8
Group 3 (decrease more than 75%)	31
Total:	48

(From Maigne JY, et al. Computed tomography follow-up study of forty-eight cases of nonoperatively treated lumbar intervertebral discal herniation. *Spine* 1992;17:1071–1074, with permission.)

TABLE 9.5. *Composition of the three groups*

Herniations	Group 1	Group 2	Group 3
Small (n = 13)	5	1	7
Medium (n = 20)	3	5	12
Large (n = 15)	1	1	13

(From Maigne JY, et al. Computed tomography follow-up study of forty-eight cases of nonoperatively treated lumbar intervertebral discal herniation. *Spine* 1992;17:1071–1074, with permission.)

the herniation. Only half of the small herniations decreased by over 75%. Conversely, the great majority of the large herniations disappeared or underwent a major shrinkage.

In a prospective study, Bush and coworkers (3) followed 111 patients with either a disc herniation ($N = 84$) or a generalized or focal bulge ($N = 27$). The second scan was done 1 year later in all patients treated conservatively with a satisfactory outcome. Of 84 herniations, 64 were resolved or improved after 1 year. Only 7 out of 27 bulging dics showed any resolution.

In 1995, Komori and coworkers (15) retrospectively studied 77 patients with lumbar radiculopathy caused by a disc herniation. All patients were examined more than twice by MRI during the conservative treatment with a mean interval of 150 days. Morphologic changes and their correlation with the clinical outcome are presented in Table 9.6. Improvement of clinical findings was usually seen before that observed on MRI. The further the herniated nucleus pulposus migrated the more decrease in size could be observed. Small herniations and protrusions showed little or no change.

The data provided by the studies previously analyzed can be summarized as follows:

1. Large and migrated herniations tend to decrease to a greater extent than protrusions or small, contained herniations, which have less tendency to spontaneous regression.
2. Morphologic changes are usually observed after 6 months and correspond to a favorable clinical outcome, although they tend to lag behind improvement of leg pain.
3. Finally, there is a group of patients who become asymptomatic without any decrease in size of their herniation. This finding raises the problem of the mechanism of the radicular pain.

TABLE 9.6. *Correlation between magnetic resonance imaging (MRI) changes and clinical outcomes*

	MRI changes	Excellent and good	Poor
45% {	Disappearance (n = 10)	10	0
	Marked decrease (n = 25)	25	0
55% {	Slight decrease (n = 14)	14	0
	No change (n = 28)	13	15
	Totals:	62 (80%)	15 (20%)

(From Komori H, et al. The natural history of herniated nucleus pulposus with radiculopathy. *Spine* 1996; 21:225–229, with permission.)

MECHANISMS INVOLVED IN THE PATHOMORPHOLOGIC CHANGES

Before the advent of CT scanning and MRI, it was generally thought that clinical improvement of patients with a positive myelography was related to decrease of the nerve root inflammation and swelling. Moreover, retraction of the annulus and of its associated herniation after extreme flexion of the spine, which is the usual position taken by patients on bed rest, was also hypothesized (21). The recent imaging findings have demonstrated that the herniated disc tissue was indeed able to decrease in size and even disappear, thus releasing the mechanical pressure on the nerve root.

Until recently little was known about the mechanisms leading to the decrease of a disc herniation. Teplick (21), who was the first to report on spontaneous regression of herniated nucleus pulposus (HNP), suggested three theoretical possibilities:

1. Dehydration and shrinkage of the HNP.
2. Regression of the HNP into the annulus via the tear in the annulus.
3. Fragmentation and subsequent sequestration at a distance from the annulus and from the nerve root.

In the case of a contained fragment behind the posterior ligament, the main mechanism may be dehydration, but this theoretical consideration remains speculative. In the case of extruded or sequestrated fragments exposed in the epidural space, recent studies have demonstrated that absorption was the mechanism of regression of the HNP.

Histologic studies (5,13) have shown the presence of a granulation tissue with an abundant neovascularization surrounding the fibrocartilage fragment. Mononuclear cells infiltrate along the margin of the necrotic and degenerated part of the disc tissue. This granulation tissue was seen in 11 of 16 extruded HNPs and three of five sequestrated HNPs in one study (5) and in 30 of 35 sequestrated HNPs in another study (13). The high vascularity of the granulation tissue explains the findings of gadolinium-enhanced MRI. The intense peripheral enhancement of the disc fragment is related to the accumulation of the contrast material in the blood vessels of the granulation tissue around the extruded or sequestrated disc (24). Gronblad and associates (9) have studied the abundant inflammatory cells present in the granulation tissue through immunocytochemistry. Using specific monoclonal antibodies, they demonstrated that macrophages were the predominant cells. In a histologic analysis of many samples from patients with extrusion or sequestration types, fibroblasts and endothelial cells were also disclosed, constituting with the macrophages the granulation tissue. Takahashi and colleagues (20) investigated samples from patients with the protrusion type. The majority of cells were chondrocytes. It is interesting to point out that many years ago, back in 1950, Lindblom and Hultquist (16) had clearly understood the absorption process. They considered that the cellular and vascular ingrowth was "eating" and destroying the disc tissue.

The intimate mechanism of the destruction of the disc tissue has not been fully elucidated. However, it has been demonstrated that at the site of lumbar disc herniation, inflammatory cytokines such as ll1, ll6, tumor necrosis factor (TNF)-alpha, and granulocyte macrophage colony-stimulating factor are produced by macrophages in extrusion and sequestration types, and by chondrocytes in the protrusion type (20). It has also been shown that cells of herniated degenerated discs produce matrix metalloproteinases, nitric oxide, and prostaglandin E2. This production is increased if the cells are stimulated by ll1 (14). An increased production of collagenase (MMP-1) and of antihuman stromelysin (MMP-3) associated with inflammatory cells in herniated discs, as well as chondrocytes, has also been demonstrated by Matsui and colleagues (18). This suggests a causal correlation of the proteinases in degradation of the disc tissue. Collagenase and stromelysin have a high specificity for cartilage proteoglycan and are effective in degrading cartilage matrix as shown by experimental studies using these proteinases as chemonucleolytic agents (12).

As previously mentioned the production of proteolytic enzymes by activated macrophages can be stimulated by cytokines including ll1 and TNF-alpha (20). Production of ll1 by the mononuclear cells might be the main starter of the cycle leading to the production of the cytokines, which in turn stimulate the production of the proteinases. However, the biochemical process is likely to be more sophisticated. Other cytokines are probably involved. For example, Haro and associates (11) have demonstrated the production by the mononuclear cells of the granulation tissue of monocyte chemotactic pro-

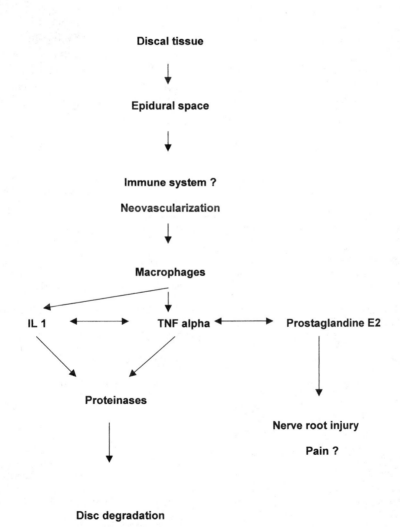

FIG. 9.1. Hypothesis for discal herniation resorption, radicular injury a pain.

tein 1 and macrophage inflammatory protein 1-alpha. Both cytokines belong to the beta-chemokine family, which further recruit and activate macrophage into the lesion. Doita and others (5) have also shown that the cells infiltrating along the margins of extruded discs express cell adhesion molecules which regulate the migration and activation of immune cells. Moreover basic fibroblast growth factor, which promotes neovascularization, is also expressed on the endothelial cells and chondrocytes of the granulation tissue. Obviously, the pathophysiology of the resorption process is extremely complex as well as the autoregulation of the cytokine network.

Figure 9.1 presents a hypothetical and rough sketch of the biological events leading to disc resorption. The main instigator that brings the cells into the lesions and starts the cycle remains hypothetical. Doita and coworkers (5) have postulated that extrusion of nucleus pulposus into the epidural space could evoke an antiimmune reaction to the antigenic components of the disc fragment considered to be foreign. This theoretical consideration has already been discussed by a few authors (8).

It is interesting to point out that ll1 and TNF-alpha produced at the site of disc herniation increase the production of prostaglandin E2 in the tissue which may result in direct stimulation of the nerve root and cause sciatic pain (14). Aoki and colleagues (1) have recently shown that TNF-alpha was the cytokine directly responsible for nerve root injury. Therapeutic use of anti-TNF-alpha to reduce the sciatic pain may interfere with the production cycle of the proteinase responsible for the HNP resorption. It can be concluded that more basic research is needed to clearly understand the complex biological scenarios leading to disc tissue resorption and radicular pain.

REFERENCES

1. Aoki Y, Rydevik B, Larson K, et al. Local application of disc-related cytokines on spinal nerve roots. Paper presented at: Annual Meeting of the International Society for the Study of the Lumbar Spine; 2000; Adelaide, Australia.
2. Bozzao A, Galucci M, Masciocchi C, et al. Lumbar disk herniation: MR imaging assessment of natural history in patients treated without surgery. *Radiology* 1992;185:135–141.
3. Bush K, Cowen N, Katz D, et al. The natural history of sciatica with disc pathology: a prospective study with clinical and independent radiologic follow-up. *Spine* 1992;17: 1205–1212.
4. Delauche-Cavallier MC, Budet C, Laredo JD, et al. Lumbar disc herniation. Computed tomography scan changes after conservative treatment of nerve root compression. *Spine* 1992;17:927–933.
5. Doita M, Kanatami T, Harada T, et al. Immunohistologic study of the ruptured intervertebral disc of the lumbar spine. *Spine* 1996;21:235–341.
6. Fraser RD. Chymopapain for the treatment of intervertebral disc herniation: the final report of a double blind study. *Spine* 1984;9:815–818.
7. Fraser RD. Chymopapain for the treatment of intervertebral disc herniation: a preliminary report of a double blind study. *Spine* 1982;7:608–612.
8. Gertzbein SD, Tile M, Grus A, et al. Auto-immunity in degenerative disc disease of the lumbar spine. *Orthop Clin North Am* 1975;6:67–73.
9. Grondblad M, Virri J, Tolonen J, et al. A controlled immunohistochemical study of inflammatory cells in disc herniation tissue. *Spine* 1994;19:2744–2751.
10. Hakelius A. Prognosis in sciatica: a clinical follow-up of surgical and nonsurgical treatment. *Acta Orthop Scand Suppl* 1970;129..
11. Haro H, Shinomya K, Komori H, et al. Upregulated expression of chemokines in herniated nucleus pulposus resorption. *Spine* 1996;21:1647–1652.
12. Haro H, Murakami S, Komori H, et al. Chemonucleolysis with human stromelysin. *Spine* 1997;22:1098–1104.
13. Ito T, Yamada M, Ikuta F, et al. Histologic evidence of absorption of sequestration type herniated disc. *Spine* 1996;21:230–234.
14. Kang JD, Stefanovic-Racic M, McIntyre LA, et al. Toward a biochemical understanding of human intervertebral-disc degeneration and herniation contributions of nitric oxide, interleukins, prostaglandin E2 and matrix metalloproteinases. *Spine* 1997;22:1065–1073.
15. Komori H, Shinomiya K, Nakai O, et al. The natural history of herniated nucleus pulposus with radiculopathy. *Spine* 1996;21:225–229.

16. Lindblom K, Hultquist G. Absorption of protruded disc tissue of protruded disc. *J Bone Joint Surg* 1950;32A: 557–560.
17. Maigne JY, Rime B, Deligne B. Computed tomography followup study of forty-eight cases of nonoperatively treated lumbar intervertebral discal herniation. *Spine* 1992;1071–1074.
18. Matsui Y, Maeda M, Nakagami W, et al. The involvement of matrix metalloproteinases and inflammation in lumbar disc herniation. *Spine* 1998;23:863–868.
19. Saal JA, Saal JS, Herzog RJ. The natural history of lumbar intervertebral disc extrusions treated non-operatively. *Spine* 1990;20:1821 –1927.
20. Takahashi H, Suguro T, Okazima Y, et al. Inflammatory cytokines in the herniated disc of the lumbar spine. *Spine* 1996;21:218–224.
21. Teplick JG. Spontaneous regression of herniated nucleus pulposus. *AJR* 1985;145:371–375.
22. Weber H. Lumbar disc herniation. A controlled prospective study with ten years of observation. *Spine* 1983;8:131–140.
23. Weber H, Holme I, Amlie E. The natural course of acute sciatica with nerve root symptoms in a double blind placebo controlled trial evaluating the effect of piroxicam. *Spine* 1993;18:1433–1438.
24. Ymashita K, Hiroshima K, Kurata A. Gadolinium DTPA enhanced magnetic resonance imaging of a sequestrated lumbar intervertebral disc and its correlations with pathologic findings. *Spine* 1994;19:479–482.

10

Silent Disc Herniation: Truth or Myth?

Norbert Boos

Disc herniation is one of the few entities in the lumbar spine where current knowledge of the pathogenesis of low back pain (LBP) and sciatica seems to be relatively good. However, the relation of structural abnormalities in the lumbar spine during aging and/or degeneration to low back and leg pain cannot be elucidated in a symptomatic population alone. Until recently, it was quite difficult and controversial to study diagnostic methods such as myelography, discography, or computed tomography (CT) on a larger scale in asymptomatic volunteers because of invasiveness and radiation exposure (8,9,15). With the advent of magnetic resonance imaging (MRI) which is presently thought to be free of biologic hazard, asymptomatic volunteers have been studied more extensively (6,12–14). Such studies have demonstrated that even pathoanatomic abnormalities, which are assumed to show a close correlation to LBP and sciatica (i.e., disc herniations), can also be found with a high prevalence in an asymptomatic population (Fig. 10.1) (1,3,10). These findings lead to significant uncertainty with regard to the importance of abnormal imaging findings in the evaluation of patients with LBP. Particularly, it is unclear whether asymptomatic disc abnormalities remain silent or become symptomatic at a later stage.

The objective of this chapter therefore is to review the literature on asymptomatic disc herniations with a particular focus on the natural history of these abnormalities.

PREVALENCE OF ASYMPTOMATIC DISC ABNORMALITIES

Because of its contrast sensitivity and multiplanar imaging capabilities, MRI provides a unique noninvasive means of viewing the lumbar spine. The anatomy of the intervertebral disc, spinal nerves, dural sac, and adjacent structures can be seen clearly by combination of imaging planes and pulse sequence parameters. In terms of morphology, MRI is thus far the most accurate means of evaluating the lumbar spine and has therefore become the gold standard for the evaluation of spinal pathology (11).

In addition, MRI makes it possible to study disc pathology in asymptomatic individuals without any known biologic hazard. This significant advance allows comparison of the prevalence of abnormal findings in symptomatic and asymptomatic individuals. In the pre-MRI era, only a few studies had been conducted on volunteers without back pain (8,9,15).

In an MRI study, Boden and colleagues (1) examined 67 asymptomatic individuals between the ages of 20 to 80 years. They found at least one herniated disc in 20% of the volunteers less than 60 years of age and at least one herniated disc in 36% of those older than 60 years. In a later study, Jensen and associates (10) reported on 98 asymptomatic individuals examined by MRI. Of these subjects, 36% had normal discs at all levels, 52% had a bulge at least at one level, 27% had a protrusion, and 1% had an extrusion. An

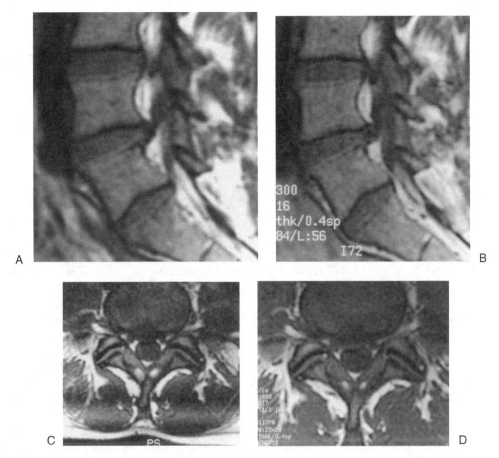

FIG. 10.1. Magnetic resonance images of a 43-year-old woman who never experienced any low back and leg pain. T_1-weighted sagittal scan (**A**) and T_1-weighted axial scan (**C**) at baseline show a sizable disc extrusion at L4-L5 compromising the exiting L5 nerve root. T_1-weighted sagittal scan (**B**) and T_1-weighted axial scan (**D**) at 5-year follow-up show a gradual increase of the extent of the disc herniation and neural compromise. However, the patient remains asymptomatic.

abnormality of more than one intervertebral disc was found in 38%. These authors concluded that people without back pain have disc bulges or protrusions, but not extrusions.

A limitation of the aforementioned studies in asymptomatic controls was that a valid comparison with a symptomatic group of patients with sciatica was not possible. Thus far, only one investigation has attempted to avoid this limitation. Boos and coworkers (3) determined the prevalence of disc herniation in a matched group of asymptomatic volunteers and assessed the diagnostic accuracy of MRI in identifying symptomatic disc herniations. Asymptomatic individuals were selected from a group of 2,000 trauma patients presenting to the university trauma clinic for minor extremity injuries. Inclusion criteria were absence of "relevant LBP" (i.e., "never seen a physician, physiotherapist, chiropractor, or other such a person because of LBP" and "never been absent from work because of LBP"), age between 20 to 50 years, full recovery without residual disability, Swiss residency, full employment, and willingness to undergo an MRI examination of the lumbar spine. In addition, data on occupational risk factors (frequent heavy lifting, twisting and bending, exposure to vibration, and predominant sedentary activity) were collected. Individuals were then matched according to age (± 5 years), gender, and occupational risk factor profile with patients ($N = 46$) requiring surgery for a symptomatic disc herniation.

This study presented evidence that an age-, gender-, and occupational risk factor-matched group of asymptomatic patients demonstrates a higher prevalence of disc herniations (76%) than generally expected and reported in other studies of unmatched asymptomatic volunteers. However, the patients requiring surgery had more severe disc herniations (disc extrusions) than the asymptomatic volunteers (35% versus 13%). There was no significant difference with regard to disc degeneration between both groups (96% versus 85%). The only substantial morphologic difference between both groups was the presence of a neural compromise (83% versus 22%), which was highly significant ($P < 0.0001$). There were additional significant differences between both groups with regard to work perception (occupational mental stress, intensity of concentration, job satisfaction, and resignation; $P < 0.027$) and psychosocial factors (anxiety, depression, self-control, marital status; $P < 0.0001$). However, the best single discriminator was the extent of neural compromise. A combination of this factor with occupational mental stress, depression, and marital status was the best predictive model. With this model, the false-negative rate (potential overtreatment of disc morphology) was reduced by more than half compared to morphologic factors (nerve root compression) alone (22% versus 11%). This study has shown that nerve root compromise plays a more important role than the extent of disc herniation per se (i.e., protrusion, extrusion, sequestration). A disc herniation should always be related to the size of the spinal canal. A large disc herniation may not cause clinical symptoms in a wide spinal canal. Conversely, a small disc protrusion into a small spinal canal can cause significant neurologic deficit.

In a related study, Boos and colleagues (2) compared symptomatic and asymptomatic disc herniation in terms of disc matrix composition as demonstrated by relaxation times measurement. Their results indicate that symptomatic disc herniations have a different matrix composition than comparable asymptomatic herniations. Thus, biochemical factors may be a reason why one disc herniation becomes symptomatic and another morphologic asymptomatic herniation remains asymptomatic.

NATURAL HISTORY OF ASYMPTOMATIC DISC ABNORMALITIES

The aforementioned findings question our morphology-based understanding of pain pathogenesis in patients with disc abnormalities. The natural history of individuals with asymptomatic disc herniations has thus far not been explored in a comprehensive manner. Furthermore, there has been a lack of prospective longitudinal trials attempting to predict LBP while simultaneously taking into account clinical, morphological, and psychological factors as well as physical job characteristics and psychosocial aspects of work.

In a preliminary communication, Borenstein and coworkers (5) report on a 7-year MRI follow-up of 67 asymptomatic individuals, 50 of whom (74.6%) returned an LBP questionnaire and 31 of whom (42.3%) were available for MRI follow-up. Twenty individuals developed LBP while only seven had an episode that lasted longer than 6 weeks without a significant correlation to lumbar spine abnormalities. From this study, the authors conclude that MRI is unable to determine those in whom LBP would develop.

Boos and associates (4) investigated the natural history of asymptomatic disc abnormalities and the predictors of future LBP, requirement for medical consultation, and absence from work in a prospective study following a group of 46 asymptomatic individuals presenting with a high rate of asymptomatic disc herniations on MRI for an average of 5 years. In terms of the morphologic alterations, disc herniations and neural compromise did not substantially worsen at follow-up. Ten individuals (24.4%) demonstrated a gradual worsening in terms of disc herniation, but this progression only led to a change from "protrusion" to "extrusion" in one case. The absolute numbers for the degree of neural compromise remained unchanged, while 12.2% demonstrated a slight increase. The authors did not observe a regression of disc herniation in any of the cases. In 17 out of 46 individuals (41.5%), disc degeneration showed a progression in at least one intervertebral disc. The authors conclude that the natural history of (asymptomatic) disc abnormalities is characterized by a gradual progression which is most pronounced for disc degeneration.

More interestingly, this study has demonstrated that approximately half of the individuals (41.3%) developed some minor episodes of LBP. This rate is comparable to that which one would expect in an unselected group of individuals (7). In six of the 46 individuals (13%), LBP became so severe that they had to consult a physician for treatment. Five of those had to stop work for 1 day to 35 months. Of note, none of the subjects developed sciatica (i.e., radicular leg pain) and none required in-hospital or surgical treatment, despite the fact that 12 people (29.3%) exhibited a minor nerve root compromise. Four of these individuals had an unequivocal compression of a nerve root (9.8%). In predicting the development of LBP-related medical consultation and work absence, MRI-identified disc abnormalities were not significant predictors. On the contrary, physical job characteristics, shift work, general job satisfaction, and the subjective impression that the job had an adverse influence on private life were significant ($P <$ 0.01) predictors of LBP-related medical consultation. Similarly, LBP-related absence from work could be best predicted by job disaffection, physical job characteristics, and shift work ($P < 0.01$).

Based on these findings, the authors hypothesize that classic occupational risk factors can result in advanced morphologic alterations of the lumbar spine, as shown in the high rate of asymptomatic disc alterations. They also play a role in predicting LBP-related medical consultation and work absence. However, when pain behavior (i.e., medical consultation and work absence) is considered rather than the mere perception of pain, psychological aspects of work may be more important even than ergonomic factors (4).

CLINICAL RELEVANCE

The current literature suggests that the explanation of LBP and sciatica by morphologic findings shown by MRI remains questionable even in disc herniations, where a close pathoanatomic relation of the visible alteration and pain is generally assumed. In particular, individuals with small disc herniations (i.e., protrusions, contained herniations) without clearly visible nerve root compromise may be at high risk that the visible morphologic alteration is not directly associated with the pain. A high percentage of matched controls (63%) have asymptomatic disc protrusions, which could lead to an indication for discectomy, if present in symptomatic patients. The natural history of asymptomatic disc alterations is characterized by a slow, gradual progression of the abnormalities. However, morphologic factors appear not to be significant predictors of LBP requiring medical consultation or work absence. In contrast, the working context considered both from a physical and psychological perspective seems to be a decisive factor when common back pain becomes disabling.

ACKNOWLEDGMENT

This work was supported by a grant from the Swiss National Science Foundation (32-52927.97).

REFERENCES

1. Boden SD, Davis DO, Dina TS, et al. Abnormal magnetic-resonance scans of the lumbar spine in asymptomatic subjects: a prospective investigation. *J Bone Joint Surg* 1990;72A:403–408.
2. Boos N, Dreier D, Hilfiker E, et al. Tissue characterization of symptomatic and asymptomatic disc herniations by quantitative magnetic resonance imaging. *J Orthop Res* 1997;15:141–149.
3. Boos N, Rieder R, Schade V, et al. 1995 Volvo Award in Clinical Sciences. The diagnostic accuracy of magnetic resonance imaging, work perception and psychosocial factors in identifying symptomatic disc herniations. *Spine* 1995;20:2613–2625.
4. Boos N, Semmer N, Elfering A, et al. Natural history of individuals with asymptomatic disc abnormalities in MRI. Predictors of low-back pain related medical consultation and work incapacity. *Spine* 2000;25:1484–1492.
5. Borenstein G, O'Mara JW, Boden SD, et al. A 7-year follow-up study of the value of lumbar spine MR to predict the development of low back pain in asymptomatic individuals. Paper presented at: 25th Annual Meeting of the International Society for the Study of the Lumbar Spine; Brussels, Belgium, 1998.
6. Buirski G, Silberstein M. The symptomatic lumbar disc in patients with low-back pain. Magnetic resonance imaging appearances in both a symptomatic and control population. *Spine* 1993;18:1808–1811.
7. Croft PR, Papageorgiou AC, Ferry S, et al. Psychologic distress and low back pain. Evidence from a prospective study in the general population. *Spine* 1996;20:2731–2737.
8. Hitselberger W, Written R. Abnormal myelograms in asymptomatic patients. *J Neurosurg* 1968;28:204–206.
9. Holt EP. The question of lumbar discography. *J Bone Joint Surg* 1968;50A:720–726.
10. Jensen MC, Brant-Zawadzki MN, Obuchowski N, et al. Magnetic resonance imaging of the lumbar spine in people without back pain. *N Engl J Med* 1994;331:69–73.
11. Kent DL, Haynor DR, Longstreth WT, et al. The clinical efficacy of magnetic resonance imaging in neuroimaging. *Ann Intern Med* 1994;120:856–871.
12. Parkkola R, Rytokoski U, Kormano M. Magnetic resonance imaging of the discs and trunk muscles in patients with chronic low back pain and healthy control subjects. *Spine* 1993;18:830–836.
13. Powell MC, Wilson M, Szypryt P, et al. Prevalence of lumbar disc degeneration observed by magnetic resonance in symptomless women. *Lancet* 1986;2:1366–1367.
14. Tertti MO, Salminen JJ, Paajanen HE, et al. Low-back pain and disk degeneration in children: a case-control MR imaging study. *Radiology* 1991;180:503–507.
15. Wiesel SW, Tsourmas N, Feffer HL, et al. A study of computer-assisted tomography. I. The incidence of positive CAT scans in an asymptomatic group of patients. *Spine* 1984;9:549–551.

11

The Clinical Presentation of Degenerative Disc Disease

Gordon Findlay

This chapter discusses the clinical presentation of cervical, thoracic, and lumbar disc disease. Patients who present with such problems may have many differing symptoms and signs depending on the nature and site of the disc herniation. To simply catalog these would produce a very long list indeed, which would be not only tedious but uninformative to the reader of this book. It is therefore intended to present this chapter in a more conceptual manner, dealing more with the approach to clinical history taking and examination and discussing the clinical consequences of disc herniation as a whole rather than on a regional or didactic basis.

It is well recognized that disc herniation may cause a variety of clinical problems but, in addition, disc protrusion may often be found on magnetic resonance imaging (MRI) in asymptomatic patients. This means that in order to correctly interpret the findings of a MRI, a complete clinical history and examination are essential. Disc herniations that do cause clinical problems may result in a pure pain syndrome with radicular pain or may be associated with neurologic signs of radiculopathy or myelopathy. Stenotic lesions in the lumbar spine may produce the clinical picture of neurogenic claudication, though it is important to note that such a syndrome may also be due to spinal cord disease from, for example, a spinal arteriovenous malformation.

In terms of achieving an accurate clinical diagnosis, the clinical history is of considerably greater importance than the actual physical examination in disc disease. Having completed the clinical history, the clinician should already have arrived at a working diagnosis or differential diagnosis. The examination merely serves to identify signs that either support that diagnosis or, more importantly, refute it. Additionally, the clinical history permits an assessment of the effect that the disc disease is having in an individual case.

An effective clinical history should evaluate the following factors:

- Pain
- Sensory symptoms
- Motor symptoms
- Sphincteric disturbance
- Degree of disability and distress

In disc disease, the most common and important symptom is pain. The first thing to establish is the site of the pain. Pain in disc disease may be axial, referred, or radicular. An accurate description of the pain should be sought, and the patient should be asked to show on their own body exactly where the pain is felt and to where it may radiate. Many clinicians find that the use of a pain drawing is helpful. Clearly it is necessary to deter-mine the duration of the pain syndrome, whether there have been previous episodes, and the periodicity of the pain. It is also important to ask whether the pain is improving, sta-tic, or becoming more severe. Factors that affect the pain such as activity and posture may be relevant as are factors that improve the pain, such as the stooped walking posture of someone with lumbar spinal stenosis.

While the features of axial and radicular pain are well recognized by all clinicians, other types of pain are less well known. Neurogenic pain implies significantly more seri-ous damage to the root or dorsal root ganglion and can also imply more central mecha-nisms of damage. The quality of this type of pain is much more of a painful sensory dis-turbance with complaints of burning discomfort and numbness or allodynia. The importance of recognizing this type of pain lies in the fact that it is resistant to narcotic-type analgesics and requires treatment with tricyclic antidepressants or related drugs. Severe lesions of the spinal cord may result in the phenomenon of "myelopathic" pain. This is indicated by a widespread regional pain disturbance often affecting the thighs and knees with an unpleasant and difficult to describe deep, gnawing pain often associated with autonomic features. Occasionally, patients will describe sharp, shooting pains like electricity. If these follow cervical flexion, they constitute the Lhermitte phenomenon indicating cervical cord pathology.

Sensory symptoms in disc disease usually constitute paresthesia or numbness in the region of an affected nerve root. In cervical myelopathy, however, proprioceptive loss results in the complaint of clumsiness of the hands and difficulty with fine finger move-ments. Major proprioceptive loss in the hands in someone with cervical disc disease often suggests a lesion at C3-C4. Proprioceptive loss in the legs results in complaints of loss of balance, falling, and unsteadiness. When eliciting sensory symptoms in the history, it is important to not only assess the region affected and the quality of sensory loss but also any resultant dysfunction that they cause. Motor symptoms fall into two categories. In radicular pathology, only the muscles affected by that nerve root will be affected. The patient may complain of foot drop or perhaps weakness of shoulder abduction if C5 is involved. Patients with myelopathy have more global weakness affecting the entire limb or limbs. It is particularly important to ask about the patient's gait. Patients with myelopa-thy will give a history of increasing unsteadiness of gait, ultimately resulting in the need to hold on to furniture or use a walking aid. Patients with lumbar spinal stenosis will give the typical history of increasing radicular pain—sometimes with developing numbness, foot drop, or even perineal numbness and rarely priapism—promptly relieved by spinal flexion.

Sphincteric symptoms are notoriously difficult to assess. With an aging population, many cases among both men and women will report some degree of urinary dysfunction. However, any sphincteric dysfunction in a patient with other neurologic symptoms should be carefully assessed. Symptoms of concern include loss of awareness of bladder filling or urethral sensation when passing urine. Constipation is a common complaint in patients taking analgesics for their pain, but loss of rectal sensation, fecal incontinence, or perineal numbness should alert the clinician to a possible neurologic cause. A patient presenting with urinary retention without abdominal pain should be considered a neuro-logic emergency until proved otherwise.

It is important when taking the history to attempt to assess what degree of disability results from the complaints. Many patients with severe pain or cord compression will have significant disability commensurate with their organic disturbance. However, it is now widely recognized that some patients with a pain syndrome will exhibit grossly abnormal levels of disability due to psychosocial factors and fear about their spinal problem. Abnormal disability patterns do not only afflict patients with lumbar degeneration. These features are often present in patients with cervical and thoracic disc disorders, though strangely not as commonly as occurs in the lumbar spine. It is essential to recognize the presence of such features as it is imperative to treat these aspects along with any coexisting organic pathology.

Before passing on to examination, it is important to obtain a full history inquiring about any previous medical conditions and to make a systematic inquiry to discover the presence of any symptoms suggestive of systemic diseases such as neoplasia or infection.

Having completed the clinical history, a full examination is required. Initially, the patient should be thoroughly examined in an effort to search for signs of systemic disease. A careful examination of the entire spine is necessary, looking for cutaneous lesions, deformity, and so forth. An assessment of any restriction of spinal movement should be made. In patients with lumbar disc disease, the objective signs of illness behavior described by Waddell should be sought, though they are less commonly present than in cases of low back pain.

Turning to the examination of the spine and neurologic system, it is this author's approach to systematically search for clinical signs that actually contradict the preliminary diagnosis reached from the history. Only then does this author look for signs that support his diagnosis. Thus, if the clinical history suggests the presence of lumbar spine pathology, the finding of upper motor signs in the legs on examination alerts the examiner and permits a reevaluation of the earlier diagnosis. Equally, signs such as a peripheral, nondermatomal sensory loss in association with absent reflexes and loss of vibration sense may suggest that the lower limb symptoms are due to peripheral neuropathy and not lumbar disc disease. In patients with cervical disc disease compressing both roots and the spinal cord, a mixed picture of either lower or upper motor signs may be found in the upper limbs with upper motor signs in the legs. Surprisingly, in some of these patients, the signs in the legs may be quite minimal and it is only when the patient's gait is observed that the real evidence of lower limb spasticity becomes apparent.

By the nature of its frequency, the most common type of disc disease to be assessed is that of the lumbar spine. Table 11.1 shows signs that, if found on clinical examination, should alert the examiner to the presence of disease other than that of lumbar disc degeneration.

Having completed the clinical history and diagnosis, the clinician should then pause to consider the situation. It may be that the evidence points clearly to a clinical diagnosis of disc disease affecting the cervical, thoracic, or lumbar spine. However, it is sensible to evaluate other possibilities. If it seems certain that the patient does have a spinal disorder, it should be considered that such a disorder may not be due to disc disease. For example, could the patient with radicular pain in the leg have a tumor of the cauda equina?

TABLE 11.1. *Signs against a diagnosis of lumbar disc disease*

Brisk reflexes
Temperature, proprioceptive or vibration loss
Peripheral sensory loss
Clonus
Severe wasting
Fasciculation
Spinal deformity

Could the patient with symptoms and signs of a cervical myelopathy actually have a metastasis? Could the patient with an apparent cauda equina lesion have a conus lesion or even a pelvic neoplasm?

Peripheral joint disease—especially in the shoulder or hip—can be surprisingly difficult to clinically differentiate from disc disease, unless the possibility is considered. Similarly, peripheral nerve entrapment can masquerade as disc pathology. In patients with apparent cervical disc disorders, thoracic outlet syndrome or brachial neuritis must be considered. Patients presenting with apparent spinal cord lesions may in fact have demyelinating disease. The list of possible differential diagnoses that must be considered is almost endless and different diseases will need to be considered for each region of the spine involved.

At this stage the clinician must establish a management plan. If after careful history taking and a thorough examination it is believed that the pathology is not that of a spinal disorder, the patient should be referred to an appropriate specialist for further evaluation. If it is decided that the disorder is spinal but there is evidence that the pathology is not discogenic, appropriate investigation should be performed to establish the diagnosis and rule out more sinister spinal pathology. If the conclusion is that the disorder is of disc pathology, then the management will depend on whether the pathology is causing axial, radicular, or myelopathic problems. However, it should be pointed out that if a clear diagnosis of a disc herniation has been made clinically, not all patients require such investigation. In particular, an MRI should only be ordered if there is a possibility of the presence of pathology more sinister than that of disc disease or to explore therapeutic options.

12

Recurrent Disc Herniation

Henry V. Crock and M. Carmel Crock

For almost 40 years, the subject of recurrent disc herniation has spawned an ever-increasing volume of literature, much of which is focused on four issues: (a) the sites and rates of recurrence; (b) the patient's psychological status and health insurance coverage; (c) the role of supplementary procedures in treatment such as intradiscal injections, spinal fusions with or without fixation, and disc replacement; and (d) the outcome after repeat surgery.

In study groups of as many as 2,500 patients (18) to as few as 16 patients (4), recurrence rates have been reported with incidences ranging between 5.9% (2) and 16% (16). The sites of recurrence include lesions arising from the original disc on the same side or from the contralateral side, herniations from an adjacent level, and, rarely, herniations from multiple discs. In 1997, Czervionke and Berquist (9) presented the following classification of disc prolapses.

(I)   Bulging—The disc margin extends diffusely in all directions
(II) Protrusion—A focal extension of nucleus and inner annulus exists, but the outer annulus remains intact
(III) Extrusion—The disc tissue penetrates through all layers to the outer annulus
(IV) Sequestration—Free fragments of disc tissue extend above or below the disc level

A study from Paris (10) analyzed the findings in 34 cases of disc sequestrations from a series of 98 surgeries for disc prolapse, but very few papers have defined the types of herniation found at surgery.

Turning to results of reoperation, Frymoyer and colleagues (11) observe that patients who had spinal fusions performed at the time of excision of the original disc herniations fare less well after surgery for recurrent herniations than those who only had simple disc fragment excisions initially. Cinotti and coworkers (3,4) conclude from their reviews that spinal fusion is not indicated as both back pain and sciatica improve after simple disc fragment excision for recurrent herniations. While some authors exclude from their computations patients with compensation claims pending, overall rates of improvement range from 40% (21) to 85% (3).

Despite the use of complex questionnaires, algorithms, and sophisticated statistical analyses, prevailing views about these issues vary widely among the different groups of people who advise and treat patients with recurrent disc herniations. Depending on the field of expertise of the treating practitioner—from physical therapy and osteopathy to general medical practice, psychology, epidemiology, neurology, rheumatology, neurosurgery, orthopedic surgery, and a small group of spinal surgeons—opinions about treatment range from outright opposition to repeat surgery to vigorous support for it.

Against this background, the purpose of this chapter is to present a practical guide for the treatment of patients presenting with recurrent symptoms after surgery for disc herniation. To deal with the problem effectively requires a breadth of knowledge in excess of what can be gained by reading isolated papers on the radiologic diagnosis of recurrent herniation or on its surgical treatment.

ESTABLISHING THE DIAGNOSIS OF RECURRENT DISC HERNIATION

The History of Symptoms

As these patients often seek further treatment from a different practitioner than the one who performed the initial surgery, the history of symptoms that existed before the first surgery should be reviewed, with particular reference to the character of pain experienced, and to findings such as limited straight leg raising on the affected side, absence or loss of reflexes in the extremities, evidence of loss of power in the limbs, or disturbance of bowel or bladder function (12). If the pain before the first surgery was of a chronic, insidiously progressive type or of excruciating character, the response to this initial surgery will almost certainly have been unsatisfactory and persistence of these symptoms will raise the possibility of unrecognized underlying benign or malignant tumors of the neural structures or vertebral column.

The Results of Preoperative Investigations

Plain films, myelography, computed tomography (CT), magnetic resonance imaging (MRI), and bone scan should be carefully examined to attempt to define the type of herniation that was originally present. The chest radiograph should be sought and the results of the previous full blood examinations and blood chemistry analyses compared with recent tests to rule out evidence of neoplastic or inflammatory lesions that may have developed since the first surgery.

Although it is often stated that, with the availability of modern imaging, plain radiographs are no longer required, those taken before surgery are nevertheless the most useful for identifying congenital abnormalities of the spine, such as spina bifida occulta, and segmentation anomalies and other lesions such as single-disc space narrowing, which is seen in patients with isolated disc resorption (20). If spina bifida occulta has not been recognized, dural injury may occur during the early stages of surgery. Segmentation anomalies of the lumbar spine are associated with varying types of disc pathology at the first mobile segment of the spine above that conjoined to the sacrum. In all cases, the disc space related to the conjoined lumbar and sacral segments is narrowed but the rudimentary disc is normal on MRI. Isolated disc resorption is an entirely separate condition which occurs in a normally segmented vertebral column and affects only one disc. These different entities, identified on plain radiographs, may play very important roles in the diagnosis and treatment of patients with back pain and sciatica, contrary to views expressed by Nachemson (15).

Notes on Surgery

Notes made at the time of the first surgery should be examined in detail, noting the position in which the patient was placed on the operating table—lateral or prone—the duration of the procedure, the record of blood loss, methods of hemorrhage control used, and information on instruments such as high-speed drills, curettes, osteotomes, surgical microscopes, endoscopes, or lasers that may have been used. Properly documented notes on surgery should contain information on how much bone was removed in approaching the interspace, for what length of time self-retaining retractors were used without release during the surgery, whether the disc hernia was easily identified or difficult to locate, whether nerve root adherence required tedious dissection to move the root from the prolapse, whether cerebrospinal fluid leakage occurred at any stage, and whether or not fat grafts were applied to the dural sac at the site of surgery. Details of this degree, if available, are of enormous value to a surgeon who is contemplating a second operation.

Response to the First Surgery

Answers to the question of the patient's response to the first surgery should be carefully considered, as these often hold the key to the diagnosis of the cause of the recurring symptoms. For example, was the sciatica immediately relieved or did the patient wake up with pain similar to or worse than that complained of before surgery? Did the patient run a temperature in the postoperative period and were there any problems with wound healing such as leakage of blood or fluid from the wound site? Were any radiographs taken after surgery? Was the postoperative course complicated by chronic pain, with loss of energy and weight loss over a period of months?

Clinical Examination

Having reviewed this body of information, a new routine clinical examination should be made and appropriate investigations ordered, including good quality anteroposterior and lateral plain radiographs of the spine, if these had not previously been obtained either before the first surgery or after it. Depending on availability, MRI with gadolinium enhancement is particularly useful for distinguishing postoperative scar tissues from recurrent herniations (14). Alternatively, CT examination with sagittal and coronal reconstructions should be obtained. These studies will provide information on segmentation of the spine, on the amount of bone removed previously at surgery, and on the degree of muscle damage sustained, and they may reveal unexpected evidence of exploration of the wrong level or of retained swabs in the wound. Previously unrecognized lesions, such as erosive arachnoid cysts of the sacrum or bony spurs of diastematomyelia, may be found and require specific attention during reexploration of the spine.

Natural History of Degenerative Disc Disease

In correlating the new information obtained on the site and nature of the herniation with the details of the first surgery, it is important to reconsider the natural history of degenerative disc disease in relation to disc herniation.

Many prolapses come from discs shown on radiographs to be of normal height. The herniations are usually small and the results following simple disc fragment excision are good. Recurrence of herniation in these circumstances is unusual but subsequent degenerative changes at the level of the herniation evolve slowly over the following years.

In patients with discs of normal height, whose pain was not relieved by excision of some disc tissue (usually from a bulging disc) but in whom it persisted and became worse, aggravated particularly by physical activity, and in whom weight loss and loss of energy has occurred in the months after the initial surgery, the cause of these recurring symptoms should be ascribed to the syndrome of *internal disc disruption* (5,6). Discography continues to be useful in confirming this diagnosis in some cases (1). In such cases, reexploration of the disc space with further excision of disc tissues will lead predictably to marked aggravation of the patient's symptoms and chronic disability. Total disc excision and interbody fusion is required. There is no place for repeating excision of any disc herniation in patients with this syndrome

In cases of disc herniation occurring where marked loss of disc height, restricted to one level, was established prior to the removal of herniated fragments, the diagnosis of *isolated disc resorption* should be considered. Sequestration of small fragments of vertebral endplate cartilage may occur in this condition, but in addition, the decrease in intervertebral space may lead to bilateral foraminal and nerve root canal stenoses. At the time of reexploration for a recurrent herniation in this condition, it is essential to excise the fragment and to perform bilateral foraminal and nerve root canal decompressions, ensuring that perineural venous refilling is observed at surgery as an indicator of the adequacy of the decompression (7) (Fig.12.1).

Patients with isolated disc resorption often present with symptoms of troublesome recurrent back pain, with bilateral buttock and leg pain radiating to the backs of the knees in the absence of neurologic findings. Occasionally these patients may present with unilateral leg pain which is due to a small subrhizal sequestration usually containing necrotic vertebral endplate cartilage. If this is removed, simply unilaterally for example, by microdiscectomy, then symptoms are likely to recur quite soon after the first surgery. The cause of referred leg pain in these patients is due to chronic obstruction of the venous drainage of the nerve roots in the narrowed foramina and nerve root canals. These patients will require reexploration of the spine for bilateral foraminal and nerve root canal decompressions without further interference with the disc space (13).

In recent years, interbody fusions with cages have been used extensively in treating patients with symptoms arising from *isolated disc resorption*. Spinal fusion should only

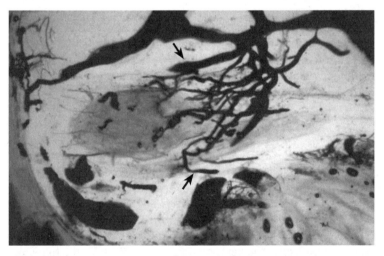

FIG. 12.1. A photograph showing details of the veins emerging from a lumbar nerve root at the level of the intervertebral foramen. (The pedicle is on the left; the intervertebral disc is at the bottom right). They drain into radicals of the anterior and posterior limbs of the internal vertebral venous plexus (*arrows*). These vessels are readily obstructed by pathologic processes in spinal stenosis. They should not be destroyed by electrocoagulation during surgery.

be recommended in patients with this form of disc disease in whom intractable back pain has been the major complaint. In the few cases where anterior interbody spinal fusion is indicated, troublesome prevertebral inflammatory changes often bind the great vessels to the anterior surface of the resorbed disc and render adequate exposure of the intervertebral disc space difficult, with the potential for serious damage to the left common iliac vein. Accordingly, laparosopic interbody fusion in such cases becomes potentially hazardous.

Where degenerative disc disease affects several levels, very large disc herniations may occur at one level, though it is difficult to anticipate from which level the herniation may arise (Fig. 12.2). In such cases, the patient may present with an acute cauda equina syndrome requiring urgent surgical treatment. By contrast, even in the presence of a very large sequestrated disc fragment arising from a single level, symptoms may be tolerable, depending on the relationship of the sequestrated fragments to the local nerve roots. The likelihood of spontaneous resorption of these fragments is now well recognized (17), and so the decision to perform further surgery in such cases must not be based on the interpretation of the imaging studies alone (Fig. 12.3).

In patients presenting with recurrent symptoms after removal of large disc prolapses or sequestrated fragments, the surgeon must pay particular attention in exposing the disc space, as the dural sac and nerve roots may be adherent to the underlying disc herniation. In this situation there is also a high risk of penetration of instruments such as curettes or pituitary rongeurs which are inserted between the vertebral bodies and which may slip into the abdomen, injuring structures such as the vena cava, aorta, or bowel.

In rare cases disc prolapses may recur seriatim at different levels over a number of years, requiring multiple surgeries. When internal fixation devices have been applied and removed in the course of dealing with these lesions, recurring herniations at higher levels are best treated by an extraperitoneal approach to the discs, allowing complete disc excision with removal of sequestrated fragments from within the spinal canal and curettage of the endplate cartilages. Spinal fusion is not required, but a plastic corset should be worn for 6 to 8 weeks in the postoperative period. Even in the presence of a cauda

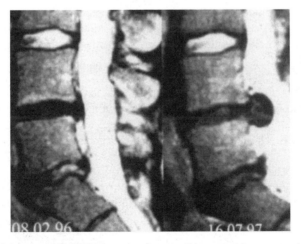

FIG. 12.2. T2-weighted sagittal MR images from a 24-year-old woman showing phases of development, between 02.96 on the left and 07.97 on the right, of a large disc herniation at the L4-L5 level and of resorptive disc changes at L5-S1.

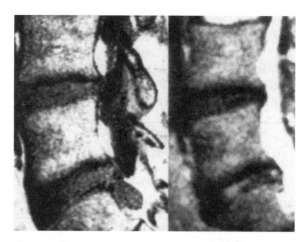

FIG. 12.3. T2-weighted sagittal MR images from a 27-year-old man showing loss of nuclear signals at L4-L5 and L5-S1 and a large sequestrated disc herniation at L5-S1 on the left, 31.03.95. Spontaneous resorption of the sequestrated herniation had occurred when the MRI of 12.08.97 was taken.

equina lesion with bladder and bowel involvement and bilateral foot drop, satisfactory recovery following this type of procedure can occur. Such a result would be unlikely if the prolapses were approached repeatedly through the spinal canal (19).

GENERAL PRINCIPLES GOVERNING ADDITIONAL SURGERIES FOR RECURRENT DISC HERNIATIONS

The general principles governing additional surgeries for recurrent disc herniations are reviewed here.

1. Prior to reexploration surgeries, appropriate instruments and fine sutures for dural repair together with biological substances such as Tisseel* should be available.
2. With the use of modern imaging techniques, the accuracy of diagnosis of recurrent disc herniations is now high. Reexplorations should therefore be directed only at the level of the pathology, avoiding hemilaminectornies or laminectomies at multiple levels (Fig. 12.4).
3. The nature of the pain described by the patient at the time of the first surgery and in the period after it should be critically assessed. Severe pain, which is described as excruciating in some cases, should raise suspicion of the possibilities of previously unrecognized malignant disease or of a chronic infective process, such as chronic epidural abscess. The latter may have persisted undiagnosed for many months after initial surgery, even in the absence of a history of discharge from the wound in the postoperative period.
4. In any case of a primary disc herniation requiring surgery, the blood supply of the paraspinal muscles must be respected during surgery by avoiding prolonged and uninterrupted use of self-retaining retractors. Even when microdiscectomy tech-

---

*Tisseel, 1 ml, 2 ml, 5 ml, Hyland Immuno, Baxter Healthcare, Ltd., Newbury, Berkshire, RGI 6 OQW England.

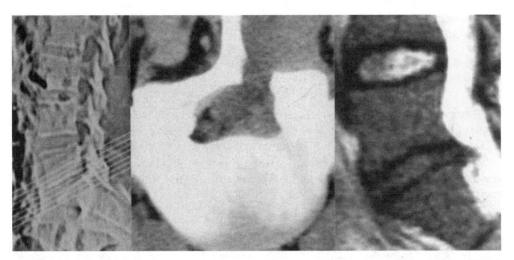

FIG. 12.4. MR images from a 37-year-old man showing disc space narrowing at L5-S1 **(left)**; an axial view of hemilaminectomy of L5 and large recurrent disc herniation 4 months after "microdiscectomy" **(center)**; and a sagittal image of isolated disc resorption at L5-S1 with fragments of recurrent disc herniation **(right)**. An excellent result followed reexploration at L5-S1 for disc fragment excision and bilateral foraminal and nerve root canal decompressions.

niques are used, the formation of dense scar tissue and ectopic bone can occur, rendering reexploration surgeries for recurrent herniations difficult and resulting in a high incidence of complications, such as dural or nerve root injury.

5. Where there is marked loss of disc height, bilateral foraminal and nerve root canal decompressions should always be performed and the perineural venous circulation respected at all times (Fig. 12.1). Bleeding from these vessels should be controlled by applying biological agents such as Spongostan* to the site of hemorrhage. Electrocoagulation should be strictly avoided.

6. In cases requiring reexploration after prior removal of large disc prolapses or sequestrations, an increased risk of injury to intraabdominal structures, such as the vena cava or aorta, or bowel, can occur if instruments should slip into the empty disc space during removal of disc remnants.

7. The use of intradiscal chymopapain has decreased considerably over the past 5 years. Some practitioners continue to recommend it however for treating recurrent herniations, particularly in adolescent patients.

8. The use of fat grafts has been shown to lead occasionally to serious complications, including cauda equina compression. Provided that the blood supply of the paraspinal muscles is protected during surgery, the naturally occurring fat found in the deep layers of this muscle mass will prevent the formation of dense scar tissue over the dura and render the use of free fat grafts unnecessary. Free fat grafts are not vascularized and, if large, they act as foreign bodies in the spinal canal (8).

9. Synchronous combined anterior and posterior fusions with internal fixation continue to be widely used in cases of recurrent disc herniation. At the present time, there is

---

*Spongostan Special (thin) and Standard ¹/₂", Johnson & Johnson, Maidenhead, Berk, SLG 3UG, England.

no scientific evidence to support the routine use of any of these complex procedures, though rising rates of complications associated with their use continue to be reported.

CONCLUSIONS

Recurrent disc herniation is not common but recurrent symptoms of spinal and limb pain after surgery to excise portions of intervertebral discs are common. To establish the diagnosis of their cause, the condition needs to be viewed in the context of a general medical problem rather than in the narrower surgical context of a recurrent simple mechanical derangement of the disc. Only in this way can the most appropriate option of medical or surgical treatment be selected for the benefit of the patient.

REFERENCES

1. Aprill CN. Diagnostic disc injection. In: *The adult spine: principles and practice*. New York: Raven Press, 1991:403–442.
2. Cauchoix J, Ficat C, Girard B. Repeat surgery after disc excision. *Spine* 1978;(3):256–259.
3. Cinotti G, Gumina S, Giannicola G, et al. Contralateral recurrent lumbar disc herniation. Results of discectomy compared with those in primary herniation. *Spine* 1999;24(8):800–806.
4. Cinotti G, Roysam GS, Eisenstein SM, et al. Ipsilateral recurrent lumbar disc herniation. A prospective, controlled study. *J Bone Joint Surg (Br)* 1998;80(5):825–832.
5. Crock HV. Internal disc disruption. In: *The adult spine: principles and practice*. New York: Raven Press, 1991: 2015–2025.
6. Crock HV. Internal disc disruption—a challenge to disc prolapse 50 years on. Presidential Address to the International Society for the Study of the Lumbar Spine 1985. *Spine* 1986;11(6):250–253.
7. Crock HV. Nerve root canal decompression. Lumbar perineural venous dilatation as an indicator of its efficacy. *Acta Orthop Scand* 1994;65(2):225–227.
8. Crock HV. Free fat grafting in lumbar spine surgery [Editorial]. *Neuro-orthopaedics* 2000;27:7–8.
9. Czervionke LF, Berquist TH. Imaging of the spine. Techniques of NIR imaging. *Orthop Clin North Am* 1997; 28(4):583–616.
10. Deburge A, Benoist M, Boyer D. The diagnosis of disc sequestration. *Spine* 1984;9(5):496–499.
11. Frymoyer JW, Hanley E, Howe J, et al. Disc excision and spine fusion in the management of lumbar disc disease: a minimum ten year follow-up. *Spine* 1978;3:1–6.
12. Jonsson B, Stromquist B. Clinical characteristics of recurrent sciatica after lumbar discectomy. *Spine* 1996;21 (4):500–505.
13. Matsuda S, Crock HV. Isolated disc resorption. In: *Lumbar spine disorders. Current concepts*, 2nd ed. New York: World Scientific Publishing Co, 1996:117–130
14. Mullin WJ, Heltoff KB, Gilbert TJ Jr, et al. Magnetic resonance evaluation of recurrent disc herniation: is gadolinium necessary? *Spine* 2000;25(12):1493–1499.
15. Nachemson AL. The lumbar spine: an orthopaedic challenge. *Spine* 1976;1:59–71.
16. O'Sullivan MG, Connolly AR, Buckley TF. Recurrent disc protrusion. *Br J Neurosurg* 1990;4(4):319–325.
17. Saal JA, Saal JS, Herzog RJ. The natural history of lumbar intervertebral extrusions treated non-operatively. *Spine* 1990;15(7):683–686.
18. Spangfort EV. The lumbar disc herniation—a computer-aided analysis of 2504 operations. *Acta Orthop Scand* 1972[Suppl]:142.
19. Tsuji H. Extra-peritoneal antero-lateral discectomy for lumbar herniated nucleus pulposus [in Japanese]. *Seikeigeka* 1984;35:795–803.
20. Venner R, Crock HV. Clinical studies of isolated disc resorption in fifty patients. *J Bone Joint Surg* 1981;63: 491–494.
21. Waddell G, Kummel EG, Lotto WN, et al. Failed lumbar disc surgery and repeat surgery following industrial accidents. *J Bone Joint Surg (Am)* 1979;61(2):201–207.

Diagnosis

13

Magnetic Resonance Imaging Examination for Degenerative Disease of the Lumbar Spine

J. Assheuer

Magnetic resonance imaging (MRI) is currently the modality of choice for visualizing spinal disorders. Tumors and specific inflammatory diseases as well as pathophysiologic changes which go along with degenerative diseases can be clearly demonstrated and diagnosed by their specific signal intensities either with or without the use of contrast media (16,18,23). Degenerative diseases of the lumbar spine cannot be regarded as a clinical diagnosis. Different pathophysiologic processes are involved in creating low back pain with or without sciatica. Some of these phenomena can be detected using MRI techniques.

NORMAL APPEARANCE OF THE DISC

In order to recognize changes in structures that are involved in degenerative diseases of the spine, especially the disc, one has to be familiar with the normal appearance under different MRI conditions and changes by aging and stress. The disc is a fibrocartilaginous organ that consists of collagen and proteoglycans. The annulus contains more collagen and the nucleus more proteoglycans. Proteoglycans can be regarded as the sponge that holds the water content of the disc (12). In the T1-weighted image the disc appears dark because of the long T1 of poorly bound water of the nucleus and of the small water content of the annulus. Moving to more T2-weighted images, the nucleus becomes brighter due to the long T2 of free water where the annulus remains dark. Because, if properly adjusted, short-time-inversion-recovery (STIR) sequences will image the free amount of water content of the disc, they give an equivalent of the water content of the disc. The gradient-echo sequence, T1-weighted with phase–contrast, can be used to measure the volume of the disc for the whole disc and appears bright. In childhood the STIR-image shows a centered nucleus with high signal intensity. The gradient-echo sequence delineates the growth-plate of the vertebra.

As we age, the disc looses its proteoglycans, the water content decreases, and signal intensity is reduced in STIR- or heavy-weighted T2 images. The disc height diminishes and a cleft appears in the nucleus (14,25). As we continue to grow older, this process continues as well (17). The intervertebral space becomes very small and the disc loses most of its proteoglycans and thereby its water. It is difficult to decide whether the dark appearance of a disc is an expression of a pathologic process or of age-related changes. One would assume a pathologic process if there is a disc that has lost its normal appearance with respect to neighboring discs. There is no correlation with patient's symptoms (Fig. 13.1A and B).

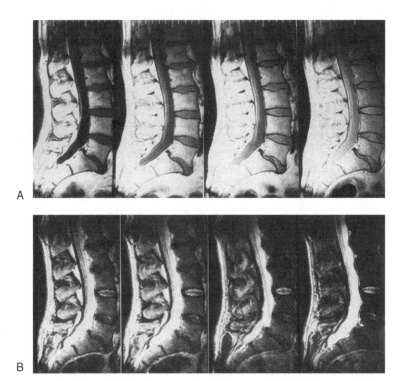

FIG. 13.1. A: Magnetic resonance (MR) appearance of the lumbar spine by spin-echo (SE) sequences going from T1-weighted images to proton–density-weighted images (SE 500/20 to SE 3,000/20). **B:** MR appearance of the lumbar spine going from proton–density-weighted images to T2-weighted images (SE 3,000/20 to SE 3,000/160). Only the disc L314 appears normal in the T2-weighted images with age-dependent cleft in the nucleus. Patient has a marked antelisthesis L5.

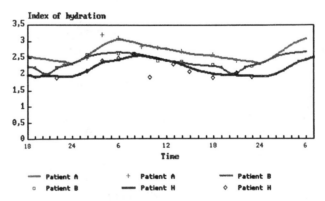

FIG. 13.2. Changes of hydration index of the discs L415 of three volunteers measured every 2 hours under stress and rest over 24 hours. Hydration index is the mean pixel signal intensity of the disc divided by mean pixel intensity of cerebrospinal fluid at the corresponding level multiplied by disc volume (ml). Pixel intensities are taken out of short-time-inversion-recovery images.

The research groups of Adams and Muir (1), Urban and McMullin (24), and Althoff and colleagues (2) point out that the disc loses water under stress. In cadaver studies the loss of water follows an exponential curve depending on the load, where light load already leads to loss of water of about 10% and a continued heavy load can lose another 3%. The changes of water content of the disc can be measured *in vivo* by MRI techniques. Loss of water and volume is about 8% in the nondegenerated disc under normal daily stress, which is consistent with the results of the cadaver studies (21). Derived from repeated measurements over 24 hours, the disc seems to lose water in 10 hours of mobility. There are no further changes to observe for the next 6 hours of mobility. Recovery takes place during the first 4 to 6 hours of rest. The percentage of water loss is higher in degenerated discs than in nondegenerated ones (4) (Fig. 13.2).

WHERE IS DEGENERATION COMING FROM?

It is supposed that overstress to the disc gives rise to microtears in the annulus, whereby nutritional pathways are destroyed and collagenous structures dissolve. In a cadaver study, Kauppilla and Tallroth (15) find new capillaries at the border of the endplates and embolized arteries more centrally at the beginning of the disc degeneration. This would allow the hypothesis that vascular disturbances occur primarily because of disc degeneration. MRI examination of perfusion of endplates shows an enlarged blood pool in about 50% of the endplates of degenerated segments and in 27% of the endplates of nondegenerated segments in patients who had one or more degenerated discs (6) (Fig. 13.3). This sup-

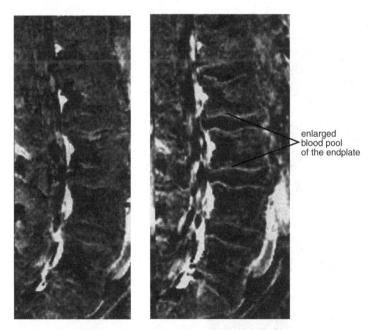

enlarged
blood pool
of the endplate

FIG. 13.3. Perfusion pattern of the lumbar spine with disc degeneration. Images are taken every 20 seconds. Gadolinium (Gd)-contrast medium is given intravenously after the second acquisition. The image before application of the contrast medium is subtracted from all subsequent images. **Left:** The image at 20 seconds. **Right:** The image at 120 seconds after application (gradient echo 50/15). The enlarged blood pool of the endplates is recognized by the high uptake of Gd-contrast medium.

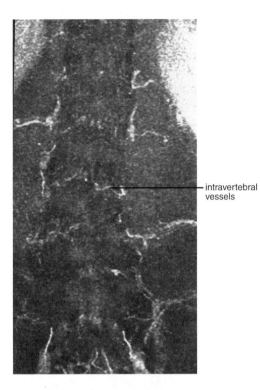

intravertebral
vessels

FIG. 13.4. Magnetic resonance angiography of the lumbar spine. This case of severe spondylosis shows a marked rarefaction of paraspinal and intervertebral vessels.

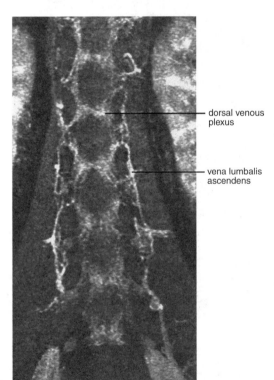

dorsal venous
plexus

vena lumbalis
ascendens

FIG. 13.5. Magnetic resonance angiography of the lumbar spine. Appearance of the paraspinal and intervertebral vessels in a normal subject.

ports the hypothesis that disturbances of perfusion of the endplates may be associated with disc degeneration. The hypothesis may further be supported by the rarefaction of the extravertebral vessels in severe spinal degenerative disease compared to the vascular system in the normal spine (7) (Figs. 13.4 and 13.5).

DISC DEGENERATION AND NONINFECTIOUS SPONDYLITIS

A marked edema of the vertebrae adjacent to the endplates is present in one-third of patients with disc degeneration. These areas are highly perfused. These changes are attributed to a noninfectious spondylitis (3). It is known that collagenous molecules have immunologically active sides when they are digested to a size of about 80,000 molecules, as may occur in disc degeneration (8,11,19), and may induce inflammatory processes when they diffuse through the endplates. In an animal study, however, noninfectious spondylitis seemed more likely to be caused by disturbed load to the endplates by loss of nuclear material in disc degeneration (5) (Figs. 13.6, 13.7, and 13.8).

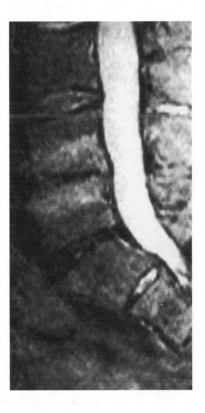

FIG. 13.6. Noninfectious spondylitis with intravertebral edema near the endplates L4 and L5 (short-time-inversion-recovery 2,000/130).

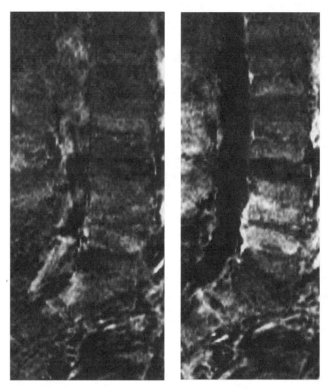

FIG. 13.7. High perfusion pattern of the vertebrae L4 and L5. **Left:** Image taken at 20 seconds. **Right:** Image taken at 40 seconds after intravenous application of gadolinium-contrast medium (gradient echo 50/15).

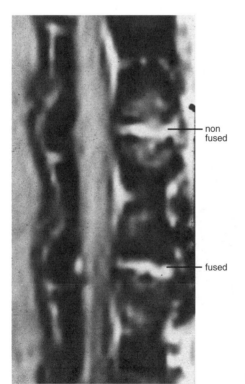

FIG. 13.8. Sagittal image of lumbar segments in a dog (short-time-inversion-recovery 1,600/125). Two weeks after nucleotomy without discectomy LWK4/5 and L5/L6 a rim of high signal intensity appears in the vertebrae L4 and L5 adjacent to the endplate. The segment LWK4/5 was not fused, the segment L5/L6 was fused.

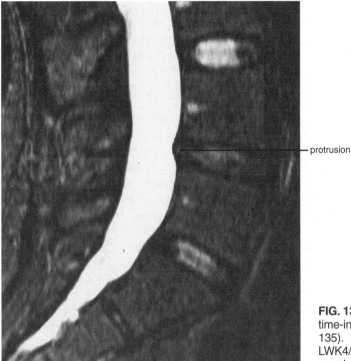

protrusion

FIG. 13.9. Sagittal image (short-time-inversion-recovery 2,000/135). Protrusion of the disc LWK4/5. The outer layer of the annulus is not disrupted.

DISC HERNIATION AND OTHER STENOSING PROCESSES

A degenerated disc is often subject to further pathologic changes, mainly herniations. Tears in the annulus are the pathways for herniation of nuclear material. It is called protrusion if the outer layer of the annulus remains intact (Fig. 13.9). If nuclear material herniates through the outer annulus it is called extrusion (Fig. 13.10). The

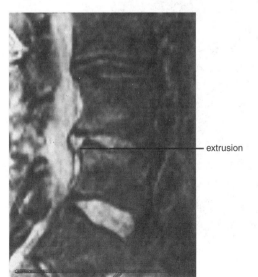

extrusion

FIG. 13.10. Sagittal image (short-time-inversion-recovery 2,000/135). Extrusion of nucleus material through the outer layer of the annulus.

extruded disc material may lose contact with its origin and migrate. This is known as a sequestrum (Fig. 13.11) (13). Experimental studies have confirmed that nucleus material induces inflammation to the neurovascular structures with concomitant edema. Hyperemia in the area of the herniation and edema can be visualized using fast MRI procedures and MR-angiography (Figs. 13.12 and 13.13). The volume of edematous tissue varies. It appears that smaller herniations have more perifocal edema than larger ones (9).

As postulated by Crock (10), processes that lead to narrowing of the spinal canal and the nerve root canal may induce circulatory disorders of the nutrient vessels and may lead to nerve damage. The narrowing may be due to osteophytes, hypertrophy of the facet joints, hypertrophy of the ligamentum flavum, or developmental spinal stenosis or disc herniation. Using fast imaging procedures after bolus injection of gadolinium (Gd)-contrast medium, MRI is able to demonstrate venous stasis of the enlarged dorsal venous plexus as well as of the nerve root canal (Fig. 13.14). The presence of venous stasis could be an indication for decompression procedures. In an animal study, Sager and Assheuer (20) demonstrate how decompression eliminates venous stasis and perifocal edema in a dog with herniation L7/S1; lameness disappeared in about 48 hours. Depending on clinical indication, herniations may require surgery. Fortunately, in most cases, patients improve postoperatively. This may be due to scar tissue enclosing the nerve root. Scar tissue is characterized by its high contrast-

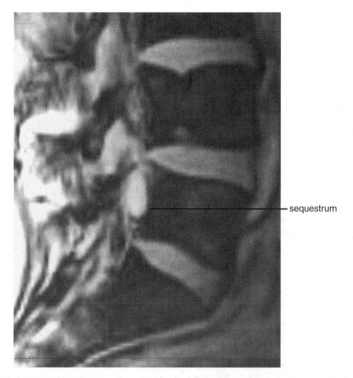

— sequestrum

FIG. 13.11. Sagittal image (gradient echo 500/11). Migration of nucleus material out of LWK4/5 dorsally to the vertebra L5.

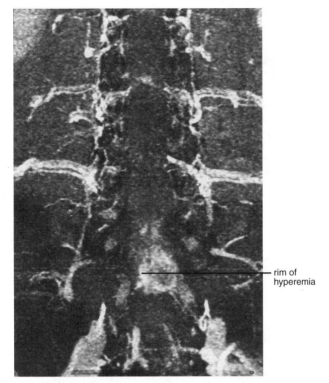

—— rim of
hyperemia

FIG. 13.12. Magnetic resonance angiography demonstrating a perifocal rim of hyperemia in a case of disc extrusion L515 right side.

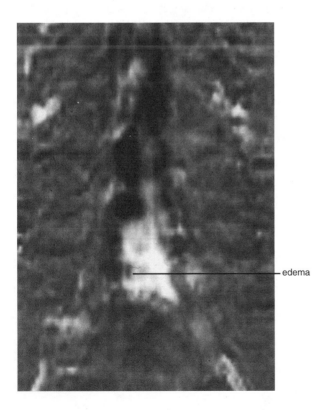

—— edema

FIG. 13.13. Coronal image 200 seconds after intravenous application of gadolinium-contrast medium (gradient echo 50/15). The perifocal edema in a case of extrusion L515 right side is visualized by the high uptake of contrast medium in the locally enlarged extracellular space.

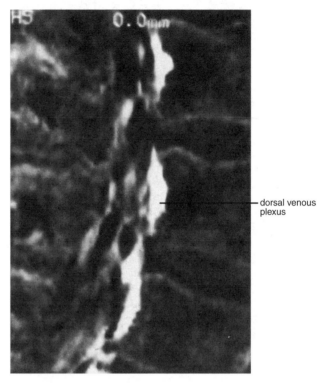

FIG. 13.14. Sagittal image (gradient echo 50/15) 80 seconds after intravenous application of gadolinium-contrast medium. The enlarged dorsal venous plexus is visualized with high signal intensity in this case of osteophytic narrowing of the spinal canal.

medium uptake (Fig. 13.15A and B) which may be due to reherniation. Disc material will not enhance after i.v. application of Gd-contrast medium which makes it able to be distinguished from scar tissue and perifocal edema (Fig. 13.16). There may be a space-occupying lesion with the appearance of scar tissue in the T1-weighted spine-echo image. After i.v. application of contrast medium it may present like reherniation using the same sequence. The T1-weighted gradient-echo sequence out of phase will demonstrate an abscess surrounded by granulation tissue because this sequence presents the fluid of the abscess with lower signal intensity than disc material (Fig. 13.17). Postoperative infection of the retrodiscal space may be demonstrated as early as 6 days after surgery (22).

Sometimes MRIs are difficult to interpret. Figure 13.18 shows a space-occupying lesion dorsal L3 enhanced by contrast-medium. The images were interpreted by ten different experts and resulted in ten different opinions. The lesion disappeared within 4 months as did the symptoms (Fig. 13.19). This was probably the best for the patient.

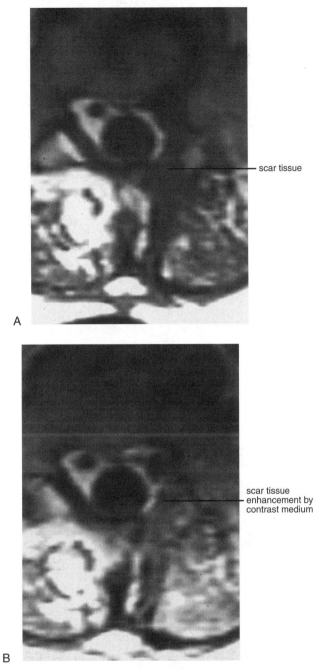

FIG. 13.15. A: Transverse image (spin echo [SE] 500/12). The scar tissue is shown with low signal intensity. **B:** Transverse image (SE 500/12) after intravenous application of gadolinium-contrast medium. Scar tissue is enhanced by the contrast medium.

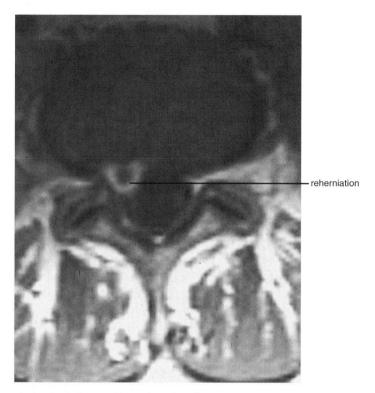

— reherniation

FIG. 13.16. Reherniation is delineated by a rim of perifocal edema with high contrast medium uptake.

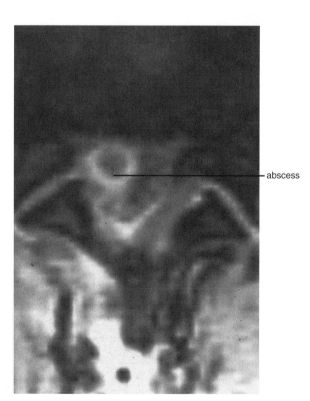

— abscess

FIG. 13.17. Transverse image (gradient echo 500/11 out of phase after intravenous application of gadolinium-contrast medium). Rim of high enhancement demarcates the abscess. The abscess fluid has a lower signal intensity than the disc material.

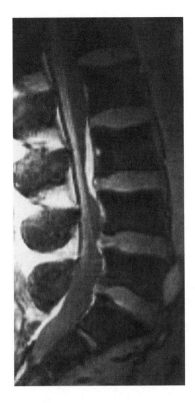

FIG. 13.18. Sagittal image (gradient echo 500/11 out of phase after intravenous application of gadolinium-contrast medium). Enhancing space-occupying intraspinal lesion.

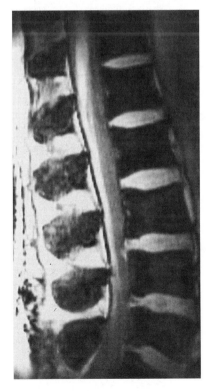

FIG. 13.19. Sagittal image (gradient echo 500/11 out of phase after intravenous application of gadolinium-contrast medium). Image taken 4 months after than image shown in Figure 13.18. The space-occupying lesion has disappeared as have the patient's symptoms.

CONCLUSION

MRI is able to visualize changes of the lumbar disc due to aging and stress. Processes narrowing the spinal canal and the nerve root canal as herniations, osteophytes, hypertrophy of the facet joints, hypertrophy of the ligamentum flavum, or developmental stenosis and scar tissue can be detected and identified. Concomitant changes in vascularity can be demonstrated.

REFERENCES

1. Adams PE, Muir H. Biochemical aspects of development and aging of human lumbar intervertebral discs. *Rheum Rehabil* 1977;16:22–29.
2. Althoff I, Brinckmann P, Frobin W, et al. *Die bestimmung der belastung der wirbelsäule mit hilfe einer präzisionsmessung der körpergröbe*. Mitteilungen aus dem Institut für Experimentelle Biomechanik, 1990:37.
3. Assheuer J, Lenz G, Lenz W, et al. Fett/Wassertrennung im kernspintomogramm. Darstellung von Knochenmarkreaktion bei degenerativen bandscheibenveränderungen. *Fortschr-Geb-Röntgenstr-Nuklearmed* 1987;147: 58–63.
4. Assheuer J, Jerosch J, Schulitz KP. Diurnal changes in water content and shape of the degenerated disc. Paper presented at: The 19th Meeting of ISSLS; 1992; Chicago.
5. Assheuer J, Sager M, Schulitz KP, et al. MR studies in models of disc resorption in dogs. Paper presented at: The 21st Meeting of ISSLS; 1994; Seattle.
6. Assheuer J, Schulitz KP, Wehling P, et al. MRI perfusion measurements of lumbar vertebra endplate and body. Paper presented at: The 22nd Meeting of ISSLS; 1995; Helsinki.
7. Assheuer J, Crock HV, Forutan F, et al. Lumbar spinal MR angiography in the normal and pathological spine. Paper presented at: The 27th Meeting of ISSLS; 2000; Adelaide.
8. Bobechko W, Hirsch C. Autoimmune response to nucleus pulposus in the rabbit. *J Bone Joint Surg* 1965;47: 574–580.
9. Castro WHM, Assheuer J, Schulitz KP. Haemodynamic changes in lumbar nerve root entrapment due to stenosis and/or herniated disc of the lumbar spine canal—a magnetic resonance imaging study. *Eur Spine* 1995;4: 220–225.
10. Crock HV. *A short practice of spinal surgery*. New York: Springer-Verlag, 1993.
11. Elves MW. (1982) Immunology of cartilage In: Haal BK, ed. *Cartilage*. Vol III. New York: Academic Press:229–266.
12. Happey F. *Studies of the structures of the human intervertebral disc in relation to its functional and aging processes. The joints and synovial fluids*. Vol II. New York: Academic Press, 1980:95–136.
13. Herzog RJ. The radiologic assessment for a lumbar disc herniation. *Spine*1996;21:19S/38S.
14. Jenkins JPR, Hickey DS, Zhu XP, et al. MR imaging of the intervertebral disc; a quantitative study. *Br J Radiol* 1985;58:705–709.
15. Kauppilla LI, Tallroth K. Postmortem angiographic findings for arteries supplying the lumbar spine: their relationship to low back symptoms. *J Spinal Dis* 1993;6:124–129.
16. Kricun R, Kricun ME. *MRI and CT of the spine. Case study approach*. New York: Raven Press, 1994.
17. Miller JAA, Schmatz C, Schultz AB. Lumbar disc degeneration: correlation with age, sex, and spine level in 600 autopsy specimens. *Spine* 1988;13:173–178.
18. Modic TM, Masaryk TJ, Ross JS. *Magnetic resonance imaging of the spine*. Chicago: Year Book Medical Publishers, 1989.
19. Naylor A, Happey F, Turner RL, et al. Enzymic and immunological activity in the intervertebral disc. *Orthop Clin North Am* 1975;6: 51–58.
20. Sager M, Assheuer J. Primary and secondary stenosating processes after disc herniation in dogs. Paper presented at: The 20th Annual Conference of the Veterinary Orthopedic Society; 1993; Lake Louise.
21. Schulitz KP, Assheuer J, Wehling P. Diurnal changes in water content and shape of the disc and vertebrae. Paper presented at: The 18th Meeting of ISSLS; 1991; Heidelberg.
22. Schulitz KP, Assheuer J. Discitis after procedures on the intervertebral disc. *Spine* 1994;19(10):1172–1177.
23. St. Amour TE, Hodges SC, Laakman RW, et al. *MRI of the spine*. New York: Raven Press, 1994.
24. Urban JPG, McMullin JF. Swelling pressure of the lumbar intervertebral discs: influence of age, spinal level, composition and degeneration. *Spine* 1988;13:179–187.
25. Videman T, Battié MC, Gill K, et al. Magnetic resonance imaging findings and their relationships in the thoracic and lumbar spine. Insights into the etiopathogenesis of spinal degeneration. *Spine* 1995;20:928–935.

14

Neurophysiologic Tests in Diagnosis of Nerve Root Compression

Jiri Dvorak

Patients with lumboradicular pain syndromes, with or without sensory motor symptoms and signs due to disc herniation, often present with discrepancies in clinical and neuro-radiologic (magnetic resonance imaging, computed tomography, myelography) findings. These discrepancies make it rather difficult to identify the particular nerve root responsible for the patient's complaints. However, as related to indications for surgical intervention, two questions are usually discussed in cases with relative indications for surgery.

- Positive predictors for surgical intervention: who are the good candidates for surgery?
- Which level or nerve root should be approached in order to perform minimally invasive surgery?

In cases where imaging and clinical findings are not in complete agreement, the surgeon may need to conduct additional tests in order to make a decision. Neurophysiologic tests can provide such information. However, the surgeon's expectations cannot always be fully satisfied due to unanswered questions related to sensitivity, specificity, and positive predictive value of a particular electrophysiologic study.

CURRENTLY USED ELECTRODIAGNOSTIC TECHNIQUES

Somatosensory-evoked potentials (SEPs) and motor-evoked potentials (MEPs) are helpful in the investigation of the central nervous system pathways including the spinal cord. Electromyography (EMG), conventional neurography (ENG), F-wave, and H-reflex studies are useful for evaluation of the peripheral segments of the sensory and motor pathways.

SEP techniques are used to evaluate the neural elements of the sensory pathways while MEPs allow for assessment of lesions that affect the upper motor neuron and lesions that affect the motor roots, plexus fibers, or peripheral nerve segments of the lower motor neuron. EMG of limb and paraspinal muscles allows the clinician to make a distinction between whether it is the motor roots that are affected or more peripheral nerve elements. ENG, F-wave, and H-reflex studies also allow for distinction between proximal root and peripheral nerve disease.

SOMATOSENSORY-EVOKED POTENTIALS

SEPs are generally recorded after electric stimulation of peripheral nerves or skin. The nerves used are: the posterior tibial, sural, or common peroneal nerves of the lower limbs.

In radicular and in spinal disease, several nerves supplied by different segments must be stimulated for a level diagnosis. This is a time-consuming investigation.

MOTOR-EVOKED POTENTIALS

The method of painless magnetoelectric transcranial stimulation of the cerebral cortex was introduced in 1985 by Barker and colleagues (1,2). They applied short magnetic pulses to the scalp, which were produced by a device designed to stimulate peripheral nerves, and recorded muscle action potentials from upper and lower limb muscles. The magnetic field passes through scalp and skull and stimulates gray matter of the cortex. Magnetoelectric stimulation is also suitable for stimulation of deep-lying proximal segments of peripheral nerves and nerve roots (3), thus allowing for evaluation of central and proximal peripheral pathways.

Muscles generally used for recording MEPs are the quadriceps, tibialis anterior, gastrocnemius, extensor hallucis, and abductor hallucis muscles (4). The segmental innervation of these muscles is used for level diagnosis. Surface recording electrodes are placed over the motor endplate.

For motor root stimulation over the lumbar spine, the intensity of the stimulator is adjusted so that a potential with a steep negative rise can be recorded. With this the onset latency is not critically dependent on the positioning of the coil or the stimulation strength (3). The excitation site of the nerve root is most likely in the region of the root exit from the intervertebral foramen (3).

In order to judge the MEP waveform it is also necessary to obtain an M-wave recording by means of conventional neurography. The M-wave is the response to a supramaximal stimulus of the peripheral nerve and provides an electric measure of muscle "size" (5). It is used as a reference signal with which transcranial stimulation MEP amplitude and duration are compared (i.e., MEP amplitude and duration are expressed as ratios of M-wave amplitude and duration.)

F-wave recordings allow for determination of a total peripheral conduction time (peripheral latency, or PL) from the anterior horn cell to the muscle, which includes the conduction over the motor root to its exit from the intervertebral foramen. Calculation of PL is especially important in lumbar spine disorders when motor roots measure 10 to 20 cm (6) and contribute considerably to PL. F-wave recordings may help localize the site of a lesion (7).

F-WAVE IN PATIENTS WITH NERVE ROOT COMPRESSION

The F-wave is usually normal in mild cases of radiculopathy. Distinct delay of the F-wave or a reduced number of F-waves after a given number of supramaximal peripheral stimuli, yet normal distal motor conduction studies, is a sign of a proximal lesion. Only in conjunction with MEPs, however, is it possible to determine conduction times for cauda fibers (i.e., motor roots) which may be affected by a disc herniation.

H-REFLEX

The H-reflex was first described by Hoffmann (8). It is a compound muscle action potential (CMAP) elicited by electric stimulation of large low threshold sensory nerve fibers, which monosynaptically excite a motor neuron pool that innervates the muscle (from which the H-wave is recorded) via the same nerve. It is a monosynaptic reflex activity comparable to the tendon jerk, bypassing the muscle spindles.

In adults, the H-wave can be recorded in a limited group of extensors, such as calf muscles (S1 root). Slight voluntary preinnervation facilitates the H-response (9). Stimulation of the tibial nerve at the knee with slowly increasing intensity from subthreshold to submaximal levels allows for recording of H-responses of growing amplitude from the soleus muscle. Further increase of stimulus intensity elicits M-waves of increasing size, while the H-reflex diminishes progressively and is eventually replaced by the F-wave with supramaximal stimulus intensity. H-reflexes and F-waves have similar latencies. Affected S1 sensory or motor roots reduce H-responses and increase their latency. Right/left latency differences are sensitive indicators of unilateral S1 radiculopathies.

Braddom and coworkers and Aiello and coworkers note a 90% to 100% true-positive rate and 0% true-negative rate in S1 radiculopathies (10,11).

ELECTROMYOGRAPHY

Electromyography (EMG) performed with concentric needle electrodes is the oldest neurophysiologic method in diagnosis of nerve root compression syndrome (12). It is an extension of the physical examination. Muscles to be tested are selected according to clinical findings (Fig. 14.1). As needle myography is not pain-free, the patient should be made fully aware of the procedure.

During the needle electromyography, the following variables are studied or observed:

- *Insertional activity*—evaluated at the time of initial placement and at each repositioning of the needle electrode in the muscle.
- *Spontaneous activity*—evaluated at rest after stationary and stable positioning of the needle electrode (Fig. 14.2).
- *Single motor unit action potentials (MUAPs)*—recorded during a mild voluntary contraction of the muscle and examined with respect to amplitude, duration, and number of phases. An average of 20 MUAPs should be calculated.
- *Motor unit recruitment* and the *interference pattern*—recorded during a gradual increase of voluntary muscle contraction and during maximal voluntary contraction (Fig. 14.3).

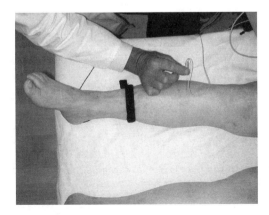

FIG. 14.1. Electromyography with concentric needle electrode from the tibialis anterior muscle.

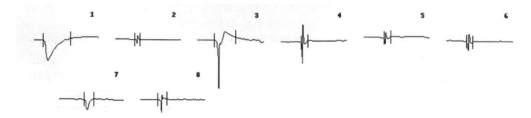

FIG. 14.2. Summary of different typical spontaneous activity from denervated tibialis anterior muscle as shown in Figure 14.1. (*1*) Sharp positive wave; (*2*) fibrillation; (*3 and 4*) fasciculation.

In normal muscles, MUAPs are elicited only in response to neural discharges. Denervated muscle fibers become unstable, as they are no longer under neural control, and individual muscle fibers will fire in the absence of neural stimuli. This uncontrolled activity results in increased insertional activity and spontaneous activity. These signs of denervation in the EMG can initially be spotted at about 14 days after the nerve lesion, first in paravertebral muscles and later in proximal and distal muscles of the leg. They are known as acute signs of denervation. The analysis of single MUAP may also reveal changes that are typical but not specific to lower motor neuron damage (e.g., radiculopathy; increased amplitude, increased number of phases, and increased duration). These changes are seen only after reinnervation or sprouting of nonaffected fibers has occurred. They are therefore termed *chronic* signs of denervation. Changes in motor unit recruitment and discharge may be seen in radiculopathy.

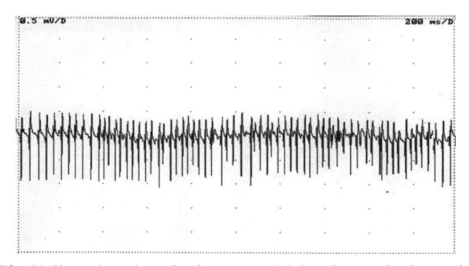

FIG. 14.3. Motor unit recruitment (interference pattern) during voluntary reduced contraction from denervated tibialis anterior muscle.

SENSITIVITY AND SPECIFICITY OF NEUROPHYSIOLOGIC ASSESSMENT

Several studies address these important measures of diagnostic ability of the neurophysiologic assessment of nerve root compression syndromes (13–15).

Tullberg and associates (13) have investigated whether comprehensive neurophysiologic testing of motor and sensory function could predict the results of surgery. In the case of EMG, a maximal voluntary contraction, motor unit analysis for occurrence of reinnervation-type potentials was used. An occurrence of spontaneous activity was also analyzed. In addition, nerve conduction velocity studies, including F-wave response by stimulation of the peroneal nerve (L5 root) and tibial nerve (S1 root) was indicated and SEPs were obtained after dermatome stimulation. In the Tullberg study, the EMG was found to be the most sensitive of the three employed methods, but the sensitivity was only 20%, which must be considered poor. This is in contrast to previous studies in which the sensitivity of EMG was 54% (16), 67% (17), and even as high as 78% (18). It must be stated, however, that the poor sensitivity of 20% was related to prediction of exact level of a root lesion. The sensitivity of pathologic EMG findings unrelated to level was 45%, possibly explained by the pleurisegmental innervation of the extremity muscles.

The sensitivity of F-wave in the presence of a root lesion has been found to be 35%, which agrees with other investigations (19–22). The results, however, are poor in terms of predicting the exact level of nerve root compression.

In the study by Tullberg and colleagues, the dermatomal SEP had a sensitivity of 40%, but the correct level was diagnosed in 15% only, a finding corresponding to a previous study by Aminoff and others (19). The authors conclude that of the three investigated neurophysiologic methods alone or in combination, none are reliable predictors of anatomic level, even if the diagnostic capacity is enhanced by using a number of tests.

It is recommended that neurophysiologic investigations be performed in patients with suspected lumbosacral radiculopathy, if radiological results and clinical symptoms are conflicting or inconclusive. Patients with normal neurophysiologic tests should be considered poor candidates for surgery (23). To be predictive of surgical outcome, complete neurophysiologic investigation must be made including tests of both motor and sensory function.

Vohanka and Dvorak (14) correlated the neurophysiologic findings with computed tomography (CT) or magnetic resonance imaging (MRI) findings of the lumbar spine not confirmed by surgery. The quantitative analysis of motor unit potentials showed a 30% sensitivity in patients with radiculopathy, but without motor deficit. The MEPs and SEPs reached sensitivities of 55%, and the MEPs had 75% false-negative findings.

The high incidence of false-negative findings indicates that neurophysiologic tests have a low reliability to confirm clinical findings. It should be repeated that in the Vohanka and Dvorak study a correlation was made between the clinical, neurophysiologic, and neuroradiologic assessment only and the diagnoses have not been confirmed by surgery.

Haig and colleagues (15) performed needle EMG of paraspinal muscles in patients with and without low back pain and radiculopathy. Normal individuals have few, if any, electromyographic abnormalities in the paraspinal musculature, which obviously contrasts to the high incidence of abnormalities found on CT and MRI (24) in asymptomatic subjects. However, persons with radiculopathy have a high degree of denervation signs in needle EMG. The authors recommend EMG studies of paraspinal muscles to rule out false-positive imaging studies.

From currently available studies it can be concluded that for patients with lumbar radiculopathy due to nerve root compression, the overall sensitivity and specificity of the neurophysiologic assessment is low. Therefore in the diagnosis of patients with radiculopathy due to disc herniation the following indications for neurophysiologic tests should be considered:

- Exclusion of more distal nerve damage (neuropathy, peripheral nerve entrapment).
- Verification of subjective muscle weakness by needle EMG in patients presenting pain inhibition or lack of cooperation.
- Recurrent disc surgery if difficult surgery is expected when documenting the preoperative muscle status (medicolegal aspects).

REFERENCES

1. Barker AT, Freeston IL, Jalinous R, et al. Magnetic stimulation of the human brain. *J Physiology* 1985;369:3P.
2. Barker AT, Jalinous R, Freeston IL. Non-invasive magnetic stimulation of the human motor cortex. *Lancet* 1985;1:1106–1107.
3. Britton TC, Meyer BU, Herdmann J, et al. Clinical use of the magnetic stimulator in the investigation of peripheral conduction time. *Muscle Nerve* 1990;13:396–406.
4. Chomiak J, Dvorak J, Antinnes J, et al. Motor evoked potentials: appropriate positioning of recording electrodes for diagnosis of spinal disorders. *Eur Spine J* 1995;4:180–185.
5. Reiners K, Herdmann J, Freund H-J. Altered mechanisms of muscular force generation in lower motor neuron disease. *Muscle Nerve* 1989;12:647–659.
6. Herdmann J, Dvorak J, Rathmer L, et al. Conduction velocities of pyramidal tract fibres and lumbar motor nerve roots: normal values. *Zent bl Neurochir* 1991;52:197–199.
7. Dvorak J, Herdmann J, Theiler R, et al. Magnetic stimulation of motor cortex and motor roots for painless evaluation of central and proximal peripheral motor pathways. Normal values and clinical application in disorders of the lumbar spine. *Spine* 1991;16(8):955–960.
8. Hoffmann P. Ueber die beziehung der sehnenreflexe zur willkuerlichen bewegung und zum tonus. *Zschr.f.Biologie* 1918;68(1111):351–370.
9. Stanley EF. Reflexes evoked in human thenar muscles during voluntary activity and their conduction pathways. *J Neurol Neurosurg Psychiatr*; 1978;41:1016–.
10. Braddom R, Joynson E. Standardization of H reflex and diagnostic use in S1 radiculopathy. *Arch Phys Med Rehabil* 1974;55:1661–1666.
11. Aiello I, Serra G, Migliore A. Electrophysiological findings in patients with lumbar disc prolapse. *Clin Neurophysiol* 1984;24(4):3313–3320.
12. Shea P, Woods W, Werden D. Electromyography in diagnosis of nerve root compression syndrome. *Arch Neurol Psychiatr* 1950;64:93–104.
13. Tullberg T, Svanborg E, Isacsson J, et al. A preoperative and postoperative study of the accuracy and value of electrodiagnosis in patients with lumbosacral disc herniation. *Spine* 1993;18(7):837– 842.
14. Vohanka S, Dvorak J. Motor and somatosensory evoked potentials in cervical spinal stenosis. Paper presented at: The 40th Congress of the Czech and Slovak Neurophysiology; 1993; Brno.
15. Haig A, LeBreck D, Powly S. Paraspinal mapping—quantified needle electromyography of the paraspinal muscles in persons without low back pain. *Spine* 1995;20(6):715–721.
16. LaJoie W. Nerve root compression: correlation of electromyographic, myelographic and surgical findings. *Arch Phys Med Rehabil* 1972;53:390–392.
17. Lane M, Tamhankar M, Demopoulos J. Discogenic radiculopathy: use of electromyography in multidisciplinary management. *NY State J Med* 1978;78:32–36.
18. Knuttsson B. Comparative value of electromyographic, myelographic and clinical–neurological examinations in diagnosis of lumbar root compression syndrome. *Arch Orthop Scand Suppl* 1961;49:1–135.
19. Aminoff M, Goodin D, Parry G. Electrophysiologic evaluation of lumbosacral radiculopathies: electromyography, late response, and somatosensory evoked potentials. *Neurology* 1985;35:1514–1518.
20. Eisen A, Hoirch M. The electrodiagnostic evaluation of spinal root lesions. *Spine* 1983;8:1(459):98–106.
21. Fisher M, Shivde A, Texeira C, et al. Clinical and electrophysiological appraisal of the significance of radicular injury in back pain. *J Neurol Neurosurg Psychiatr* 1978;41:303–306.
22. Tonzola R, Ackil A, Shahani B, et al. Usefulness of electrophysiological studies in the diagnosis of lumbosacral root disease. *Ann Neurol* 1981;9:305–308.
23. Kimura J. *Electrodiagnosis in diseases of nerve and muscle: principles and practice*, 2nd ed. Philadelphia: FA Davis Co, 1989.
24. Boden S, McCowin P, Davis D, et al. Abnormal magnetic resonance scans of the cervical spine in asymptomatic subjects. *J Bone Joint Surg* 1990;72-A(8):1178–1184.

Conservative Treatment Modalities

15

Importance of Sensitivity and Specificity of Diagnostic Tests

Björn Rydevik and Helena Brisby

The majority of patients with low back pain have a favorable natural course and no specific underlying cause for the disease can be found. However, some patients with back pain syndromes may have diagnoses such as cancer, infection, spondylolisthesis, or disc herniation. Such conditions may require surgical therapy, making careful diagnostic evaluation of the patient very important. In the management of these patients, the weak associations between clinical symptoms, pathologic changes, and radiologic findings create challenges for the treating clinician (1,5).

SENSITIVITY AND SPECIFICITY: ACCURACY OF DIAGNOSTIC TESTS

In order to understand the accuracy of any diagnostic test, one must assume that we know the ultimate truth about the presence or absence of the disease in the patient (2,7,13). Thus some kind of "gold standard" for the diagnosis is required. The gold standard is regarded as a definitive diagnosis obtained by autopsy, biopsy, surgery, long-term follow-up, or some superior diagnostic test. None of these so-called gold standards are without limitations, but in the clinical management we must assume that there is some gold standard which is reasonably acceptable. For patients with low back pain syndromes, the situation may be further complicated due to the fact that many diagnoses do not have widely agreed upon definitions or criteria. Examples of such clinical diagnoses where controversy remains include fibrositis, sacroiliac disorders, disc degeneration, facet joint syndrome, trigger point syndromes, and spinal instability (8,9,11).

If we assume that there is an acceptable gold standard, the next question is how a diagnostic test will compare with the results of the gold standard. Evaluation of the accuracy of a diagnostic test requires that a so-called 2 × 2 table is created (Table 15.1). This involves categorizing the patients in question into four groups. As an example we may consider a positive straight leg raising (SLR) test to be positive for disc herniation. Since this test (and many other tests) are not perfect, one may typically have four groups of patients when applying the test:

- True-positives (TP) are patients with the disease and a positive test result (positive SLR and a disc herniation).
- True-negatives (TN) are patients without the disease and a negative test (negative SLR and no disc herniation).
- False-positives (FP) are patients without disease, but in whom the test is positive (positive SLR but no disc herniation).

TABLE 15.1. *Comparison of magnetic resonance imaging (MRI)*
test to a "gold standard" (HNP)

| | Gold standard | | |
Result	Patient has HNP	Patient does not have HNP	Total
MRI			
Positive	*(a)* true positives	*(b)* false positives	*a + b*
Negative	*(c)* false negatives	*(d)* true negatives	*c + d*
Totals:	*a + c*	*b + d*	*a + b + c + d*

HNP, herniated nucleus pulposus.
Stable properties:
   Sensitivity = *a/(a + c)*
   Specificity = *d/(b + d)*
Frequency or prevalence-dependent properties
   Predictive value of a positive test *a/(a + b)*
   Predictive value of a negative test *d/(c + d)*
Prevalence of disease in the sample: *(a + c)/(a + b + c + d)*
(Modified from Deyo R. Understanding the accuracy of diagnostic tests. In: Weinstein JN, et al., eds. *Essentials of the spine.* New York: Raven Press, 1995:55–69, with permission.)

- False-negatives (FN) are patients with disease, but with a negative test result (negative SLR but a disc herniation).

In Table 15.1 the total number of patients who have a disc herniation are *(a+c)*. The *a* patients have a positive magnetic resonance image (MRI). Those in category *c* have the disease but have a false-negative test. The sensitivity of the test is defined as

$$a/(a + c)$$

and is often expressed as a percentage value. Thus, a test that is good at detecting the disease in patients is a highly sensitive test. To help remember the definition of sensitivity the term PID (Positive In Disease) has been introduced (5).

In order to be of clinical value, a diagnostic test must not only be positive when the disease is present, but also be negative when the disease is absent. The ability of a diagnostic test to correctly identify patients without the disease is called specificity. For calculation of specificity, one can use the data in Table 15.1. Patients in category *d* have true negative results, while those in category *b* have no disease but false-positive test results. Specificity is calculated as

$$d/(b + d)$$

To help remember the definition of specificity, the term NIH (Negative In Health) can be used (5).

Sensitivity and specificity of a test, as presented in Table 15.1, are sometimes referred to as vertical properties. It is often regarded that sensitivity and specificity are stable properties of a test, which means that they do not vary with disease prevalence and other related factors (1,5).

Sensitivity and specificity values for various diagnostic tests are thus useful characteristics but may not fully reflect how the test results are used in clinical practice. It should be pointed out that since we usually do not have the results of a gold standard, we must rely on the less definitive diagnostic tests. When evaluating the individual patient, the most important aspect is to know the probability that the patient has the disease if the test result is positive, rather than how likely the test is to be positive if the patient has the disease. The so-called *predictive value* of a test is obtained by calculating horizontally in Table 15.1 rather than vertically. The predictive value can answer the question, "Given a positive result, how likely is it to be a true-positive finding?" A positive predictive value of a test is shown in Table 15.1 by the value

$$a/(ab)$$

In a corresponding way the predictive value of a negative test is calculated as

$$d/(c+d)$$

Predictive values can be expected to vary to a large extent according to the prevalence of the disease, in contrast to sensitivity and specificity, which are regarded as stable properties. The prevalence of disease in the patients shown in Table 15.1 can be calculated as

$$(a+c)/(a+b+c+d)$$

ACCURACY OF MEDICAL HISTORY, PHYSICAL EXAMINATION, AND RADIOLOGIC TESTS

A patient's medical history can be of considerable value in helping to rule out various diseases such as cancer as the cause of back pain (6). For example, previous history of cancer has very high specificity (0.98) for back pain and therefore such patients should be considered to have cancer in the spine until proven otherwise. However, the sensitivity of this finding is rather low (0.31).

Disorders of the lumbar spine can involve neurologic abnormalities in the lower extremities, often caused by disc herniation but also as a result of spinal stenosis, infection, or cancer. The absence of sciatic pain indicates that clinically important disc herniation is very unlikely. The SLR test is commonly used and can be defined as positive if it reproduces sciatic pain at less than 60 degrees of leg elevation. Based on such assumption one can calculate the sensitivity and specificity of this test for lumbar disc herniations. The data presented in Table 15.2 indicate that the SLR test has a fairly high sensitivity (0.80) but a rather low specificity (0.40) in the diagnosis of a herniated disc. The crossed SLR test (straight leg raising is performed on the patient's nonsymptomatic leg and pain is elicited in the symptomatic leg) has a low sensitivity (0.25) but a high specificity (0.90). This means that ipsilateral SLR test is mostly effective as a "rule-out" test while crossed SLR test is more effective as a "rule-in" test (5,10).

TABLE 15.2. *Estimates of test accuracy for diagnosis of herniated discs*

Test	Sensitivity	Specificity
Ipsilateral SLR	0.80	0.40
Crossed SLR	0.25	0.90
Impaired ankle reflex (HNP at L5-S1)	0.50	0.60
Plain CT	0.90	0.70
CT myelography	0.90	0.70
MRI	0.90	0.70

CT, computed tomography; HNP, herniated nucleus pulposus; MRI, magnetic resonance imaging; SLR, straight leg raising.

(Modified from Deyo R. Understanding the accuracy of diagnostic tests. In: Weinstein JN, et al., eds. *Essentials of the spine.* New York: Raven Press, 1995:55–69, with permission.)

The data summarized here regarding the clinical evaluation of patients with suspected disc herniation indicate that MRI and computed tomography (CT) should be used selectively, usually for surgical planning. Since abnormal findings are common in asymptomatic persons, it is of major importance to always correlate the imaging findings with the medical history and physical examination. Several investigations have shown that asymptomatic individuals without back pain and sciatica may have a high prevalence of spinal abnormalities on CT and MRI images (3,4,14). For example, disc herniation has been reported in 20% to 76% of asymptomatic individuals. Such findings should be regarded as true anatomic abnormalities without clinical relevance. This means that for clinical decision-making purposes these abnormalities can be regarded as false-positive results and this fact reduces the specificity of these imaging tests.

In Table 15.2, several investigations regarding the sensitivity and specificity of various diagnostic tests for lumbar disc herniation are summarized. It is important for the clinician to consider these data when managing patients with suspected lumbar disc herniation. It should be noted that the data indicate that CT, MRI, and CT–myelography have approximately the same values of sensitivity and specificity. This means that factors such as availability and cost may influence the choice of imaging method (5,12).

CONCLUSION

Available data regarding sensitivity and specificity of medical history, physical examination, and radiologic tests should be implemented when evaluating patients with low back pain and sciatica in order to obtain the best possible diagnostic accuracy in identifying patients with disc herniation.

REFERENCES

1. Andersson GBJ, Deyo RA. History and physical examination in patients with herniated lumbar discs. *Spine* 1996;21(24s):10s–18s.
2. Andersson GBJ, Deyo RA. Sensitivity, specificity and predictive value: a general issue in screening for disease and in interpretation of diagnostic studies in spinal disorders. In: Frymoyer JW, ed. *The adult spine: principles and practice*, 2nd ed. New York: Raven Press, 1996.
3. Boden SD, Davis DO, Dina TS, et al. Abnormal magnetic resonance scans of the lumbar spine in asymptomatic subjects: a prospective investigation. *J Bone Joint Surg (Am)* 1990;72A:403–408.
4. Boos N, Rieder R, Schade V, et al. The diagnostic accuracy of magnetic resonance imaging, work perception and psychosocial factors in identifying symptomatic disc herniations. *Spine* 1995; 20(24):2613–2625.
5. Deyo R. Understanding the accuracy of diagnostic tests. In: Weinstein JN, Rydevik BL, Sonntag VH, eds. *Essentials of the spine*. New York: Raven Press, 1995:55–69.
6. Deyo RA, Diehl AK. Cancer as a cause of back pain: frequency, clinical presentation, and diagnostic strategies. *J Gen Intern Med* 1988;3:230–238.
7. Deyo RA, Haselkorn J, Hoffman R, et al. Designing studies of diagnostic tests for low back pain or radiculopathy. *Spine* 1994;185:2057s–2065s.
8. Deyo RA, Rainville J, Kent DL. What can the history and physical examination tell us about low back pain? *JAMA* 1992;268:760–765.
9. Garvey TA, Marks MF, Wiesel SW. A prospective randomized double-blind evaluation of trigger point injection therapy for low back pain. *Spine* 1989;14:962–964.
10. Kortelainen P, Puranen J Koivistor E, et al. Symptoms and signs of sciatica and their relation to the localization of the lumbar disc herniation. *Spine* 1985;10:88–92.
11. Sackett DL. A primer on the precision and accuracy of the clinical examination. *JAMA* 1992;267:2638–2644.
12. Thornbury JR, Fryback DG, Turski PA, et al. Disk-caused nerve compression in patients with acute low-back pain: diagnosis with MR, CT myelography, and plain CT. *Radiology* 1993;186:731–738.
13. Waddell G, Main CJ, Morris EW, et al. Normality and reliability in the clinical assessment of backache. *Br Med J* 1982;284:1519–1523.
14. Wiesel SW, Tsourmas N, et al. A study of computer assisted tomography: I. The incidence of positive CAT scans in an asymptomatic group of patients. *Spine* 1984;9:549–551.

16

Physical Medicine:
Traction, Exercise, and Revalidation

Margareta Nordin and Marco Campello

Physical medicine in general implies pain relief and treatment focusing on improving function. Current update of randomized controlled trials has forced the health care provider to revalidate more traditional treatments such as traction, ultrasound, heat, and other passive modalities. The recently published findings of the Paris Task Force included a literature review of exercise efficacy for the patient with nonsurgically treated sciatica (1). This chapter provides an update on traction and exercise treatment in patients with sciatica related to lumbar disc herniation.

Patients with sciatica pain may or may not have pain in the lumbar spine. Sciatica is defined as pain that radiates down the leg, with dermatomal distribution and perhaps additional neurologic deficits. Pain radiating below the knee is documented as a sign of disc involvement and nerve compromise (7). This pain can range from very modest to very severe. Few patients have no radiating pain down the leg but do show a neurologic deficit. The efficacy of two selected noninvasive physical medicine/physical therapy modalities will be explored as this chapter will focus on the choice of passive or active treatment with a special emphasis on lumbar spine traction and exercises for patients with sciatica.

TYPE OF TREATMENT

Active or Passive Treatment

The health care provider treating patients with sciatica with or without low back pain can choose between passive and active treatment in physical medicine (Fig. 16.1).

Common passive treatments include bed rest, therapeutic heat/cold, transcutaneous laser treatment, electrotherapy, traction, and massage. Bed rest has proven negative effects on the cardiovascular and musculoskeletal systems (5,8,9). Nordin and Campello (13) reviewed the proposed physiologic response, common use, and evidence of efficacy and patient satisfaction for the above modalities. Few studies are aimed at patients with sciatica; most studies concern patients with low back pain with or without leg pain. Although passive treatment may give short-term relief of sciatic pain, it has no long-lasting effect for pain reduction and long-term passive treatment may reinforce a perception of severe sickness and illness behavior (4,21).

There is strong evidence against long-lasting passive treatment. It is detrimental for the individual's well being and recovery for patients with low back pain. However there is only moderate evidence of the benefits of active treatment for patients with acute sciatica and sparse evidence for patients with chronic sciatica (1). The consensus among spe-

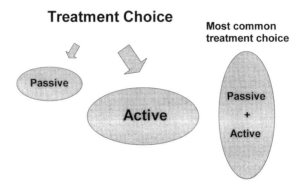

FIG. 16.1. The choice of passive (bed rest or passive modalities) or active (active exercises) treatment affects the outcome for patients with low back pain and sciatica. In clinical practice both are commonly used. Passive treatment should be minimized, however, and not encouraged.

cialists is generally that activity is more beneficial for the individual with sciatica than passive treatment (1).

TRACTION

Traction was first used in ancient times (21). Medical texts from Hippocrates to Sculleti in the seventeenth century have described traction in combination with manipulation. Traction is still used in some parts of the world but progressively less for patients with low back pain and sciatica. Common types of traction treatment are shown in Table 16.1.

The proposed physiologic response to traction is "Vertebral joint distraction; prevention of adhesion within the dural sleeves, nerve roots, and adjacent capsular structures; reduction of compression and irritation of the nerve root and discs; and reduction of pain, inflammation, and muscle spasm" (16). The scientific proof for these physiologic responses is weak at best and the efficacy of traction treatment for patients with sciatica is poor (18). Potential reported harm to patients subjected to traction is low. However, we should not underestimate the harm of prolonged bed rest when traction, bed rest, and hospitalization are combined and the potential reinforcement to the patient that he or she is sick (8,21). Inverted traction is reported to increase blood pressure. The cost for traction

TABLE 16.1. *Examples of traction treatments given for patients with low back pain and sciatica with no proven long lasting effect*

The Lumbar Spine and Available Types of Traction Treatment
• Manual Traction
• Mechanical Traction
Intermittent (7 to 60 seconds)
Vertebral Axial Decompression (VAX-D) (10 to 20 decompression)
Sustained (static) Traction (10 to 30 minutes)
Continuos Traction (20 to 40 hours)
• Autotraction
• Gravity or Inversion Traction
• Other

treatment is generally low to moderate when traction is given on an outpatient basis and high when the patient is hospitalized (4). In fact, the recent guidelines from different countries are against the use of traction for patients with low back pain and sciatica (4,17,22).

Despite these recommendations traction treatment continues. It gives patients false hope about a cure, inactivates the patient, and uses health care dollars for ineffective nonevidence-based treatment.

ACTIVE TREATMENT

Exercise Efficacy for Patients with Sciatica Treated Nonsurgically

Active treatment such as exercises and activity modification is proven beneficial for the patient with subacute and chronic low back pain (1). There is moderate evidence for patients with sciatica. Type of exercise and activity modification and their efficacy is not well known and needs to be further studied. Vroomen and colleagues (19) studied the effectiveness of bed rest in patients with sciatica. They randomly assigned patients ($N =$ 183) to either strict bed rest for 2 weeks or "watchful waiting." Patients assigned to the "watchful waiting" group were instructed to be up and about but to avoid straining the back or provoking pain. They were allowed to go to work but bed rest was not prohibited.

The primary outcome was the independent investigator's and the patient's global assessment of improvement at 2 and 12 weeks. Secondary outcome measures were changes in functional status, pain scores, work absenteeism, and need for surgical intervention. There was no difference in outcomes between the two groups. The Paris Task Force (1), in their extensive literature review, only partially supports these findings. They state, "Patients whose pain is intense enough to justify bed rest must be referred for a specialized back pain evaluation if they have not begun to progressively resume their daily activity after 10 days of strict bed rest (getting up only to go to the bathroom) and adequate pain therapy." This discrepancy may be explained by the fact that the Vroomen (19) study was not included in the extensive literature review because it was not available at the time. Another explanation may be difference in clinical practice. The Paris Task Force was made up predominantly of experts in France and the traditional treatment and clinical practice for severe sciatica in France was (is) bed rest and hospitalization. The consensus of bed rest for acute severe sciatica may therefore be influenced by cultural clinical practice.

Four additional recommendations from this review were put forward (1). Exercise recommendations for acute sciatica are as follows: "The prescription of active physical exercises or re-education is contraindicated in the first week in all cases of low back pain including sciatica. Dynamic, active exercises, in particular are contraindicated." This supports the findings of watchful waiting (19). Exercise recommendations for patients with intermittent, subacute (4 to 12 weeks of duration), and chronic sciatica (longer than 12 weeks' duration) are as follows: "Given the absence of specific data in the literature, these programs are authorized but not recommended" (1). Many patients with sciatica do improve with an exercise program. However, the Paris Task Force found no strong evidence for exercises in patients being nonsurgically treated for sciatica. Manniche, et al. (11,12) showed that patients can tolerate an exercise program and even improve with all the secondary benefits thereof after surgery.

The Task Force also wanted to evaluate whether of not certain specific exercises were superior to others (1). The review included 1,141 articles with an in-depth review of 150 studies concerning exercises for low back pain including sciatica. It appears that the key to success is the physical activity itself (i.e., activity of any form rather than a specific activity). The Task Force recommendation based on the review concluded that there is scientific evidence in favor of programs combining strength training, endurance training, stretching, and fitness. However it should also be mentioned that there was no study directly related to sciatica. This evidence was derived mainly from studies including patients with low back pain with or without leg pain.

In summary "watchful waiting," activity modification, and progressive exercise treatment including muscle strengthening, stretching, and aerobic fitness has a longer lasting effect for patients being nonsurgically treated for sciatica. Studies, however, are sparse.

Exercise Efficacy in Patients with Surgically Treated Sciatica

Exercise after surgical treatment for sciatica has been studied in randomized controlled trials by several authors (2,6,10,12,15). Supervised exercise and home training were reviewed (6,10). Conventional exercises compared to high-intensity exercises with or without hyperextension of the lumbar spine were studied by Manniche and associates (11,12). A rehabilitation program with and without horseback riding was studied by Rothaupt and coworkers (15). All patients who received physical training seemed to benefit from the exercises, both those with chronic pain after lumbar disc surgery and those who were still recovering from recent surgery. Chronic patients (less than 1-year post-surgery) experienced significantly more pain relief at 3 months' follow-up, however, this effect did not remain after 1 year. Exercise intensity did not yield better results (6,10–12). Most programs used strengthening and endurance training for the trunk muscles, flexibility, and fitness training. It was not possible to determine from these studies whether one type of exercise was superior to another.

PHYSICAL ACCOMMODATIONS

Abenhaim and colleagues (1) and Nordin and Balague (14) have discussed work resumption and ergonomic adaptation of the workplace. Waddell and Burton (20) recently published occupational health guidelines for patients with low back pain at work. Again, given the absence of specific data in the literature, the maintenance of progressive resumption of occupational activities is authorized in acute and subacute cases of sciatica and is recommended in patients with chronic sciatica. Chronic severe sciatica leads to an increase in perceived disability (3). Ergonomic adaptation of the work site can be very helpful in these cases. Ergonomic adaptation, administrative cooperation, and even retraining may be necessary for patients with chronic and severe sciatica to remain productively employed.

CONCLUSIONS

Acute or chronic severe sciatica may be related to a substantial decrease in function. Chronic severe sciatica may lead to permanent disability. The literature indicates that "watchful waiting" and activity modification in acute sciatica is as effective as bed rest. Progressive exercises such as strengthening, stretching, and aerobics are more effective alternatives for the subacute and chronic patient with surgically or nonsurgically treated sciatica than passive long-term treatment. Accommodations of work and leisure tasks are reported helpful on empirical bases for patients with chronic sciatica.

REFERENCES

1. Abenhaim L, Rossignol M, Valat JP, et al. The role of activity in the therapeutic management of back pain. *Spine* 2000;25(4):IS–33S.
2. Alaranta H, Hurme M, Eionola S, et al. Rehabilitation after surgery for lumbar disc herniation. Results of a randomized clinical trial. *Int J Rehabil Res* 1986;9:247–57.
3. Balague F, Nordin M, Sheikhzadeh A, et al. Recovery of severe sciatica. *Spine* 1999;24(23):2516–2524.
4. Bigos SJ, Bowyer OR, Braen GR, et al. *Clinical Practice Guideline No.14: Acute low back problems in adults.* Rockville, MD: Agency for Health Care Policy and Research, US, Department of Health and Human Services; December 1994:1–60. AHCPR Publication No. 95-0642.
5. Conventino VA, Bloomfield SA, Greenleaf JE. An overview of the issues: physiological effects of bed rest and restricted physical activity. *Med Sci Sports Exerc* 1997;29:187–90.
6. Danielsen JM, Johnsen, R, Kibsgaard SK, et al. Early aggressive exercise for postoperative rehabilitation after discectomy. *Spine* 2000;25(8):1015–1020.
7. Deyo RA, Loeser JD, Bigos SJ. Herniated intervertebral disk. *Ann Intern Med* 1990;112: 598–603.
8. Dittmer DK, Teasell R. Complications of immobilization and bed rest. 1. Musculoskeletal and cardiovascular complications. *Can Fam Physician* 1993;39:1428–1432;1435–1427.
9. Ferrando AA, Stuart CA, Brunder DG, et al. Magnetic resonance imaging quantitation of changes in muscle volume during 7 days of strict bed rest. *Aviat Space Environ Med* 1995;66:976–981.
10. Johanssen F, Renzvig L, Kruger P. Supervised endurance exercise training compared to home training after first lumbar discectomy. *Clin Exp Rheumatol* 1994;12:609–614.
11. Manniche C, Skall HF, Braenholt L, et al. Clinical trial of prospective dynamic back exercises after first lumbar discectomy. *Spine* 1993;18:92–97.
12. Manniche C, Asmussen K, Lauritsen B, et al. Intensive dynamic back exercises with or without hyperextension in chronic back pain after surgery for lumbar disc protrusion: a clinical trial. *Spine* 1993;18:560–567.
13. Nordin M, Campello M. Physical therapy. Exercises and the modalities: when, what and why? *Neurolog Clin North Am* 1999;17(1):75–89.
14. Nordin M, Balague F. Biometrics and ergonomics in disk herniation accompanied by sciatica. In: Weinstein JN, Gordon SL, eds. *Low back pain—a scientific and clinical overview.* Rosemont, IL: American Academy of Orthopedic Surgeons, 1996:23–48.
15. Rothhaupt D, Laser T, Ziegler H, et al. Die orthopädische abt. klinik Dr. Erler GmbH, Nürnberg. *Sportverl Sportschad* 1997;11:63–69.
16. Tan JC. *Practical manual of physical medicine and rehabilitation.* New York: Mosby, 1998:145–148.
17. Teasell R, Dittmer DK. Complications of immobilization and bed rest. 2. Other complications. *Can Fam Physician* 1993;39:1440–1442,1444–1446.
18. van der Heijden GJ, Beurskens AJ, Koes BW, et al. The efficacy of traction for back and neck pain: a systematic blinded review of randomized clinical trial methods. *Physical Ther* 1995;75:93–104.
19. Vroomen P, de Krom, M, Wilmink JT, et al. Lack of effectiveness of bed rest for sciatica. *N Engl J Med* 1999;340(6):418–423.
20. Waddell G, Burton AK. *Occupational health guidelines for the management of low back pain at work evidence review recommendations.* London: Faculty of Medicine of Occupational Medicine, 2000.
21. Waddell G. *The back pain revolution.* Edinburgh: Churchill Livingstone, 1998.
22. Waddell G, Feder G, McIntosh A, et al. *Low back pain evidence review.* London: Royal College of General Practitioners, 1996.

17

Single-Blind Randomized Controlled Trial of Chemonucleolysis and Manipulation in the Treatment of Symptomatic Lumbar Disc Herniation

A. Kim Burton, K. Malcolm Tillotson, and John Cleary

Back pain with associated leg pain is a common complaint, although the lifetime prevalence of lumbar radicular syndrome probably affects no more than 5% of the population (7). For these patients, however, this is a particularly painful and distressing experience. Although the predominant complaint regarding this syndrome is leg pain, most patients report concomitant back pain with associated disability. The natural course of acute cases is favorable, and conservative management strategies usually are sufficient (17). However, for some patients the pain will be unremitting and other therapeutic options need to be considered.

Manipulation is an accepted primary care treatment for back pain (15). Although osteopathic and chiropractic texts suggest manipulation is also a safe and effective treatment for sciatica due to lumbar disc herniation (5,12), there is little beyond anecdotal evidence for its efficacy and it is considered to be contraindicated by some authorities (17). Nevertheless, osteopaths and chiropractors do treat many cases of lumbar radicular syndrome, and serious complications such as cauda equina syndrome seem to be rare (2). Investigations into its efficacy are, therefore, desirable to inform clinical practice. The manipulative techniques used vary from one clinician to another, but the main elements are soft tissue stretching maneuvers, passive techniques to articulate the lumbar spine throughout its ranges of motion (sometimes known as "mobilization"), and side posture high-velocity rotatory thrusts (sometimes termed "manipulation") (5,12). The term "manipulation" is used in this chapter to cover the range of manual techniques used by osteopaths, and not as a synonym for thrust-type techniques.

The two most common orthopedic interventions for a lumbar radicular syndrome due to disc herniation are partial discectomy and chemonucleolysis. Conventional discectomy involves a spinal surgical procedure, with removal of a varying proportion of the disc material. Chemonucleolysis involves injection of an enzyme (chymopapain) into the nucleus to reduce the water-binding capacity of its proteoglycans, and thus reduce the amount of nuclear material. A recent systematic review has concluded that chemonucleolysis is an effective treatment, but that it is less effective than discectomy, with up to 30% of patients subsequently requiring surgery (9). Chemonucleolysis can be considered an intermediate between conservative management and open surgery, which avoids the accepted, but rare, complications of a surgical procedure and its high health care costs.

A consensus summary of a recent focus meeting on disc herniation (1) outlines some of the problems with current management. While discectomy and chemonucleolysis can be accepted as proven treatments, there is concern about differential surgery rates, the optimal type of intervention, its timing, and the selection of appropriate patients. It was also felt that noninvasive interventions, such as manipulation, are of unknown efficacy due to the lack of prospective randomized trials. The present trial was proposed to address this latter issue.

The hypothesis to be tested was that manipulative treatment provides at least equivalent 12-month outcomes when compared with treatment by chemonucleolysis for patients with sciatica due to confirmed lumbar disc herniation, where chemonucleolysis is taken as a procedure known to be more effective than placebo (9). It was also hypothesized that manipulation produces a more rapid improvement, particularly for disability and back pain.

MATERIALS AND METHODS

The trial participants were recruited from the orthopedic department of a hospital in the north of England. They were patients complaining of unremitting sciatica, diagnosed due to a lumbar disc herniation, for whom there was no clinical indication for surgical intervention.

The study design was a prospective randomized controlled trial to determine 2-week, 6-week, and 12-month outcomes from manipulation compared with chemonucleolysis, where chemonucleolysis acted as the control. Local ethical committee approval was obtained for random allocation to treatment either by chemonucleolysis or osteopathic manipulation. Blinding of patients and treating clinicians to the treatment allocation was clearly not possible, but a blinded independent observer performed baseline and follow-up assessments, supplemented by validated self-report questionnaires.

Specific entry criteria were similar to those described elsewhere (3,13). All patients displayed the following:

Age range: 18 to 60 years
Unilateral unremitting sciatica (with leg pain worse than back pain)
Positive straight leg raising test with positive nerve root tension signs, radiculopathy limited to a single nerve root

In addition, there was unequivocal evidence of single-level nonsequestrated lumbar disc herniation on either computed tomography (CT) or magnetic resonance imaging (MRI), where imaging findings were consistent with the clinical picture. Exclusion criteria were:

Sequestrated herniation
Multiplelevel marked lumbar degenerative changes
Previous lumbar surgery
Previous chemonucleolysis
Previous manipulative treatment for the present complaint
Involvement in litigation

Following diagnosis (and consideration of exclusion criteria) patients were informed of the nature of the trial and asked to sign a consent form. The randomization sequence was generated by computer and balanced over order. A blinded envelope system was used to allocate patients to treatment. Those patients randomized to manipulation were contacted by the research team and given an appointment to see a private osteopathic manipulator (A.K.B.), while those randomized to chemonucleolysis were put on the waiting list of an orthopedic surgeon (J.C.).

The manipulative treatment comprised a number of 15-minute treatment sessions over a period not exceeding 12 weeks, with the bulk of the sessions occurring in the first 6 weeks. The treatments followed a typical protocol for osteopathic management of sciatica (12). Briefly, the procedures included soft tissue stretching of the lumbar and buttock muscula-ture, low-amplitude passive articulatory maneuvers of the lumbar spine, and judicious use of high-velocity thrusts to one or more lumbar articulations (5). (A high-velocity thrust is a manipulative technique that delivers a low-amplitude, high-velocity movement within the physiologic range intended to be perpendicular to a specific lumbar zygapophysial joint.) Any or all of these procedures were performed on each occasion at the clinical discretion of the manipulator. Advice was given to continue normal daily activity as much as possi-ble, while early return to work (for those employed) was encouraged.

The chemonucleolysis was administered as an in-patient procedure under general anesthesia. A single injection of chymopapain (Chymodyactyl) was given. An 18-gauge spinal needle was placed into the center of the nucleus of the disc under biplanar radi-ographic control, and a discogram was performed with 0.5-ml contrast medium. Then, 2-ml (4,000 units) chymopapain was gradually injected. Finally, the needle was retracted to clear the posterior spinal elements, and 10 ml of 0.25% bupivacaine was injected. Patients recovered overnight and were discharged the following day to the usual care of their family doctor.

Baseline data for all patients were obtained immediately before treatment by a senior physiotherapist at the hospital who was blinded to the treatment allocation. The same physiotherapist performed the follow-up assessments (barring holidays, when a deputy stood in). Patients were asked not to reveal their treatment allocations. Clinical assess-ments were conducted to a simple structured protocol, supplemented by a booklet of questionnaires that was returned to the research office, where a blinded research assistant entered them into a computer database. The clinical variables included measures of lum-bar flexion, lumbar side bending, and straight leg raising, along with details of the his-tory of the complaint and work status. Disability was measured with the Roland Disabil-ity Questionnaire (RDQ) (14), while the extent of pain was measured with seven-point "annotated thermometer" rating scales for leg pain and back pain (14). Baseline psycho-logical parameters were checked using additional questionnaires. Distress was estimated by the Distress and Risk Assessment Method (11), which involves measures of depres-sion and somatic perceptions.

At each follow-up point, the clinical assessments were as at the pretreatment assessment, with additional questions concerning complications and other treatments being sought. Outcomes at each point were assessed from self-reported disability (measured by the RDQ) along with pain ratings for back pain and leg pain (measured by the pain scales).

A total of 40 patients were recruited (20 in each group). Their mean age was 41.9 years (standard deviation [SD] 10.6) and 19 were male. Twenty-five patients were allocated to treatment strictly through the randomization protocol, but administrative difficulties, caused by movement of key hospital staff, resulted in 15 patients being allocated to treat-ment outside the randomization sequence. A comparison between the baseline data of the properly randomized group and the remainder revealed no statistically significant differ-ences; investigation of the recruitment patterns revealed no systematic bias. All 40 patients were available for follow-up at 2 weeks, while 37 (93%) were available at 6 weeks, and 30 (75%) at 12 months. The loss to follow-up rate was the same in both treat-ment groups.

The average length of the presenting spell of similar leg pain at the point of diagnosis was 30 weeks (SD 34) for the manipulation group and 32 weeks (SD 36) for the injected group. A previous history of low back trouble was reported by 15 manipulated patients and 12 injected patients, with a previous history of sciatica being reported by 13 and 10 patients, respectively. Seven manipulated and six injected patients were off work at baseline. None of these differences between groups were statistically significant. The mean delay before commencement of manipulative treatment in the manipulator's office was 3 weeks (SD 3.6), while the mean delay for chemonucleolysis, performed at the hospital, was 12.9 weeks (SD 7.8).

The data were variously suitable for statistical analysis by two-tailed Student's t tests, chi-square tests, and multiple regression. Repeated measures analysis with general linear modeling was used to study trends and the influence of covariates. The level of statistical significance was set at 5%.

RESULTS

There were no instances of major complications from either treatment, but a number of patients required additional orthopedic intervention (between 6 weeks and 12 months) due to persisting symptoms; these we have termed "therapeutic failures." Four of the manipulated patients received chemonucleolysis and one required lumbar discectomy. Three of the injected patients received epidural steroid injections and one of these also underwent manipulation under anesthetic.

The outcome data (means and standard deviations of scores for leg pain, back pain, and disability) from baseline through 12 months are given in Table 17.1. For ease of interpretation of the patterns of response, the data are shown in the form of graphs in Figures 17.1 through 17.3. By 12 months, both treatment groups showed statistically significant improvement for mean scores on all three measures, with no statistically significant differences between groups, although there were between-group differences during the first few weeks.

Both treatment groups followed a similar pattern of steady improvement in leg pain over time, with no statistically significant difference between the groups (Fig. 17.1). There was a statistically significant benefit from manipulation over chemonucleolysis for back pain at both 2 weeks and 6 weeks (Fig. 17.2). In contrast to the manipulation group, the chemonucleolysis group did not show a significant improvement in mean back pain

TABLE 17.1. *Means (SD) for the main outcome variables from baseline though 12 months by treatment group*

	Baseline (n = 20/20)	2 weeks (n = 20/20)	6 weeks (n = 19/18)	12 months (n = 15/15)
Leg pain				
Manipulation	4.00 (0.85)	3.20 (1.51)	2.68 (1.60)	2.13 (1.92)
Chemonucleolysis	3.65 (1.59)	3.26 (1.52)	2.72 (1.02)	2.27 (1.75)
Back pain				
Manipulation	3.79 (1.62)	3.16 (1.34)	2.68 (1.60)	2.27 (1.53)
Chemonucleolysis	4.05 (1.28)	4.00 (1.15)	3.58 (0.97)	2.87 (1.36)
RDQ				
Manipulation	11.90 (5.48)	10.15 (4.53)	7.79 (6.65)	5.87 (5.96)
Chemonucleolysis	11.95 (5.83)	13.90 (5.99)	11.00 (5.69)	7.27 (6.65)

(n = manipulation/chemonucleolysis; RDQ = Roland Disability Questionnaire)

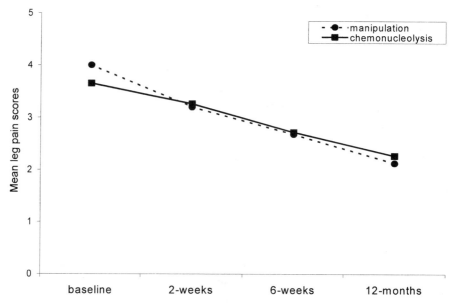

FIG. 17.1. Graph of the mean leg pain scores from baseline though 12 months by treatment group. Over time, the improvement was statistically significant from baseline to 2 weeks for the manipulated patients, and from baseline to 6 weeks for the injected patients. Between groups, the differences were not statistically significantly different at any assessment point.

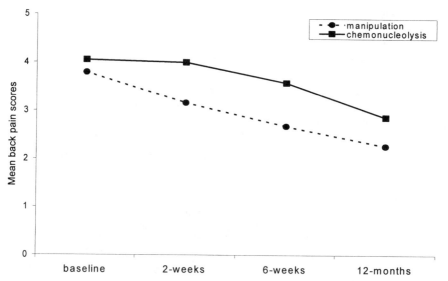

FIG. 17.2. Graph of the mean back pain scores from baseline though 12 months by treatment group. Over time, the improvement was statistically significant from baseline to 6 weeks for the manipulated patients, and from baseline to 12 months for the injected patients. Between groups, the difference was statistically significant both at 2 weeks and 6 weeks.

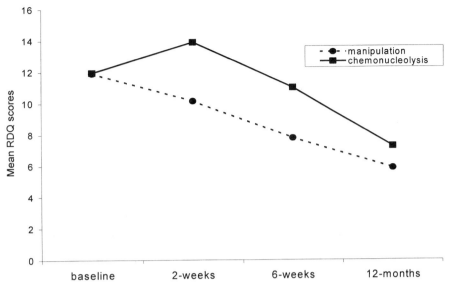

FIG. 17.3. Graph of the mean Roland Disability Questionnaire (RDQ) scores from baseline though 12 months by treatment group. Over time, the improvement was statistically significant from baseline to 2 weeks and from 2 weeks to 6 weeks for the manipulated patients, and from 2 weeks to 6 weeks and from 6 weeks to 12 months for the injected patients. Between groups, the difference was statistically significant only at 2 weeks.

score (compared with baseline) during the first 6 weeks. There was a statistically significant benefit from manipulation for mean disability score at 2 weeks compared with chemonucleolysis. At this point, the manipulation group had significantly improved on this measure, but the chemonucleolysis group had deteriorated somewhat. By 6 weeks, there was no significant difference between the groups for mean disability scores; the manipulated patients, however, had significantly improved over baseline, but the chemonucleolysis group had not (Fig. 17.3).

Covariates (age, sex, initial degree of straight leg raising, and lumbar mobility) had minimal and nonsignificant influences on marginal means for the outcome measures. Of the other baseline variables, higher baseline depression scores predicted a poorer prognosis in terms of pain but not disability, and a longer history of symptoms predicted an inferior prognosis only in respect of back pain.

Possible confounding influences were explored. There was no statistically significant difference in baseline scores for any of the outcome measures (leg pain, back pain, and disability) between the patients undergoing manipulation and those receiving chemonucleolysis, despite the average 9-week further delay between randomization and commencement of treatment for the latter group. A subgroup analysis was performed to determine whether the breakdown in the randomization procedure had any influence on the results. Comparing the properly randomized patients with the remainder revealed that the patterns of responses across all three follow-up points for all three outcome variables were statistically indistinguishable.

A formal cost analysis was not included in the study design but, in view of the interest in this measure, the crude treatment costs were estimated for patients who provided 12 months of data. The average number of treatment sessions given to the manipulated group was 11 (range 6 to 18). None of the injected patients remained in hospital beyond 24 hours. The manipulator's fee was $28 per session, while the cost of the chemonucle-olysis (inclusive of all drug and hospital costs) was $1,120. A total of 165 manipulative sessions were given, at a total cost of $4,620. This can be compared with the overall cost for the 15 injections, at $16,800. The costs incurred for treating therapeutic failures must be added to these figures. Our best estimates for these, in this cohort, suggest that the extra principal costs incurred over 1 year for treatment by chemonucleolysis rather than manipulation would be of the order of $420 per patient.

DISCUSSION

This study was a randomized controlled trial comparing osteopathic manipulative treat-ment with chemonucleolysis for symptomatic lumbar disc herniation confirmed by clinical criteria and imaging. Taking chemonucleolysis as an effective treatment (9), the trial sought to determine whether manipulation is a comparably safe and effective treatment option. As far as we are aware, it is the first report of a prospective randomized trial comparing manip-ulation with a proven effective treatment for this diagnosis. It may be argued that partial dis-cectomy would have presented a more suitable control treatment, but the intention was to test the value of manipulation as an option in patients for whom there was no clear-cut clin-ical indication for surgical intervention (bearing in mind the favorable long-term prognosis [16]). In addition, it would have been exceedingly difficult to obtain patient consent to ran-domization if the options were surgery or a nonsurgical procedure.

The trial protocol was designed, as far as reasonably possible, to avoid sources of bias. While it was impossible to blind either the patients or the clinicians to the randomized treatment, the measures of outcome were assessed independently. Precautions were taken to ensure that the trial participants represented a homogeneous diagnostic category. There were no identifiable baseline differences between the two treatment groups, and the fol-low-up period was of sufficient length to reveal failures in both treatment arms.

Nevertheless, there are certain limitations that should be discussed. The most obvious problem is that some of the patients were not randomized according to the predetermined order, which was an unfortunate consequence of administrative difficulties. However, there were no discernible baseline or follow-up differences between the correctly and incorrectly randomized groups; we found no reason to believe the breakdown in the ran-domization procedure exerted any systematic bias on the results. Due to local factors gov-erning the provision of hospital services that were beyond the control of the investigators, the patients receiving chemonucleolysis experienced an extra 9 weeks delay on average between diagnosis and commencement of treatment compared with the patients under-going manipulation. In view of the similar baseline scores for both groups, the differen-tial delay is unlikely to have exerted any bias on the results.

The primary result was that osteopathic manipulation was no less effective than chemonucleolysis in reducing self-reported pain and disability when assessed at 12 months, and the number of therapeutic failures was not significantly different. In addi-tion, the improvement for the patients undergoing manipulation occurred sooner and did not show the tendency for increased disability at 2 weeks seen in the injected patients, and there was some indication that there will be a moderate cost benefit. Manipulation can thus be considered an effective option for treatment of symptomatic lumbar disc her-niation. This patient population was relatively chronic and, since the length of history had some predictive value, it would be logical in future trials to explore the possibility that earlier manipulative intervention could have an enhanced effect.

The mechanism through which manipulation may exert an effect is unknown. Manipulative treatment is generally directed toward improving spinal mobility (5), but increases in mobility are found in only about half of back pain patients following lumbar manipulation (4), and were not statistically significant covariates here. Any effect is unlikely to be due to a reduction in the size of the herniation, because the CT appearance of the disc is unchanged by manipulation in most cases (5). The mechanism of symptomatic improvement with chemonucleolysis is also unclear. There is certainly a permanent reduction in disc height in most cases (10), but this does not necessarily result in a reduction of the herniation (8); any change in the size of herniation seems to depend largely on the natural history of the condition (6). Lumbar disc herniation (in the absence of clear indications for surgery) has a favorable long-term prognosis under conservative therapy (16). Therefore, it may be that treatments such as chemonucleolysis and manipulation are effective through some as yet unknown influence on pain mechanisms rather than by any physical effect on the herniation.

CONCLUSIONS

This randomized controlled trial of manipulation and chemonucleolysis for unremitting lumbar radicular syndrome has shown no statistically significant difference in outcomes between the two treatments at 12-months' follow-up, although there was a small statistically significant short-term benefit from manipulation for back pain and disability (though not for leg pain). The therapeutic failure rates did not differ between the treatment groups. There was an overall crude cost saving from manipulation, and no evidence was found to question its safety. We conclude, therefore, that osteopathic manipulation can be considered a safe and effective treatment option for patients with a lumbar radicular syndrome due to disc herniation, at least in the absence of clear clinical indications for surgical intervention.

ACKNOWLEDGMENTS

Sincere thanks are due to Alison Sharp, MCSP, for undertaking the patient assessments during the trial. The contribution of Rebecca Burt, Bsc, for administrative management and data entry is gratefully acknowledged. The study was funded by the NHS Executive, Northern and Yorkshire, UK (Project No. ND0020 T367).

This chapter is reprinted with permission from Burton AK, Tillotson KM, Cleary J. Single-blind randomised controlled trial of chemonucleolysis and manipulation in the treatment of symptomatic lumbar disc herniation. *Eur Spine J* 2000;9:202–207.

REFERENCES

1. Andersson GBJ, Brown MD, Dvorak J, et al. Consensus summary on the diagnosis and treatment of lumbar disc herniation. *Spine* 1996;21:755–785.
2. Assendelft WJJ, Bouter LM, Knipschild PG. Complications of spinal manipulation: a comprehensive review of the literature. *J Fam Pract* 1996;42:475–480.
3. Benoist M, Bonneville J-F, Lassale B, et al. A randomized, double-blind study to compare low-dose with standard-dose chymopapain in the treatment of herniated lumbar intervertebral discs. *Spine* 1993;18:28–34.
4. Burton AK, Tillotson KM, Edwards VA, et al. Lumbar sagittal mobility and low back symptoms in patients treated with manipulation. *J Spinal Disord* 1990;3:262–268.
5. Cassidy JD, Thiel HW, Kirkaldy-Willis WH. Side-posture manipulation for lumbar intervertebral disk herniation. *J Manipulative Physiol Ther* 1993;16:96–103.
6. Castro WHM, Halm H, Jerosch J, et al. Long-term changes in the magnetic resonance image after chemonucleolysis. *Eur Spine J* 1994;3:222–224.

7. Clinical Standards Advisory Group. *Epidemiology review: the epidemiology and cost of back pain*. London: HMSO, 1994.

8. Fraser RD, Sandhu A, Gogan WJ. Magnetic resonance imaging findings 10 years after treatment for lumbar disc herniation. *Spine* 1995;20:710–714.

9. Gibson JNA, Grant IC, Waddell G. The Cochrane review of surgery for lumbar disc prolapse (Cochrane review) and degenerative lumbar spondylosis. *Spine* 1999;24:1820–1832, and the Cochrane Library, Issue 1. Update Software, Oxford (www.update-software.com/ccweb/cochrane/cdsr.htm)

10. Leivseth G, Salvesen R, Hemminghytt S, et al. Do human lumbar discs reconstitute after chemonucleolysis? A 7-year follow-up study. *Spine* 1999;24:342–348.

11. Main CJ, Wood PL, Hollis S, et al. The distress and risk assessment method: a simple patient classification to identify distress and evaluate the risk of poor outcome. *Spine* 1992;17:42–52.

12. McClune T, Clarke R, Walker C, et al. Osteopathic management of mechanical low back pain. In: Giles LGF, Singer KP, eds. *Clinical anatomy and management of low back pain*. Vol 1. Oxford: Butterworth Heinemann, 1997:358–368.

13. Nordby EJ, Fraser RD, Javid MJ. Chemonucleolysis. *Spine* 1996;21:1102–1105.

14. Roland M, Morris R. A study of the natural history of back pain. I. Development of a reliable and sensitive measure of disability in low-back pain. *Spine* 1983;8:141–144.

15. Royal College of General Practitioners. *Clinical guidelines for the management of acute low back pain*. London: Royal College of General Practitioners, 1996.

16. Weber H. Lumbar disc herniation. A controlled prospective study with ten years of observation. *Spine* 1983;8:131–140.

17. Weber H. The natural history of disc herniation and the influence of intervention. *Spine* 1994;19:2234–2238.

18

Chemonucleolysis

Robert Deutman

Chymopapain, by direct injection into the intervertebral disc, causes dissolution of the nucleus pulposus without effect on the surrounding tissues. The first two patients treated in this manner were given these injections secretly by Lyman Smith in 1963 in Vienna. He reported promising results of the first ten patients treated with chymopapain in the United States in 1964 (29). However, in the years since, the enzymatic treatment of patients with a herniated disc has been the subject of a fierce debate between supporters and opponents of this method. This discussion was largely based on emotions in the past ("We are carpenters, what the hell is a mucopolysaccharide?") (30), and still can be today ("...not even on their worst enemy ...") (25) and does not always take into account the clinical and scientific facts. Readers with an interest in history are referred to an eye-opening review by Ford written in 1977 (9).

Approximately 100,000 patients were treated by chemonucleolysis in the United States after the Food and Drug Administration (FDA) released chymopapain for clinical use in November 1982. In the years following, the favorable effects of this treatment were over-shadowed by complications reported to the FDA. As a result the use of chymopapain decreased significantly, although while analyzing these complications it became evident that the complications had nothing to do with the enzyme itself, but with an inadequate injection technique (24).

In our hospital, the number of patients undergoing chemonucleolysis has been kept at the same annual level since the first patients were treated in April 1980. Studies published in the literature as well as data on more than 2,000 patients treated in our clinic will form the basis for this chapter.

EFFECT OF CHYMOPAPAIN

Chymopapain hydrolyzes the cementing protein of the nucleus pulposus (32), reducing its water-binding capacities, resulting in disc narrowing and, temporarily, affecting its mechanical behavior. Chymopapain is neutralized immediately after injection by binding to the acid proteoglycans, although some residual chymopapain activity has been demonstrated in dogs at 2 weeks. The effect on the nucleus pulposus is dose-related. There is an increase of serum levels of keratan sulfate during the first 5 days after injection (20). It has been shown that a lower dose (2,000 units of enzyme) is as effective as a higher dose (4,000 units of enzyme), which was advised by the manufacturer originally.

In a prospective computed tomography (CT) study we have shown that the compression of the herniated disc was reduced in two-thirds of the patients after 3 months, and in nearly all patients after 12 months. Chymopapain did not cause epidural fibrosis (Fig. 18.1). The reduction in disc height was on average one-fourth of the original disc height (15). On mag-

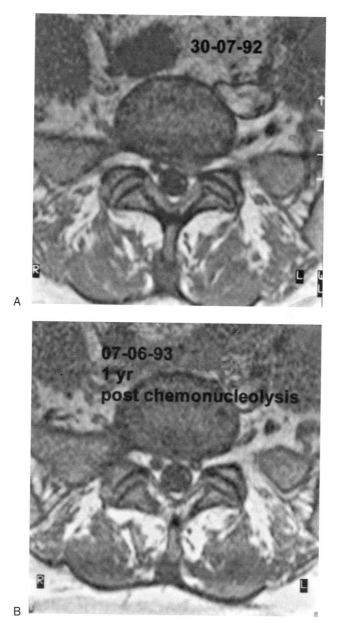

FIG. 18.1. Magnetic resonance image of a 43-year-old woman with a left-sided herniation at the L5-L1 level. Before treatment (**A**) and 10 months after treatment (**B**). No herniation is visible after treatment and no epidural fibrosis is observed.

netic resonance imaging (MRI) scans a complete loss of the signal of the nucleus, due to loss of its water content can be seen after 6 weeks and corresponds to a maximum reduction in disc height (34). In young animals, an injected, healthy disc may regenerate (4). In clinical practice this reexpansion of the disc to some degree is an inconsistent phenomenon. Apart from the influence on nuclear size it has been shown that chymopapain exhibits anti-inflammatory properties, inhibiting phospholipase A_2 activity (27).

Chymopapain in itself is not neurotoxic, but if chymopapain is injected into the sub-arachnoid space it causes a rapid rise in cerebrospinal fluid (CSF) pressure. This probably occurs because of capillary bleeding and in time the microcirculation of nerve tissue may be interrupted.

EFFICACY

A high level of scientific evidence regarding the efficacy of chymopapain is available.

In an impeccable double-blind, randomized prospective study, Javid and associates show the superiority of chymopapain in comparison with placebo (13). A similar study demonstrates that the therapeutic effect was sustained up to the 10-year follow-up evaluation (10). Based on these studies and many clinical studies thereafter, a multidisciplinary consensus meeting in the Netherlands in 1995 reached the following conclusion: "Chemonucleolysis is a proven effective treatment for a herniated disc, with after one-year results equal to those of operative treatment" (31).

INDICATIONS

Chymopapain, if used properly, is indicated in the treatment of incapacitating radicular pain, caused by a herniated disc. There is no sound evidence that the prognosis of a paresis is improved by surgery or chemonucleolysis. The ideal patient for chymopapain chemonucleolysis is also the ideal candidate for surgical discectomy. The radicular pain typically dominates back pain and during physical examination there will be root tension signs and/or neurologic signs like a decreased knee or ankle reflex and/or weakness of muscles corresponding to the nerve roots involved. The only absolute contraindication is the rare cauda equina syndrome with sphincter disturbances.

There is also a place for treatment with chymopapain in selected patients with isthmic spondylolisthesis and unilateral radiculopathy.

Repeat chemonucleolysis is an option in patients with recurrent radiculopathy provided that they initially had a good response to the first injection.

At present there is sufficient clinical evidence to recommend the use of chymopapain for patients suffering from a herniated cervical disc.

PREOPERATIVE TESTS AND TECHNIQUE

It is mandatory to order plain radiographs and blood tests to exclude other causes of pain like tumors and infections. Thereafter a CT scan—or preferably MRI—must confirm the clinical diagnosis of the herniated disc. One has to realize that the main indication for performing a scan is to exclude a (neurogenic) tumor and to locate the exact level of the herniation. If imaging does not confirm a herniated disc, Lyme disease should especially be excluded. In our region of the world this is presently a common reason for radiculopathy.

We have always performed the procedure in the x-ray department under general anesthesia. We never performed skin testing. Prescreening or skin testing for immunoglobulin E (IgE)-specific antibodies has never been proven to be a reliable indicator for a possible anaphylactic reaction. Promethazine (an H_2-receptor blocker) is given as premedication. During the procedure the patient has an intravenous infusion with corticosteroids. The patient is positioned in a secured left lateral decubitus position using an inflatable cushion in the flank to straighten the spine. Via a lateral approach, starting at

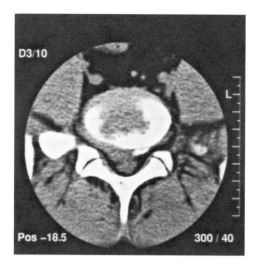

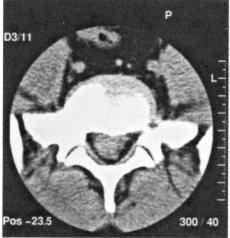

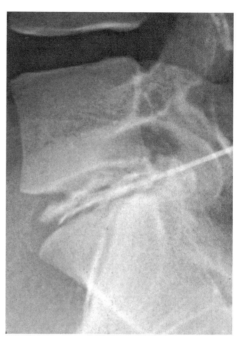

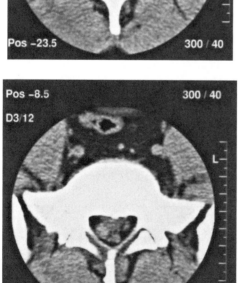

FIG. 18.2. A: Computed tomogram of a 31-year-old man with a severe radicular syndrome. The straight leg raising test on the right side was restricted to 40 degrees with an absent Achilles tendon reflex. **B:** Discogram confirms the continuity between the nucleus and the big herniation. The patient had excellent results after chemonucleolysis. His irradiating pain disappeared 2 weeks after treatment.

least 8 cm from the midline, the intervertebral disc is reached with an 18-gauge needle. With this approach the dura is protected by the intervertebral joints. Flexion of the hips facilitates the approach to the L5-L1 disc. A discogram of the symptomatic level is performed and recorded on a video (Fig. 18.2). Epidural leakage is no contraindication for the administration of chymopapain, but one has to realize that intrathecal injection is highly toxic and dangerous. When the correct needle position is assessed, 2,000 U of chymopapain (Chymodiactin) is slowly injected during a 3-minute period. Although opinions in the literature differ about the preferred form of anesthesia, we feel very comfortable with this controlled setting with the patient optimally conditioned. Many surgeons prefer local anesthesia with supplemental intravenous sedation. In the event of a systemic allergic reaction the treatment of choice is the immediate infusion of epinephrine (starting dose, 0.2 to 0.3 mL of 1:10,000 dilution).

POSTOPERATIVE CARE

Patients are mobilized as soon as they feel up to it. Most patients notice the difference in the level of pain compared to their preoperative situation immediately. Sciatic pain is absent or has significantly decreased, although in some cases the sciatica can reappear for a couple of days. Much has been written about paravertebral back spasm after chemonucleolysis, but today this is not seen as a clinical problem anymore. This is probably due to the lower dose of enzyme injected today in comparison to the early days. Patients are discharged from the hospital as soon as they feel comfortable enough to go home. This is often within 24 hours. Pain medication (ibuprofen 200 mg, 3 dd) is prescribed routinely for 10 days, but its use depends on the amount and length of postoperative pain. Although patients are permitted to resume all normal activities and nothing is forbidden, they have to realize that the healing process takes 6 to 12 weeks. Sitting up is often not well tolerated in the beginning, while riding a stationary bicycle is very well tolerated. As a consequence this activity should be started as soon as it can be tolerated. It is one of the simplest ways to increase the physical endurance in the healing process. A physiotherapy program is prescribed routinely; in this program stretching exercises are not recommended for the first 4 to 6 weeks. Returning to work is advised after 6 to 12 weeks depending upon the type of occupation. However, many (self-employed) patients resume their work activities within 6 weeks.

COMPLICATIONS

Complications in chemonucleolysis are short-term and limited to the surgical and immediate postoperative period. Based on a survey in the United States of approximately 135,000 patients treated between 1982 and 1991, serious complications (fatal anaphylaxis, infections, hemorrhage, neurologic and miscellaneous events) occurred in 0.0815%, with a mortality rate of 0.019%. Apart from the anaphylactic reactions the causes of the other complications are unlikely to have been due to the enzyme itself, but are the consequence of poor needle placement (24). Based on the literature of the past 30 years one can conclude that injection of chymopapain is 3 to 20 times safer than surgery (5).

The complications of our first 2,000 patients have been followed prospectively and are categorized in eight significant and 21 less significant complications (Tables 18.1 and 18.2). There was no mortality. One female patient developed a severe type III ana-

TABLE 18.1. *Significant complications of chemonucleolysis*

Mortality	0
Anaphylactic reaction	1[a]
Gastric bleeding (NSAID)	1
Neurologic deficit (S1 root)	1
Hysteric paraplegia	1
Discitis	3
Lung embolism	1
Total:	8

NSAID, nonsteroidal antiinflammatory drug
[a]Of more than 3,000 patients treated in our hospital since 1980 on both neurosurgical and orthopedic wards, there was only one other case with a type III anaphylaxis, also in a woman. She was treated promptly and appropriately without sequelae. This makes the overall rate of severe anaphylaxis in our region 1:1,500. There was no mortality and there were no other significant neurologic events in those other 1,000 patients.

phylactic reaction. She recovered fully after adequate treatment. She experienced a good clinical outcome of her treatment. One male patient, who was treated for an L4-L5 disc herniation, developed a paralysis of the triceps surae. He was treated conservatively and although after 5 years his walking distance was unlimited he still could not tiptoe on his affected leg. Three patients received antibiotic treatment because they developed symptoms and signs of a spondylodiscitis, although in one patient the diagnosis was equivocal.

Less significant complications included seven cases of type I or II sensitivity reactions, all of whom quickly responded to the treatment of histamine blockers; and one case of a allergic dermatitis. This female patient had to be readmitted after 1 week; she recovered within 2 weeks. In one male patient we had suspicions of a spear injury of the spinal root. After 6 weeks he presented with the clinical syndrome of a causalgia, but within another 4 weeks he was cured by a witch doctor. A temporary decrease of motor functions of the (big) toe or foot extensors was noted in some patients postoperatively, but in other patients with an existing weakness the function improved immediately postinjection. Recently, we saw one female patient who did spectacularly well after chemonucleolysis in the past. She returned after many years with a new herniation at another level. This time she developed contralateral sciatic pain immediately after chemonucleolysis, which did not respond over time. A new MRI showed a contralateral herniation at the recently treated level. This patient subsequently underwent open surgery with a favorable outcome.

TABLE 18.2. *Less significant complications of chemonucleolysis*

Bladder retention	2
Allergic dermatitis	1
Sensitivity reaction, type I	5
Sensitivity reaction, type II	2
Causalgia	1
Transient (increased) paresis	9
Contralateral herniation	1
Total:	21

RESULTS

A compilation of long-term results of chemonucleolysis in 3,130 patients shows satisfactory results in 77% of patients (23). In two studies performed in the Netherlands and presented in a thesis, it appeared that at 1 year the leg pain had disappeared in 74% and 79% of all patients. There was still some slight irradiating pain in 11% and about 15% of patients complained of back pain (8,17). In a third thesis, the results of our first 200 patients were analyzed after a mean period of 7 years. No patient was lost to follow-up. Of these 200 patients, 152 (76%) were in a satisfactory condition (14).

In 1987 a questionnaire was sent to the first 500 patients who we had treated. The follow-up period was 0.5 to 5 years. An excellent or good result was reported in 77%, a fair result in 14%, and a poor result in 9% of all cases. A secondary intervention (open surgery or repeat chemonucleolysis) was performed in 19 patients (4%). Although most of these 19 patients were (again) satisfied after this secondary intervention, they were scored as having a poor result. Nearly 80% had returned to work and 20% were receiving worker's compensation. Six percent used pain medication on a regular basis and 15% were at the time of this follow-up study in a (para)medical program because of their back problems.

From 1980 onward other clinical studies were performed on our material, all by observers not involved with the treatment (Table 18.3). Results of treatment of patients under the age of 20 are rewarding. None of these adolescents treated required open surgery afterward; however, five patients had repeat injections with chymopapain. Two patients had a second treatment at the same level after an asymptomatic period of 7 and 10 years, respectively. Two other patients had a second treatment at another level after 2 and 8 years. One patient had a total of three chemonucleolysis procedures in a 12-year period (first at the L4-L5 level, 6 years later at the L5-L1 level, and 12 years later at the L4-L5 level again because of a recurrence). As a consequence, we believe that there is no longer any place for open surgery in this age group (7). At the other end of the spectrum highly satisfactory results were obtained in older adults over 60 and even over 75 year of age. Other authors had similar findings (3). This is important to know because many authors state the belief on theoretical grounds that there is no place for chymopapain in older adults. Chymopapain is also effective in the treatment of the herniated L3-L4 disc (12).

McCulloch (19) proposes an anatomic staging concept wherein each anatomic segment can be viewed as a three-story house. In this concept a contained disc protrusion is

TABLE 18.3. *Results in different subgroups*

	Year of study	N	Follow-up period	Good/excellent	Secondary intervention
First 200 patients	1990	200	7 years	152 (76%)	26 (13%)
First 500 patients	1987	500	0.5–5 years	384 (77%)	19 (4%)
Adolescents	1993	55	7 (0.5–12.5) years	42	5
Patients over 60 yrs of age	1988	21	44 (9–76) months	18 (85%)	1 (5%)
Patients over 75 yrs of age	1998	10	36 (5–115) months	8	0
Herniation of the L3-L4 level	1991	16	39 (6–80) months	15	0
Lateral herniation	1999	38	1–4 years	32	2
Physicians	1995	20	92 (16–152) months	17	2
Contained discs	1985	31	7.5 months	24	1
" "	1992	31	84 months	27	1
Extruded discs	1985	12	7.5 months	9	1
" "	1992	12	84 months	9	1
Spondylolisthesis	1995	63	54 months	41	13

located at the level of the disc space, the first story. Disc extrusions and sequestrations mostly are located above (story two) or below (story three) the level of the disc. The common thought was that there is no place for chemonucleolysis for herniations that have migrated to story two or three (Fig. 18.3). However, in a CT study performed by a neuroradiologist from our hospital and other doctors not involved in the treatment, it was shown that at 7 and 84 months there was no difference in result between chemonucleolysis of contained discs (story one) and herniations migrated to story two or three! This was corroborated later by the results obtained in the lateral herniation (mostly located in story two) (Fig. 18.4). To understand these findings it is important to realize that in most extruded discs there is still continuity between the center of the disc and the herniated part and that apparently a remaining sequestrated fragment—undigested by the enzyme—as a cause of persistent leg pain is rare. Likewise, French investigators have not found a significant correlation between results and the size of the herniation or the morphology of the spinal canal (1).

In 1995, a very interesting study was performed on our request by C. Bouwsma, an unbiased consultant neurologist from our hospital on 20 patients (who all happened to be

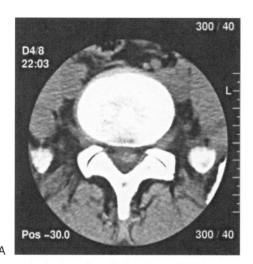

FIG. 18.3. A: A 29-year-old man presented with unremitting left-sided sciatica 1-week before his marriage. The straight leg raising test was restricted to 20 degrees bilaterally. The computed tomogram showed a herniated L5-L1 disc with indication of sequestration. **B:** After the first day of treatment, the irradiating pain in his leg had disappeared, and 1 week after the chemonucleolysis the man danced at his wedding. **C:** The result of treatment remained excellent at 2-year follow-up, by which time he was the proud father of a daughter.

A

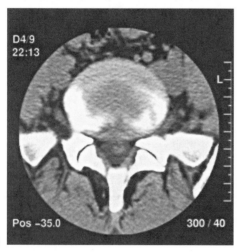

B

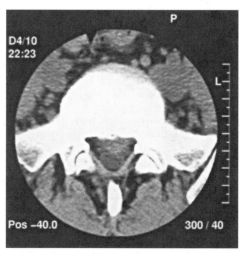

C

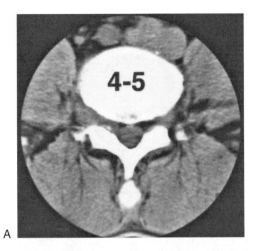

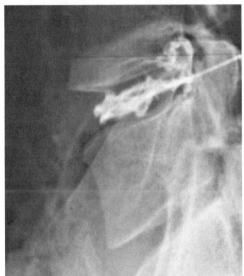

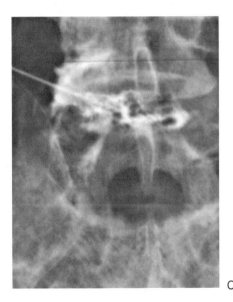

FIG. 18.4. A: Computed tomogram of a 51-year-old man with right-sided L4 radiculopathy caused by a foraminal herniation. This herniation is corroborated on the discogram. **B:** Lateral view. **C:** Anteroposterior view. The patient had an excellent outcome; he had no pain 1-year after treatment and was working without restrictions as a bartender.

physicians). Dr. Bouwsma independently interviewed and examined all 20 patients from our series who had undergone chemonucleolysis. The mean follow-up period was 7.5 years. Dr. Bouwsma concluded (to his—but not our—surprise) that even after such a long follow-up period the results remained good in 85% of the patients. One patient was a physician from internal medicine who had a repeat chemonucleolysis after 4 years because of a recurrent herniation. He has been asymptomatic since. A general practitioner who had undergone surgery at the same level 10 years prior to chemonucleolysis, had a second open surgery after another 10 years.

To analyze the time it takes for irradiating pain to disappear, which is the main reason to perform the procedure, a study was performed in 2000 by a junior doctor. He reviewed the posttreatment course of 100 randomly selected patients. Seventy-nine patients had no—or virtually no—leg pain at the first follow-up visit after 6 weeks (Table 18-4). If the pain persisted or rebounded during the first couple of weeks, the patients mostly noted a very sudden change with a rapidly disappearing sciatica in 1 day. Seventeen of the

TABLE 18.4. *Disappearance of the sciatic pain after chemonucleolysis (N = 100)*

On discharge	14
At 1 week	11
At 2 weeks	7
At 3 weeks	12
At 4 weeks	3
At 5 weeks	2
At 6 weeks	30
At 12 weeks	11
Total:	90
Still radiculopathy at 12 weeks	6
Lost at 12 weeks	4
Total:	10

(On discharge through At 3 weeks bracketed as 79)

remaining 21 patients were seen at 3 months. Eleven patients no longer had any irradiating pain and six patients still complained of radiculopathy. One female patient had a surgical decompression elsewhere later on as second procedure of no avail. Four patients were discharged at 6 weeks and they were not seen at 12 weeks.

FAILURE OF TREATMENT

Failures do occur. According to a survey of the literature, on average, 1 in 10 patients require open surgery in the same year as chemonucleolysis. It is interesting to note by analyzing these failures that a sequestrated fragment as a cause of persisting root compression is a rare event, and that in nearly half of the failures no explanation of the failure can be given. A consistent finding, however (when active enzyme is used), is an empty disc. In all cases of persistent symptoms that we have explored surgically, the disc or a loose fragment never was found to be the cause of persistent pain; in those cases, a relative lateral recess stenosis could have been the reason of persistent symptoms. Our statistics indicated in 1993 that a second procedure in the same year, for whatever reason, was performed in 3% of 550 patients treated in a 5-year period. According to many studies and our own experience, the final result of surgery is not influenced in a negative way by prior chymopapain treatment.

There is a place for chemonucleolysis in the treatment of patients with a lytic spondylolisthesis and unilateral irradiating pain. Satisfying results have been reported by Nordby (22) in 11 of 13 patients who were treated for this condition. Although a herniated disc at the level of a pars defect is considered rare, it does occur. In such a case one has to distinguish patients with or without tension signs. During the years, supported by results in patients with tension signs, we have treated some patients with an unstable segment. It became apparent that without the existence of tension signs the results were mostly poor. In these patients a fusion was needed to obtain a satisfactory result. Nevertheless, from a group of 15 patients good or excellent results were seen in 11 patients after a mean follow-up period of 19 months (26).

In another study covering a larger group with a mean follow-up period of 4.5 years, 41 of all 63 patients treated with the enzyme had a good or excellent outcome according to the Prolo scale. The first patient of this group was treated in 1982 and we became fascinated because of the pathology and the final result. At 16 years of age this boy had severe sciatica for more than 6 months. During examination he had a list and the straight leg raising (SLR) test was restricted on the right side to 40 degrees. He had a spondylolisthesis of nearly 50% and a myelography showed a herniated disc at the level of the slip.

The patient underwent chemonucleolysis and has been asymptomatic ever since, thus having been the subject of many follow-up studies. In 2000, he had no complaints; he has lived a normal life without any restrictions. Radiographically, the spondylolisthesis was unchanged with a slightly narrowed disc.

A spontaneously fused segment as described by Nordby (22) in one of his patients was seen in one of our female patients treated for a disc herniation at the level of a pars defect.

RECURRENCES

Recurrences of a herniated disc in a treated patient do occur. This is true for herniations treated conservatively, after surgery, and after chemonucleolysis. For a long period of time repeat chemonucleolysis was considered contraindicated because of the fear of an increased risk of sensitivity. Sutton, however, strongly recommends chemonucleolysis as the last stage of conservative treatment in case of a recurrence (33). Based on a worldwide survey on repeat chemonucleolysis, a task force of the International Intradiscal Therapy Society concluded in 1997 that a repeat injection of chymopapain under controlled circumstances (intravenous line, standby of an anesthesiologist) is safe. Pretreatment with H_1 and H_2 receptor blockers is recommended. Thus far we have pretreated such patients for 3 days orally, but based on experiments in animals probably the best way to block the release of histamine is to give those blockers intravenously 30 minutes before the (second) injection.

From 1980 until 1996, 66 patients from our series received a second injection at the level previously treated after an interval of 57 (range, 2 to 127) months. There were no life-threatening complications. After a follow-up period of 57 (range, 2 to 143) months two patients were lost to follow-up, four patients had open surgery and three patients received a third injection with chymopapain with a good outcome. Of the remaining 57 patients, 51 had a good or excellent outcome (36).

The longer the follow-up period, the more recurrences are noted; this applies to all treatments. In a prospective study of microsurgery, complaints of recurrent ipsilateral radicular pain occurred in 8.5% of patients within 3 years leading to a second surgery in 7.4% (6) (18% after 5 to 10 years) (18).

With a follow-up of 1 to 19 years, the number of known secondary procedures at the same level primarily treated in our series increased to approximately 10%. (Of these 170 patients, 85 had a repeat chemonucleolysis, 69 a decompressive surgery, and 16 a fusion.) Quite a few of these secondary procedures occurred after the first 10 years. Thirty-six patients had treatment at another level. Of the first 200 patients treated, the number of secondary procedures had increased to 20% (35 patients same level, five patients another level). This equals the number of second surgeries at 10 years as seen in a prospective study of 100 discectomies (18).

CHEMONUCLEOLYSIS VERSUS OPEN SURGERY

Open surgery is considered the gold standard in the treatment of patients with symptoms due to a herniated disc. In two prospective, randomized controlled studies the outcome after 1 year showed no significant difference. In both studies the outcomes at 6 weeks and 3 months were better for the surgery group, and in both groups more patients required additional surgery after chemonucleolysis. However, in analyzing these studies more carefully it became apparent that failure after chemonucleolysis was followed by surgery much more often than failure after surgery in one study (35), and in the other study (21) no mechanical abnormality could be found during exploration in the majority of patients. In both studies the rate of additional surgery in the patients treated with chemonucleolysis was six to eight times higher than the 3% in our series. In other studies the rate of improvement after chemonucleolysis and open discectomy was similar after the first 6 weeks, and in a review of the literature on patients treated by surgery or chemonucleolysis a similar success rate of 77% was found. In 1992, French researchers calculated that compared to surgery, chemonucleolysis gives 52 extra days of good health per patient over a 7-year period and is less costly (16). That chemonucleolysis is less costly than open surgery was also demonstrated by British investigators (37). There is no evidence today that the results of open surgery have improved with more minimal invasive surgical techniques. In many studies it has been shown that in time results after chemonucleolysis remain stable, whereas results have the tendency to deteriorate in time after open surgery (23).

Apart from these considerations, one has to realize that in all of these studies the majority of patients treated with chemonucleolysis have avoided open surgery and its inherent complications.

CERVICAL CHEMONUCLEOLYSIS

We have no personal experience with cervical chemonucleolysis. Several centers however have reported on the efficacy of this procedure and its safety. Gomez-Catsresana obtained 34 good/excellent results in group of 40 patients after a follow-up of 21 (range, 3 to 43) months. There were no complications. Three patients required fusion. Postinjection MRI performed in 18 patients confirmed the complete disappearance of the herniation in 13 cases (11). Recently the remarkable efficacy of cervical chemonucleolysis was confirmed by Benoist and coworkers (2). With a follow-up of 4 years these researchers obtained excellent or good results in 116 (90.5%) in a group of 141 patients. There were no complications. Four patients underwent immediate surgery. Disappearance of the radicular pain was obtained in the first 2 weeks in 80% of the successful results. Ninety percent of the patients were back to work within 38 (range, 8 to 90) days.

NEWER ENZYMES

Of all the enzymes used in the past, only chymopapain has withstood the test of time. Newer enzymes have thus far been used in animal experiments. Chondroitin sulfate ABC has been studied most thoroughly. This enzyme is a disaccharide. It effectively depletes the proteoglycans of the nucleus pulposus in animals, and it decreases disc height in the period after injection. It does not cause capillary bleeding and as such it is potentially safer than chymopapain. Clinical studies recently have been started in Goteborg, Sweden. Thus far no clinical results are available.

CONCLUSION

Chemonucleolysis is an effective treatment for patients with symptoms due to a herniated disc. Even today this treatment remains the ultimate in miniaturized surgery (28). It is an attractive alternative for open surgery because there is no occurrence of epidural fibrosis and there is a lower rate of complications. It deserves to keep its place in today and, therefore, requires renewed support from the medical establishment and pharmaceutical industry.

REFERENCES

1. Benoist M, et al. Chemonucleolysis: Correlation of results with the size of the herniation and the dimensions of the spinal canal. A prospective study. Paper presented at: Eleventh Annual Meeting of the International Intradiscal Therapy Society; May 1998; San Antonio, Texas.
2. Benoist M, et al: Chemonucleolysis for herniated cervical disc. Paper presented at: Thirteenth Annual Meeting of the International Intradiscal Therapy Society; June 8–10, 2000; Williamsburg, Virginia.
3. Benoist M, et al. Lumbar disc herniation in the elderly: long term results of chymopapain chemonucleolysis. *Eur Spine J* 1993;2(3):149–152.
4. Bradford DS, Cooper KM, Oegema TR Jr. Chymopapain, chemonucleolysis, and nucleus pulposus regeneration. *J Bone Joint Surg (Am)* 1983;65(9):1220–1231.
5. Brown MD. Update on chemonucleolysis. *Spine* 1996;21:62–68.
6. Cinotti G, Roysam GS, Eisenstein SM, et al. Ipsilateral recurrent lumbar disc herniation. A prospective controlled study. *J Bone Joint Surg* 1998;80B(5):825–832.
7. Deutman R. Chemonucleolysis in the treatment of adolescent lumbar disc herniations. In: Wittenberg RH, ed. *Chemonucleolysis and related intradiscal therapies.* New York: Thieme, 1994.
8. Dekker M. *Chemonucleolysis* [thesis]. Groningen, the Netherlands: University of Groningen; 1987.
9. Ford LT. [Letter to the Editor]. *Clin Orthop* 1977;122:367–373.
10. Gogan WJ, Fraser RD. Chymopapain: a 10-year, double blind study. *Spine* 1992;17(4):388–394.
11. Gomez-Castresana FB, Vasquez Herrero C, Baltes Horche JL. Cervical chemonucleolysis. *Orthopedics* 1995;18(3):237–242.
12. Hofstra L, van Woerden HH, Deutman R. Chemonucleolysis in the herniated L3-4 disk. *Clin Orthop* 1991;269:151–156.
13. Javid MJ, et al. Safety and efficacy of chymopapain (Chymodiactin) in herniated nucleus pulposus with sciatica. Results of a randomized, double blind study. *JAMA* 1983;249(18):2489–2494.
14. Konings JG. *Chemonucleolysis, anatomical, radiological and clinical aspects* [thesis]. Groningen, the Netherlands: University of Groningen.
15. Konings JG, Williams FJ, Deutman R. Computed tomography (CT) analysis of the effects of chemonucleolysis. *Clin Orthop* 1986;206:32–36.
16. Launois R, et al. Analyse coût-utilité à 7 ans du traitement de la hernie discale lombaire. *J déconomie Méd* 1992;10:307–325.
17. van Leeuwen RB. *Chemonucleolysis* [thesis]. Utrecht, The Netherlands: University of Utrecht, 1989.
18. Leweis, Wier, et al. Prospective study of 100 lumbosacral discectomies. *J Neurosurg* 1987:67;49–53.
19. McCulloch JA, et al. Surgical indications and techniques. In: Weinstein JN, Wiesel SW, eds. *The lumbar spine.* Philadelphia: WB Saunders, 1990.
20. Muralikuttan KP, Adair IV, Roberts G, et al. Serum keratan sulfate level following chemonucleolysis. *Spine* 1991;16 (9):1078–1080.
21. Muralikuttan KP, et al. A prospective randomized trial of chemonucleolysis and conventional disc surgery in single level lumbar disc herniation. *Spine* 1992;17(4):381–387.
22. Nordby EJ. Eight- to 13-year follow-up evaluation of chemonucleolysis patients. *Clin Orthop* 1986;206:18–24.
23. Nordby EJ, Fraser RD, Javid M. Spine update chemonucleolysis. *Spine* 1996;21(9):1102–1105.
24. Nordby EJ, Wright PH, Schofield SR. Safety of chemonucleolysis. *Clin Orthop* 1993;293:122–134.
25. Postacchini F. Presidential address. *Spine* 1999;24(10):1991–1995.
26. Rijk PC, Deutman R, De Jong T, et al. Spondylolisthesis with sciatica. Magnetic resonance findings and chemonucleolysis. *Clin Orthop* 1996;326:146–152.
27. Sawin PD, et al. Chymopapain-induced reduction of proinflammatory phospholipase A2 activity and amelioration of neuropathic behavior changes in an in vivo model of acute sciatica. *J Neurosurg* 1997;86(6):998–1006.
28. Sciatica—management by chemonucleolysis versus surgical discectomy. *Neurosurg Rev* 1986;9:103–107.
29. Smith L. Enzyme dissolution of the nucleus pulposus in humans. *JAMA* 1964;187:137.
30. Smith L. Personal communication.
31. Stam J. Consensus on diagnosis and treatment of lumbosacral root entrapment syndromes. *Ned Tijdschr Geneeskd* 1996;140(52):2621–2626.
32. Stern IJ. The biochemistry and toxicology of chymopapain. In: Brown JE, Smith L, eds. *Chemonucleolysis.* Thorofare: Slack Inc, 1985.
33. Sutton JC Jr. Repeat chemonucleolysis. *Clin Orthop* 1986;206:45–49.
34. Szypryt EP, Gibson MJ, Mulholland RC, et al. The long-term effect of chemonucleolysis on the intervertebral disc as assessed by magnetic resonance imaging. *Spine* 1987;12(7):707–711.
35. Van Alphen HA, et al. Chemonucleolysis versus discectomy: a randomized multicenter trial. *J Neurosurg* 1989;70(6):869–875.
36. Van de Belt H, Franssen S, Deutman R. Repeat chemonucleolysis is safe and effective. *Clin Orthop* 199;363:121–125.
37. Wardlaw D. Experience with chemonucleolysis. In: Aspden RM, Porter RW, eds. *Lumbar spine disorders: current concepts.* World Scientific Publishing Co, 1995.

19

Neuromodulation in Failed Back Surgery:
A Neurosurgical Overview

L.E. Augustinsson

Despite the fact that neuromodulation has been used for almost 30 years, it is still not very well known within the medical domain. Historically, the procedure goes back to 1965 when Melzack (neurosurgeon) and Wall (neurophysiologist) presented their so-called "gate control theory," which states that electric stimulation of the large I-A afferents closes the "gate" for pain impulses propagated by the thin C fibers. This somewhat primitive neurophysiologic model has been revised and refined many times over the years, however the scientific work of Melzack and Wall began a push for science in neuromodulation and later even in movement disorders. Few other disciplines have more publications than algology, which today is an area consisting of all kinds of investigations from pure clinical work to molecular biology. Neurosurgeons, and above all those who focus on functional and stereotactic neurosurgery, have contributed profoundly to the science of neuromodulation. Today there are both international and national societies for neuromodulation as well as a journal titled *Neuromodulation*.

DEFINITIONS

Firstly, what does failed back surgery mean? It means nothing but chronic pain in the back and/or the leg(s) from previous open lumbar surgery. It says nothing about strict diagnosis, anatomy and pathophysiology which all will be discussed more profoundly later in this chapter. Secondly, how is neuromodulation defined? It is not so easy to do this in a few words but basically it means that the central, autonomic, or peripheral nervous systems are supplied with electric impulses or chemical substances in a way that nervous domains and effector organs will be activated or inhibited. Neuromodulation is considered as nondestructive and minimally invasive. The autonomic or peripheral systems are less used for direct neuromodulation. However, the so-called transcutaneous electric nerve stimulation (TENS) is widely used for pain treatment including the failed back surgery syndrome, but will not be evaluated in this chapter because of its weak relationship to this headline. The central nervous system dominates in neurologic neuromodulation and both the brain and the spinal cord are modulated depending on the symptoms and signs that are to be treated.

NEUROMODULATION BY ELECTRICITY

The most common symptom to treat is chronic pain. It was here it all started with rereference to the Melzac-Wall gate theory. Both the brain and spinal cord can be stimulated, but the spinal cord is much more common. Movement disorders are also used as an indication for electric stimulation. For example, Parkinson's disease is successfully treated today by implantation of electrodes in the nucleus subthalamicus. Further, epilepsy can be treated with electric stimulation of the vagus nerve at the level of the neck.

This chapter focuses only on stimulation of the spinal cord in order to relieve severe chronic pain in the low back and/or the legs from failed back surgery syndrome. Another indication that is very useful for spinal cord stimulation is chronic stable angina pectoris, which originates from nociceptive myocardial ischemia.

The common abbreviation for spinal cord stimulation in the literature is SCS. A prerequisite for all electric stimulation is that the areas in pain must be covered with stimulation-produced paresthesias, otherwise it will not work. We still do not know after all these years whether or not the paresthesias per se have a pain relieving effect or are just a paraphenomenon.

Surgical Technique

The dorsal epidural space is punctured in the lumbar area and two to four thin multipolar electrodes are placed with the tip somewhere between T9 and T11, depending on pain localization. Percutaneous testing is performed for 1 to 4 weeks. When pain relief is successful (at least 40% pain reduction on the subcutaneous visual analog scale [VAS] scale), a fully implantable and telemetrically programmable pulse generator is connected to the electrode via an extension cable. The pulse generator is placed subcutaneously, usually in the left ilium fossa.

Surgery is performed under local anesthesia with the patient in a prone position. Fluoroscopy is mandatory in this procedure because it is necessary to see where the electrode moves at intraoperative manipulation. A normal surgery—all sequences together—seldom takes more than 1 hour.

Complications

Severe complications such as epidural hematoma or abscess are extremely rare. Mild complications such as electrode tip migration and superficial infections are more common and show a variation of about 5% to 20% in the literature.

NEUROMODULATION BY DRUGS (MORPHINE)

Direct impact on the central nervous system with drugs for pain relief is a method that was developed much later than the use of electric neuromodulation for the same purpose. Technically this type of neuromodulation is based on very sophisticated drug pumps that were initially developed for treatment of spasticity with intrathecal infusion of baclofen (which is a γ-aminobutyric acid agonist). During the last 10 years, it has become more accepted to use intrathecal morphine for nonmalignant pain conditions that also carry components of neurogenic pain. The benefit is that only a small fraction of the systemic doses of morphine can be given intrathecally. Pain from failed back surgery is one of the best indications for this method.

Surgical Technique

In pain it is always advisable first to implant a common epidural catheter set, however, here it is done subarachnoidally for a test infusion of morphine for a period of 1 to 2 weeks. The catheter is removed after testing and, at successful pain relief, the definitive catheter will be implanted intrathecally some weeks later and in the same session connected to the drug pump which is placed in the left fossa subcutaneously. The surgery can be done either locally or under general anesthesia. The pump is filled with morphine intraoperatively due to a certain paradigm.

Surgical Complications

Severe complications such as intraspinal hematoma or abscess are extremely rare in both methods of neuromodulation. However, mild complications such as electrode or catheter migration with loss of clinical effect or superficial infections are more common and have been reported in the literature to be present in 5% to 20% of cases. These later complications are usually easy to correct. It is also important to follow the filling instructions from the manufacturers of the pumps, as overdose of morphine can lead to coma.

PHYSIOLOGY

Semantically, pain related to failed back surgery is termed chronic lumbago–sciatica, which means ache in the lumbosacral domain as well as in the legs. However leg pain is radicular pain (one or more segments) and thus considered neuropathic pain while back pain can be of both nociceptive and neuropathic character. This is important to consider when the adequate method of neuromodulation is chosen. Generally it can be said that neuropathic pain is suitable for electric stimulation while nociceptive pain is suitable for morphine. However, there are exceptions.

CLINICAL CONSIDERATIONS

Perhaps as many as 150,000 to 200,000 spinal cord stimulators have been implanted over the years because of intractable pain after failed back surgery. The conclusion must be that a vast majority of these patients have undergone incorrect surgical procedures prior to receiving spinal cord stimulators. Unclear indications, unskilled or inexperienced surgeons, and in many cases multiple surgeries have been catastrophic for patients. The spine is very sensitive to open surgery and the indications for spinal surgery must be crystal clear. Luckily, the access to neuromodulation has helped many of these patients lead a normal life. The question is which type of neuromodulation should be recommended in a single case. This depends on which type of physiology the actual pain condition presents.

If radicular leg pain is the only symptom, the first line of treatment should always be SCS. If leg pain and back pain are the case, with leg pain dominating, SCS should also be tried first. If only back pain exists, the results with SCS are not that good. It is possible to try bilateral epidural electrodes, but it is difficult if not impossible to create paresthesias solely in the back. Therefore, many neurosurgeons prefer to start with a trial of intrathecal morphine.

PSYCHOSOCIAL CONSIDERATIONS

Not only are etiology and genesis of failed back surgery heterogenous, but also the whole group of patients that constitute the domain of patients who suffer from failed back surgery syndrome. It cannot be emphasized enough that there are many patients who demonstrate massive functional symptoms and problems in the syndrome. Therefore, it is mandatory for all patients to undergo solid investigations at pain clinics or pain cen-

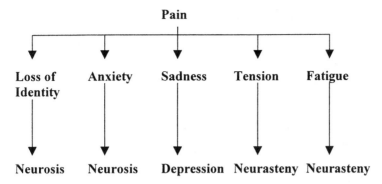

FIG. 19.1. Psychiatric aspects of chronic pain. (Reprinted from Lindquist G, personal communication.)

ters before surgical neuromodulation is suggested. Eventual psychosocial problems have to be brought into perspective and treated. In many cases surgical intervention can be avoided after this step is taken.

The algorithm in Figure 19.1 mirrors schematically what chronic pain can lead to from a psychiatric perspective. The endpoint might be neurosis, which is a psychiatric diagnosis and must be treated correctly and professionally. After this is done, surgery might be performed. All patients who are approved for neuromodulation have to be thoroughly informed and supplied with the realistic information of not having too high of expectations. A patient who says, "Doctor, you can do anything and I will be healed" has not understood the information from the physician about the surgical procedure of neuromodulation.

RESULTS

Results achieved through SCS and intrathecal morphine infusion can be broken down as follows.

Spinal Cord Stimulation

1. *Only leg pain:* In thoroughly selected patients, a 60% to 65% response to treatment after 1 year or more is reported in the majority of the literature.
2. *In leg and back pain*: Somewhat lower results are reported under the prerequisite that the leg pain is dominating and that back pain is of minor degree.
3. *Back pain*: It is very difficult to get adequate paresthesias focused solely on the back; thus, SCS has poor results in this scenario.

Only one prospective randomized study comparing SCS and open additional surgeries in failed back surgery has been designed. It was performed by Richard North at Johns Hopkins University Medical Center, Department of Neurosurgery in Baltimore. A 6-month follow-up report was published, followed by abstracts on 2- and 5-year follow-up. At each follow-up point, SCS has proven to be superior to additional surgeries.

Intrathecal Morphine Infusion with Fully Implantable Drug Pumps

This method has been developed during the last 10 to 15 years. The success rate regarding intrathecal morphine infusion is significantly lower than SCS, which has been routinely used over the last 30 years in failed back surgery syndrome. However, several papers have been published showing more or less the same results as with SCS. On average, 50% to 60% of patients respond favorably to intrathecal morphine infusion with fully implantable drug pumps.

CONCLUSION

Neuromodulation in chronic lumbago–sciatica from failed back surgery is a treatment modality, lenient to the patient, and significantly effective in the long-term follow-up. Although the equipment necessary for the treatment is initially expensive, neuromodulation has been shown to be cost-effective, and above all the pain relief leads to a better quality of life for the patients. Neuromodulation is thus strongly recommended for cases of failed back surgery syndrome.

SUGGESTED READING

Spinal Cord Stimulation

Bell G, Kidd D, North R. Cost-effective analysis of spinal cord stimulation in treatment of failed back surgery syndrome. *J Pain Sympt Mgmt* 1997;12(5)286–295.

Burchiel K, et al. Prognostic factors of spinal cord stimulation for chronic back pain and leg pain. *Neurosurgery* 1995;36:1101-1111.

Burchiel K, et al. Prospective, multicenter study of spinal cord stimulation for relief of chronic back and extremity pain. *Spine* 1996;21(23)2786–2794.

De Laporte C, Van de Kelft E. Spinal cord stimulation in failed back surgery syndrome. *Pain* 1993;52:55–61.

Devulder J, De Laat M, Van Bastelaere M, et al. Spinal cord stimulation: a valuable treatment for chronic failed back surgery patients. *J Pain Sympt Mgmt* 1997;13(5):296–301.

Devulder J, et al. Spinal cord stimulation in chronic pain therapy (includes FBS). *Clin J Pain* 1990;6(1)51–56.

Dumoulin K, et al. A psychoanalytic investigation to improve the success rate of spinal cord stimulation as a treatment for chronic failed back surgery syndrome. *Clin J Pain* 1996;12:43–49.

Hassenbusch S, Stanton-Hicks M, Covington E. Spinal cord stimulation versus spinal infusion for low back and leg pain. *Acta Neurochir* 1995;64[Suppl]:109–115.

Kumar K, Nath R, Wyant G. Treatment of chronic pain by epidural spinal cord stimulation: a 10-year experience (includes FBS). *J Neurosurg* 1991;75:402–407.

Law J. Targeting a spinal stimulator to treat 'failed back surgery syndrome.' *Appl Neurophysiol* 1987;50(1–6): 437–438.

LeDoux M, Langford K. Spinal cord stimulation for the failed back syndrome. *Spine* 1993;18(2):191–194.

North R, Bakshi S. The failed back: augmentative pain procedures. *Semin Spine Surg* 1996;8(3):239–244.

North R, Kidd D, Lee M, et al. A prospective, randomized study of spinal cord stimulation versus reoperation for failed back surgery syndrome: initial results. *Stereotact Funct Neurosurg* 1994;62:267–272.

North R, et al. Failed back surgery syndrome: 5-year follow-up in 102 patients undergoing repeated operation. *Neurosurgery* 1991;28(5)685–691.

North R, et al. Failed back surgery syndrome: 5-year follow-up after spinal cord stimulator implantation. *Neurosurgery* 1991;28(5)692–699.

Rossi U, Ralbar J. Spinal cord stimulation in the failed back syndrome: a reappraisal. *Am Pain Soc,* 1994.

Turner J, Loeser J, Bell K. Spinal cord stimulation for chronic low back pain: a systematic literature synthesis. *Neurosurgery* 1995;37(6):1088–1096.

Intrathecal Morphine Infusion

Anderson VC, Burchiel KJ. A prospective study of long-term intrathecal morphine in the management of chronic nonmalignant pain. *Neurosurgery* 1999;44:289–300.

Bennett G, et al. Evidence-based review of literature on intrathecal delivery of pain medication. *J Pain Sympt Mgmt* 2000;2:12–36.

Bennett G, et al. Clinical guidelines for intraspinal infusion: report of an expert panel. *J Pain Sympt Mgmt* 2000; 2:37–43.

Follett KA, Hitchon PW, Piper J, et al. Response of intractable pain to continuous intrathecal morphine: a retrospective study. *Pain* 1992;49:21–25.

Hassenbusch SJ, Stanton-Hicks M, Covington ED, et al. Long-term intraspinal infusions of opioids in the treatment of neuropathic pain. *J Pain Sympt Mgmt* 1995;10:527–543.

Onofrio BM, Yaksh TL. Long-term pain relief produced by intrathecal infusion in 53 patients. *J Neurosurg* 1990;72: 200–209.

Paice JA, Penn RD, Shott S. Intraspinal morphine for chronic pain: a retrospective, multicenter study. *J Pain Sympt Mgmt* 1996;11:71–80.

Penn RD, Paice JA. Chronic intrathecal morphine for intractable pain. *J Neurosurg* 1987;67:182–186.

Tutak U, Doleys DM. Intrathecal infusion systems for treatment of chronic low back and leg pain of noncancer origin. *South Med J* 1996;89:295–300.

Winkelmuller M, Winkelmuller W. Long-term effects of continuous intrathecal opioid treatment in chronic pain of nonmalignant etiology. *J Neurosurg* 1996;85:458–467.

SECTION 5

Surgical Treatment Modalities

20

General Principles: When to Operate

Michael Sullivan

Different general principles must apply to different pathologies within the disc. They present differently and therefore require different treatments. Also one needs to define what constitutes surgery. Most practitioners would agree that open laminectomy and laminotomy would definitely be classified as operations, as would microdiscectomy. However, this becomes somewhat more problematic when one gets into the realm of minimal intervention surgery. Tube surgery, using either a dorsal, lateral, or foraminal approach would also be considered surgery, and chemonucleolysis would fall in this category as well. The most difficult to categorize are dorsal nerve root blocks and either lumbar or caudal epidurals. Both of these procedures require the patient's consent and both carry a very small complication rate in that the local anesthetic and steroid can be administered intrathecally (4). For the purpose of this chapter, I refer to root blocks as surgical procedures, but not epidurals, particularly as they are done in the caudal approach.

When to operate depends on the diagnosis (i.e., the pathology that is presented) and also on the complication rate of the procedure that is to be undertaken. As an example, most practitioners would prefer to offer a caudal epidural than an open laminectomy.

There seem to be six different problems that must be addressed, each in a different way prior to determining whether or not to operate. In any of these situations there may be degenerative change of the lumbar spine and therefore a degree of stenosis. This will only make the symptoms worse, but the principles of when and when not to operate essentially remain the same. The six problems that need to be addressed are:

1. Soft disc prolapse affecting the traversing nerve root;
2. Soft disc affecting the exiting nerve root;
3. Progressive neurologic dysfunction;
4. Cauda equina lesion;
5. The adolescent disc;
6. Recurrent disc herniation.

Each of these will command a different treatment and a different degree of urgency as to when to operate.

SOFT DISC HERNIATION AFFECTING THE TRAVERSING NERVE ROOT

This is a common pathology among younger patients, usually those between 20 to 45 years of age who present with back and leg pain and limited straight leg raising. One must assume there is no cauda equina involvement, in which case one should not contemplate performing surgery until 6 weeks after diagnosis. Between 60% and 70% of patients will spontaneously improve over that period and not require any surgical intervention. During that period it is unreasonable not to give any treatment modality and the patient, if in severe pain, can be allowed 2 to 3 days' bed rest but no more than that. Epidural injections can be given as well as nerve root blocks. Nerve root blocks to the L5 root and above (Fig. 20.1) need to be done under image intensification. The S1 nerve root is injected under computed tomography (CT) guidance (Fig. 20.2). During this period it is wise to give adequate analgesics and physiotherapy and, although there is not a great deal of evidence that this in fact changes the pathology, it is certainly good for the well being of the patient.

If the pain or paresthesia remains severe at 6 weeks, surgery should be discussed. Patients should be very well aware of the fact that if nothing is done they will come to no great harm but they will continue to have pain over the course of the next 2 to 4 years (13). That is to say, they will have pain but at 4 years they will be no worse off than patients who have undergone surgery. If patients are totally against surgery and understand that they will have to endure their current symptoms, they should be given this option. Assuming that the symptoms are not acceptable to the patient and the two things that they do not like are pain and paresthesia, then surgery should be undertaken. Patients seem to tolerate loss of muscle function much more easily than pain or paresthesia. With the understanding that surgery at 6 weeks is not going to make any difference to their long-term recovery but in the short term (up to 2 years) they will be considerably better off with surgical intervention, they must make their own decision.

This is the time when it is necessary to explain to the patient the pros and cons of different treatment modalities and the complication rate of each treatment. At this stage of our knowledge it is probably best to refer to the Cochrane Library as to which is the best treatment modality (6). In the Cochrane Library different null hypotheses are tested. The types of outcome measures for disc surgery that are taken into account are:

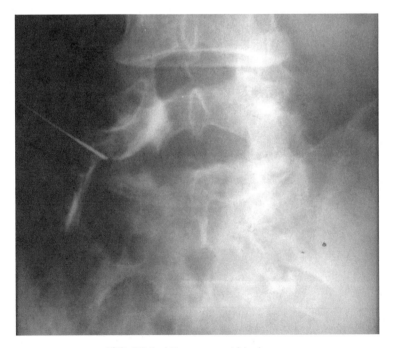

FIG. 20.1. L5 nerve root block.

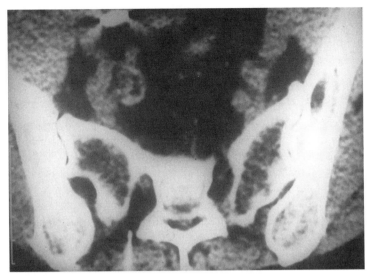

FIG. 20.2. S1 computed tomography-guided nerve root block.

1. The proportion of patients recovering according to both themselves and their clinician;
2. Improvement in pain;
3. Improvement by disability or quality of life scale;
4. The ability to return to work;
5. The economics of the treatment and the economics of returning the patient to a work status;
6. The rate of additional surgery with the type of procedure performed.

Also taken into account must be the adverse reactions, which for disc surgery are:

1. The early complications
   a. Cauda equina damage
   b. Nerve root damage
   c. Vascular damage
   d. Infection
2. The late complications
   a. Chronic pain
   b. Instability
   c. Arachnoiditis
   d. Nerve root dysfunction
   e. Myelocele.

Taking all these into account and looking at the Cochrane null hypotheses, one can offer a 95% chance of success with open disc surgery. There is no evidence that the results are any different between the standard operation of laminectomy or microdiscectomy. Chemonucleolysis offers a 70% to 75% success rate with a very low complication rate. Unfortunately, in the Cochrane Library, both laser discectomy and tube surgery have not come out well and should still be considered as experimental. Probably in the very near future, papers will come out to show the usefulness of tube surgery, especially for foraminal and extraforaminal disc prolapses. At the present time, one should not offer tube surgery for traversing nerve root pathology from a prolapsed disc. This applies to both intradiscal and foraminal tube surgery. If paresthesia is causing the patient major problems, the best option is open surgery.

SOFT DISC PROLAPSE AFFECTING THE EXITING NERVE ROOT

This usually occurs at the L4-L5 level, occasionally at L3-L4, and infrequently at L5-S1. The vast majority of the patients are middleaged men with involvement of the exiting L4 nerve root. They present with profound anterior thigh pain with or without loss of a knee jerk. Of all discogenic pain, this appears to be by far the worst and it is absolutely mandatory to provide some form of treatment. Bed rest has no place as it does not alleviate the symptoms. As the patients often have a positive femoral stretch as well as limitation of straight leg raising, they are more comfortable sitting up. They need immediate powerful analgesia. As soon as the diagnosis has been made on magnetic resonance image (MRI), scanning a nerve root block is extremely helpful, as it will get patients through the very painful first 2 to 3 weeks (14). The nerve root block may need to be repeated two or three times during the first 6 weeks. At the end of that period, if patients still have symptoms, the question then arises as to whether they should have surgery. The classic teaching is a lateral approach down to the foramen using a microscope (5) but this has been superseded by tube surgery (8), which is the surgical modality of choice. Tube surgery at the lumbosacral level can be extremely difficult and may require a tangential approach (10). However, for the past 6 years, the author has treated all patients whose conservative treatment failed (11) with chemonucleolysis; over that 6-year period not one patient required surgery. This is one of the three good uses of chemonucleolysis, the other two being the adolescent disc and recurrent disc, which will be discussed later in this chapter.

PROLAPSED DISC AND PROGRESSIVE NEUROLOGIC LOSS

If over the course of the first week or two the patient experiences increasing muscle and reflex loss, one should seriously consider a more sinister diagnosis. There is often increase in pain and sensory disturbance, but if power and reflex changes continue to get worse, then one should undertake further investigation to determine if there is not some higher lesion. Assuming this is not the case, then this problem should be treated in the normal way for 6 weeks to see whether it resolves with conservative treatment of nerve root blocks, epidurals, analgesia, and physiotherapy.

Occasionally there is severe pain and then sudden loss of function with a complete foot drop, but also with complete loss of pain. This indicates a large sequestrated disc fragment. The question then arises as to whether one should operate at once or await recovery of the foot drop. We do not perform surgery in these cases. We give the patient a foot drop splint and if there is no recovery or only minimal recovery at 18 months, the foot drop is treated with tendon transfers around the foot or hindfoot stabilization.

CAUDA EQUINA SYNDROME

The cauda equina syndrome presents in two ways, chronic and acute. In the former patents experience slow, insidious increase of back pain, leg pain, weakness, followed by loss of bladder function; they are then found to have saddle anesthesia. These patients, whose problem comes on slowly, have a much better prognosis than the next group, who experience sudden acute pain, loss of bladder function, and loss of saddle sensation. This is almost invariably due to a large central disc prolapse and the treatment is immediate decompression and removal of the disc fragments and ensuring that there is no stenotic element to the spine. The main question arises as to when this operation should be undertaken. There have been two large series, that of Kostuick and colleagues (9) from Toronto and that of Gleave and MacFarlane (7) from Cambridge, England. Between the two series there were 1,400 back operations, of which 64 were cauda equina lesions. It would appear that the most important factor for a good result is the length of time that it took for the symptoms to come on. Those who had acute onset had a much worse prognosis, especially with return to function of the bladder. Surgeries were undertaken at between 1 and 3 days and there seemed to be no difference in outcome whether it was performed at day 1 or day 3.

Cauda equina lesions can occur postoperatively after routine disc surgery, either due to a large further fragment of disc material or a hematoma. If these are operated on within 6 hours, prognosis is very good. One could extrapolate this finding to cauda equina lesions presenting in clinical practice, and thus one could hypothesize that the ideal situation would be to operate within 6 hours of the onset of symptoms. This is probably unrealistic in terms of getting patients into the hospital, being examined, having MRI scans, and moving to the operating theater. If 24 hours have gone past it probably does not matter whether the surgery is performed in 1 day or in 3 days.

THE ADOLESCENT DISC

If one uses age as the criterion of adolescence (i.e., patients under the age of 20), then there are three presentations of an adolescent disc (12).

1. The vertebral rim fracture.
2. The typical adult disc prolapse presenting in a patient under 20 years of age.
3. A true adolescent disc.

The rim fracture (Fig. 20.3) presents with patients having back pain and a certain amount of leg pain but quite marked paresthesia. The diagnosis is easily made on CT scanning,

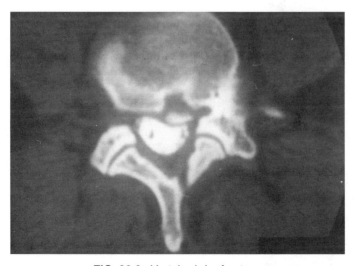

FIG. 20.3. Vertebral rim fracture.

which yields a better bone definition than MRI but, if one is aware of the possibility of a rim fracture, MRI will show the fracture line. Patients have limited straight leg raising, and they have pain, paresthesia, and perhaps a muscle and reflex loss in the distribution of the nerve root affected. There is no evidence that conservative treatment is going to be helpful in terms of paresthesia although undoubtedly the pain resolves but the treatment of choice is to operate and remove the fragment, this being done at the patient's convenience.

The young adult disc is effectively exactly the same as the disc affecting a traversing nerve root. The patients are younger than the age of 20 but essentially have the same pathology as that of a 25-year-old patient. On MRI a single level disc prolapse is seen and after 6 weeks of conservative management the same questions can be asked as would be asked of a 25-year-old with a traversing nerve root lesion. There is a tendency toward chemonucleolysis rather than surgery because of the age of the patient. The results however are exactly the same as in an adult disc prolapse.

The true adolescent disc has a completely different clinical and pathologic picture. The patients are children who present with a very stiff back (Fig. 20.4). They experience

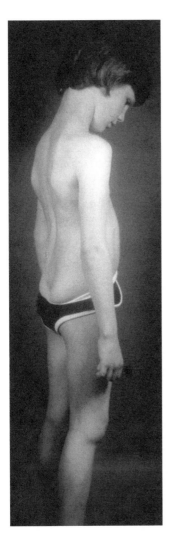

FIG. 20.4. True adolescent disc patient.

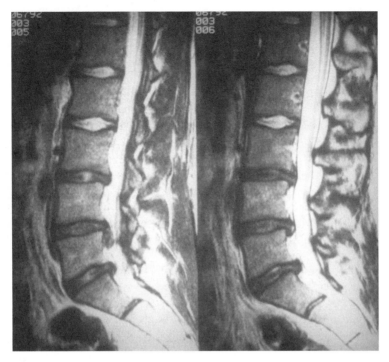

FIG. 20.5. Magnetic resonance image scan of true adolescent disc prolapse.

remarkably little in the way of pain and neurologic deficit is not common. However, these patients do have such marked stiffness that they can be lifted up by their heels so that they rest on the back of their neck with comparatively little complaint. On MRI scanning they have multiple level disc degeneration but only one is of the symptomatic level (Fig. 20.5). Because of the young age of these patients and the fact that they are experiencing very little pain, there is a tendency to treat them conservatively with physiotherapy and hope that the symptoms will improve. However, they have a marked disability in that they cannot sit down at school and they cannot play any sport. These symptoms do not improve. In most series, the time from diagnosis to treatment is 1 year, although there is no evidence that there is any point in continuing conservative treatment after 6 weeks. The treatment of choice in this age group is chemonucleolysis (1); surgery does equally well but has no advantage. The one thing that the practitioner need not consider is multiple level treatment, as there is only one symptomatic level.

RECURRENT DISC HERNIATION

Recurrent disc herniation can occur on the contralateral side at the same level as the previous surgery or at a different level, in which case it is treated in the same way as any other primary disc affecting a traversing nerve root (2). With ipsilateral recurrence at the same level as previous surgery, the tendency is to be more conservative than in primary surgery. There is less need for bed rest but analgesics and nerve root blocks are very helpful for pain and also for diagnosis during the first 6 weeks. Nerve root blocks are far superior to epidurals in this situation because the epidural seems to go to all parts except that to which they are directed because of the fibrosis around the nerve root. At 6 weeks, if symptoms have improved to an acceptable degree, no further treatment should be undertaken. However, if symptoms are still profound, as they often are, these patients need an MRI scan but very little attention needs to be placed on the degree of fibrous tissue.

All surgeries form fibrous tissue and because of that the nerve root will, to some degree, be bound down to the disc in front. Even a small disc prolapse can cause profound pain. Secondary surgery should be undertaken when the patient has unacceptable symptoms that have plateaued for 3 weeks after the original 6 weeks. The results of subsequent surgery are not much different from those of primary surgery (3) and are unrelated to the amount of fibrous tissue present. Another means of dealing with a recurrent disc prolapse is to withdraw the fragment back into the disc space and remove it that way. Unfortunately, there is an element of fixation of fragment to the annulus. One method that has been tried is to inject the disc with chymopapain thus freeing the collagenous fragment, which could then be pulled down into the disc space by means of tube surgery and removed (15). This surgery can be undertaken at exactly the same time as repeat surgery, which will be somewhere between 6 and 10 weeks after symptoms recur.

It cannot be too strongly emphasized that patients must always be made aware that if they do not have bladder or bowel dysfunction, they have a pathology that, if they wait long enough, will resolve and give as good a result as any surgical intervention. Patients must make their own decision when and if they want to have surgical intervention.

REFERENCES

1. Bradbury N, Wilson LF, Mulholland RC. Adolescent disc protrusions. A long-term follow-up of surgery compared with chymopapain. *Spine* 1996;21(3)372–377.
2. Cinotti G, Gomina S, Giannicola G, et al. Contralateral recurrent lumbar disc herniation. Results of discectomy compared with those in primary herniation. *Spine* 1999;24 (8)800–806.
3. Cinotti G, Roysam GS, Eisenstein SM, et al. Ipsilateral recurrent lumbar disc herniation. A prospective controlled study. *J Bone Joint Surg* 1998;80(5)825–832.
4. Cuckler JM, Bernini PA, Wiesel SW, et al. The use of epidural steroids in the treatment of lumbar radicular pain. A prospective randomised doubleblind study. *J Bone Joint Surg* 1985;67(1):63–66.
5. Darden BV, Wade JF, Alexander R, et al. Far lateral disc herniations treated by microscopic fragment excision. Techniques and results. *Spine* 1995;20(13):1500–1505.
6. Gibson JNA, Grant IC, Waddell G. *The Cochrane Library* 2000;Issue 3.
7. Gleave JR, MacFarlane R. Prognosis for recovery of bladder function following lumbar central disc prolapse. *Br J Neurosurg* 1990;4 205–209.
8. Kambin P, O'Brien E, Zhou L, et al. Arthroscopic microdiscectomy and selective fragmentectomy. *Clin Orthop* 1998;(347):150–167.
9. Kostuik JP, Harrington I, Alexander D, et al. Cauda equina syndrome and lumbar disc herniation *J Bone Joint Surg* 1986;68A:386–391.
10. Muller A, Reuben HJ. A paramedian tangential approach to lumbosacral extraforaminal disc herniations. *Neurosurgery* 1998;43(4):854–861.
11. Rust MS, Olivero WC. Far lateral disc herniation: the results of conservative management. *J Spinal Disord* 1999; 12(2):183–140.
12. Sullivan MF. The adolescent disc. In: Findlay G, Owen R, eds. *Surgery of the spine.* Blackwell Scientific, 1992: 733–736.
13. Weber H. Lumbar disc herniation: a controlled prospective study with ten years of observation. *Spine* 1983;8: 131–140.
14. Weiner BM, Fraser RD. Foraminal injection for far lateral lumbar disc herniation. *J Bone Joint Surg* 1997;79(5): 804–807.
15. Yeung A. Use of chymopapain in recurrent disc. Personal communication, 1999.

21

Disc Herniation: Are Recent Surgical Developments Also Recent Advances?

Gordon Waddell and Alastair Gibson

Surgeons, by nature, are mechanics and inventors. We are excited by new tools and techniques in our trade and so it is perhaps of no surprise that spinal surgery is replete with new gadgetry and innovative treatments. The important question, however, is whether recent developments in disc surgery really are advances, and whether they do deliver the progress we seek.

The original case series by the proponents of any new surgical technique usually show a success rate of anywhere from 70% to 97%. Other enthusiasts soon present similar or slightly lower success rates. Over a number of years, sometimes a surprising number of years, more critical authors suggest the results may not be quite as good. Such personal series and case reports are of course uncontrolled and open to bias. Sometimes the complications and failures of the technique become so blatant over time that the procedure becomes discredited and is discarded. This has happened to many procedures over the decades, as demonstrated in any history of spinal surgery. The only truly objective scientific evidence, to either prove or disprove a procedure, comes from randomized controlled trials (RCTs), as has been advocated for many years by Alf Nachemson and is now embodied in the Cochrane Library reviews (4). Whether we like it or not, we now live in an era of evidence-based medicine. Both the purchasers and the consumers of our services are increasingly likely to demand proper evidence of the efficacy of our procedures, particularly when they are expensive and carry significant risk.

This chapter will begin with a discussion of open discectomy, in all its varieties, as the gold standard. There is still only one RCT that directly compares surgical discectomy with conservative treatment (15), but there is a wealth of other evidence summarized in the Cochrane Library review (4). That concluded that there is considerable evidence on the clinical effectiveness of discectomy for carefully selected patients with sciatica due to lumbar disc prolapse that fails to resolve with conservative management. It provides faster relief from the acute attack, although any positive or negative effects on the lifetime natural history of disc problems are unclear. There is lack of evidence on the long-term outcomes and on occupational outcomes.

There is now scientific evidence from RCTs on a number of more recent, alternative techniques for lumbar disc herniation including:

- Microdiscectomy
- Chemonucleolysis
- Arthroscopic microdiscectomy
- Automated percutaneous discectomy
- Laser discectomy

Microdiscectomy and chemonucleolysis have both, to varying degrees, survived the tests of time, wide clinical experience, and critical scientific evaluation in RCTs. This is based more, however, on earlier rather than recent advances.

Microdiscectomy is now an established and widely used technique, and many surgeons advocate the benefits of improved vision and illumination when operating within a confined space. There are two RCTs (5,9) and one comparative trial (7) comparing microdiscectomy with standard discectomy. These trials suggest that use of the microscope lengthens the operative procedure, but no differences were observed in perioperative bleeding, length of inpatient stay, or the formation of scar tissue. The two RCTs provide clinical outcome data (5,9) which are not directly comparable and are difficult to combine, but clinical outcomes and duration of sick leave with microdiscectomy seem broadly similar to those of standard discectomy. It is not possible to draw any firm conclusions about complication rates from the trials. It should also be noted that it is now 5 years since the publication of the most recent of these trials and during that time surgeons have become increasingly familiar with use of the operating microscope when performing surgery on the spine and elsewhere. Indeed, microdiscectomy is now the preferred method of treatment of lumbar disc prolapse in many major centers.

Chemonucleolysis initially faced powerful surgical opposition, but despite that there is now strong evidence from five RCTs that chemonucleolysis is more effective than placebo and strong evidence from another five RCTs that it is not quite as effective as surgical discectomy (4). The Cochrane Library review concluded that the scientific evidence supports chemonucleolysis as a possible therapeutic option. It may be considered as a minimally invasive, intermediate stage between conservative management and open surgical intervention. It has a lower complication rate and might save about 70% of patients from requiring open surgery. However, the final outcome of chemonucleolysis followed by surgery if chemonucleolysis fails, remains poorer than the outcome of primary discectomy. It is then a matter of debate for the individual case about the relative balance of possibly avoiding surgery, relative risks and complication rates, clinical outcomes over the next year or so, and the unknown impact of chemonucleolysis or surgery on the lifetime natural history of degenerative disc disease.

But what about more recent developments? There are now RCTs on three alternative techniques: arthroscopic microdiscectomy, automated percutaneous discectomy, and laser discectomy. It is particularly important that the safety, clinical outcome, and cost-effectiveness of such innovative procedures should be compared with established forms of treatment.

There are now two RCTs of arthroscopic microdiscectomy. Hermantin and colleagues (6) report approximately similar "satisfactory outcomes" compared with open discectomy, and Chung (3) finds the same compared with microdiscectomy. However, both of these trials have weaknesses and the full report from Chung (3) is still awaited.

There are several nonsystemic reviews that consider the relative merits of microdiscectomy and automated percutaneous discectomy. In both treatments, smaller wounds are said to promote faster patient recovery with earlier hospital discharge (7,12). There are now four RCTs of automated percutaneous discectomy. Two trials compared automated percutaneous discectomy with microdiscectomy. These trials were not directly comparable, as one used modified forceps and an automated cutter with suction, while the other used an automated suction nucleotome alone. Mayer and Brock (11) show that clinical outcomes are comparable to microdiscectomy, but consider that only 10% to 15% of patients requiring surgical treatment might be suitable for automated percutaneous lumbar discectomy (APLD). In contrast, Chatterjee and associates (1) report only 29% satisfactory results for APLD compared with 80% for microdiscectomy. Two trials compared APLD with chemonucleolysis. In a study of only 22 patients, Krugluger and Knahr (8), report a similar improvement in Oswestry score following both treatments at 1 year, but by 2 years the patients treated by APLD were worse (although no figures were given). In a much larger series of 134 patients, Revel and coworkers (13) find that APLD is markedly inferior, with one-third of subjects requiring open surgery within 6 months.

A 78% good or fair result was reported in the first clinical series of 420 patients who had laser discectomy, but there was no control group and outcome assessment was nonblinded (2). Since then, some reports have suggested similar success rates but others have shown much poorer results. There are now two RCTs of laser discectomy, though both were very small and only preliminary results are presently published. Steffen and associates (14) find that a holmium:yttrium-aluminum-garnet (YAG) laser discectomy produces 31% excellent/good results compared with 53% for chemonucleolysis. Livesey and colleagues (10) find no significant difference between potassium titanylphosphate (KTP) laser discectomy and epidural steroid injection, but only nine patients received laser therapy.

There is no acceptable scientific evidence presently available on intradiscal electrothermal therapy (IDET), despite it being strongly promoted and currently fashionable in some countries.

On the evidence presently available, we may conclude that:

1. There is now wide clinical experience and moderate scientific evidence from RCTs that the clinical outcomes of microdiscectomy are comparable to those of standard discectomy.
2. There is strong scientific evidence from RCTs that chemonucleolysis produces better clinical outcomes than placebo, but there is also strong scientific evidence from RCTs that the clinical outcomes are not as good as those of surgical discectomy.
3. There is limited scientific evidence from RCTs that arthroscopic microdiscectomy gives comparable results to standard or open microdiscectomy.
4. There is moderate scientific evidence from RCTs that automated percutaneous discectomy produces poorer results than microdiscectomy or chemonucleolysis.
5. There is limited scientific evidence from RCTs that laser discectomy is no more effective than epidural steroids and less effective than chemonucleolysis.
6. There is no scientific evidence on IDET.

Microdiscectomy is now a well-established alternative to standard discectomy. Chemonucleolysis and arthroscopic microdiscectomy may be considered as alternative options to either micro- or standard discectomy in appropriately trained and experienced hands for appropriately selected patients. Automated percutaneous discectomy, laser discectomy, and IDET should be regarded as experimental techniques that cannot be advocated for routine use unless—or until—better scientific evidence of their effectiveness is provided by their proponents.

In this age of evidence-based medicine, it is no longer acceptable to promote new surgical techniques and devices purely on the basis of personal series by their advocates, who are inevitably biased and sometimes have a commercial interest. Such personal series are obviously, and quite reasonably, the first step in the development and reporting of a new surgical breakthroughs. It may then be reasonable to have a second case series, undertaken by one or more independent observers, to confirm the inventor's findings. After that, within a few years and before the procedure is promoted widely for routine use, there should be a properly designed and conducted RCT published in a peer-reviewed journal. Anything else is simply unacceptable and is likely to be open to increasing question from health care purchasers and consumers in this age of evidence-based medicine and managed care.

The authors will be pleased to receive information about any other RCTs on surgical treatment for lumbar disc prolapse (or degenerative lumbar spondylosis) to add to the next update of the Cochrane Review.

REFERENCES

1. Chatterjee S, Foy PM, Findlay GF. Report of a controlled clinical trial comparing automated percutaneous lumbar discectomy and microdiscectomy in the treatment of contained lumbar disc herniation. *Spine* 1995;20(6): 734–738.
2. Choy DS, Ascher PW, Saddekni S, et al. Percutaneous laser disc decompression. A new therapeutic modality. *Spine* 1992;17:949–956.
3. Chung J-Y. A prospective randomized study of arthroscopic and microdiscectomy in protruded type lumbar disc herniation. Paper presented at: ISSLS Proceedings; 1999.
4. Gibson JNA, Grant IC, Waddell G. Surgery for lumbar disc prolapse. The Cochrane Library. Oxford: Update Software. 2000; Issue 4.
5. Henrikson L, Schmidt V, Eskesen V, et al. A controlled study of microsurgical versus standard lumbar discectomy. *Br J Neurosurg* 1996;10(3):289–293.
6. Hermantin FU, Peters T, Puartararo L, et al. A prospective randomized study comparing the results of open discectomy with those of video-assisted arthroscopic microdiscectomy. *J Bone Joint Surg* 1999;81A:958–965.
7. Kahanovich N, Viola K, McCulloch JA. Limited surgical discectomy and microdiscectomy: a clinical comparison. *Spine* 1989;14(1):79–81.
8. Krugluger J, Knahr K. Chemonucleolysis and automated percutaneous discectomy—a prospective randomized comparison. *Int Orthop* 2000;24:167–169.
9. Lagarrigue J, Chaynes P. Comparative study of disk surgery with or without microscopy. A prospective study of 80 cases. *Neurochir* 1994;40(2):116–120.
10. Livesey JP, Sundaram S, Foster L, et al. Laser discectomy versus lumbar epidural steroid injection: a randomised comparative study of two treatments for sciatica. *J Bone Joint Surg* 2000;82B[Suppl 1]:74.
11. Mayer HM, Brock M. Percutaneous endoscopic discectomy: surgical technique and preliminary results compared to microsurgical discectomy. *J Neurosurg* 1993;78(2):216–225.
12. Onik G, Mooney V, Maroon JC. Automated percutaneous discectomy: a prospective multi-institutional study. *Neurosurgery* 1990;2:228–233.
13. Revel M, Payan C, Vallee C, et al. Automated percutaneous lumbar discectomy versus chemonucleolysis in the treatment of sciatica. *Spine* 1993;18:1–7.
14. Steffen R, Luetke A, Wittenberg RH, et al. A prospective comparative study of chemonucleolysis and laser discectomy. *Orthop Trans* 1996;20:388–389.
15. Weber H. Lumbar disc herniation. A controlled, prospective study with ten years of observation. *Spine* 1983;8: 131–140.

22

The Reduction of Peridural Fibrosis

Nick Boeree

Surgery in the lumbar spine may fail for a wide variety of reasons, the underlying problem for the patient in all cases being significant persisting or recurrent pain, either in the back, in the leg, or both. Peridural fibrosis, the development of scar tissue around the nerve root and dura, is recognized as one of the possible causes of the failed back syndrome. As such, the prevention or reduction of fibrosis must be considered a desirable aim. Indeed, as a pathologic process, peridural fibrosis may represent one of a limited number of causes of failure in lumbar surgery, which it is at least possible to influence either by surgical technique or some other form of intervention. Many of the other causes of failure are more related to the actions of the surgeon, for example, poor patient selection, incorrect diagnosis, wrong level, or inadequate surgery, and as such cannot be prevented, except arguably through improved training and education. Peridural fibrosis occurs outside the dura and is distinct from arachnoiditis or intradural fibrosis, which are inflammatory responses occurring within the piaarachnoid and resulting in clumping of the roots forming the cauda equina. The causes, clinical effects, and management of this particular problem will not be considered here.

Peridural fibrosis can occur even in the absence of any surgical intervention, in response to pathologic changes in the spine. When related to inherent pathology in the spine, the generation of fibrosis is probably caused by certain chemical mediators (1,2). Loose fibrinous adhesions may form around the nerve root, for example after a disc protrusion, or more dense fibrotic tissue may intimately involve and tether the root. Such changes may be recognized on radiologic imaging and are certainly commonly encountered by the spinal surgeon, although fortunately it rarely presents a significant technical problem. It may, however, be a cause of a less satisfactory outcome for the patient. Some understanding of the possible chemical mediators is now emerging, although it is still unclear why some patients should develop a considerable fibrotic reaction while others with apparently similar pathology have very little. Nonetheless, knowledge of the etiologic factors offers the potential of therapeutic modulation of this process and with it some improvement in clinical results. The extent of fibrosis that forms may be related to the duration for which the underlying pathology continues, and as such presents an argument for avoiding undue delay where surgery is indicated.

While fibrosis occurring in response to pathology such as a disc prolapse may occasionally result in a rather tedious mobilization of an involved nerve root, the surgeon is rarely presented with any particular difficulties as a result of this problem. In contrast most surgeons approach revision exploration of a nerve root with some trepidation, anticipating a tedious, painstaking, and difficult dissection which will be associated with some risk to the involved nerve root. The common, although by no means invariable, experience is of dense scar tissue enveloping and tethering a nerve root to adjacent structures.

Any natural tissue planes tend to be obliterated and normal anatomic landmarks are often obscured. The procedure is generally time consuming and, in our experience, undertaken with a sense of foreboding that the scar tissue, and at least some of the clinical problems, will recur within a relatively short period of time. This is certainly supported by reported experience (3).

It is likely that some degree of fibrosis will always occur where there is surgical ingress to the spinal canal. Peridural fibrosis principally originates from the migration of fibroblasts derived from the dedifferentiation of overlying detached muscle. The same response will occur at any site where muscle is stripped from bone. It may be viewed as part of the normal healing response, the fibroblastic proliferation and migration initially forming a loose fibrinous network which matures and contracts into a dense adherent layer. This ensures reattachment of the traumatized muscle, ultimately facilitating functional restoration. The problem of peridural fibrosis is thus a direct consequence of our surgical intrusion into the spinal canal, an iatrogenic problem resulting from the removal of the natural barrier of the lamina and ligamentum flavum, leaving the underlying dura and nerve root exposed. This is illustrated schematically in Figure 22.1.

Fortunately, most patients will not experience any apparent symptoms as a result of the fibrosis that will almost certainly follow surgical exposure of the spinal canal. Regrettably, however, some undoubtedly do. It may well be that the true incidence of attributable symptoms is higher than generally appreciated and dependent upon how hard one looks. Reports in the literature suggest that of those whose outcome following lumbar spinal surgery is unsatisfactory, the principal cause is peridural fibrosis in 6% to 24% (4,5). The patient experiences a return of lumbar or radicular symptoms after a period of time, often a matter of months. However, in the normal clinical situation when the patient is reviewed following excision of a disc prolapse in a busy outpatient clinic, the relief and satisfaction that they report in losing their previous severe sciatica is documented as a

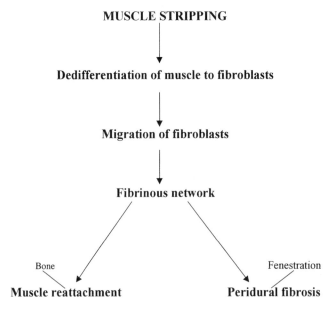

FIG. 22.1. Schematic representation of the pathogenesis of peridural fibrosis secondary to surgical intrusion into the spinal canal.

successful outcome. Comparatively, mild residual symptoms may not be reported, or if they are, the patient is often simply treated expectantly with advice and reassurance. The patient is often discharged at an early stage, before recurrent symptoms due to fibrosis will have become apparent. The spinal surgeon may believe that he or she can feel secure in the knowledge that the patient should be referred back if significant symptoms recur. Regrettably this cannot necessarily be relied upon. Taking all these factors together, it is perhaps not surprising that surgeon-reported results after discectomy suggest a good or excellent outcome in 85% to 95% of patients, while independent evaluation suggests that up to 40% of patients experience residual or recurrent symptoms of leg pain sufficient to limit activity after discectomy (6).

Residual or recurrent symptoms due to peridural fibrosis after spinal surgery may be due to compression of the nerve root by fibrotic tissue, constriction, tethering, or probably most importantly, ischemia (7). The amount of fibrosis will certainly vary from one individual to another, for reasons that are not yet clear. Nonetheless, there is good evidence now (8–10) to suggest a statistically significant relationship between the extent of peridural fibrosis and symptoms, specifically recurrent radicular pain and activity-related pain ($P = 0.02$). The correlation is not particularly close; the severity of clinical symptoms often proving very different for comparable degrees of fibrosis when assessed radiologically. Gadolinium diethylenetriamine (Gd-DTPA)-enhanced magnetic resonance imaging (MRI) is regarded by many now as the gold standard for assessment of peridural fibrosis (9,11,12).

Perhaps as a consequence of the imprecise correlation at first inspection between the radiologic extent of fibrosis and clinical symptoms, some clinicians may cast doubt on whether the problem really exists. The evidence, of course, is there and such arguments are rarely taken beyond the hypothetical. In the surgical environment the same clinicians, mindful of the possibility of peridural fibrosis, will adopt surgical techniques with the aim of reducing the risk and extent of scarring (13–15).

Careful surgery is undoubtedly a sensible precaution, and should involve minimal muscle stripping and trauma and the use of minimally invasive techniques. Within the canal the nerve roots and dura should be handled gently, where possible preserving the epidural fat and avoiding unnecessary damage to peridural structures, particularly, for example, the periradicular venous plexus (7). The surgeon should ensure meticulous hemostasis and utilize lavage periodically, particularly at the end of the procedure, to remove residual blood and debris. Consideration may be given to the use of local or systemic antiinflammatory agents (16). However, while these various surgical techniques are now widely adopted, it is frustrating that peridural fibrosis remains a problem.

Recognizing that fibrosis originates from the migration of fibroblasts derived from overlying detached muscle, many surgeons attempt to create a barrier to fibroblastic migration using a free fat graft (17). There is a small risk associated with this technique from migration of the fat graft, which can result in radicular symptoms or even a cauda equina syndrome (18,19). This risk, although small, must be considered against whatever benefits might be gained from free fat grafts. Several studies certainly cast doubt on these benefits. While fat graft techniques may perhaps reduce adhesions between overlying muscle and dura, peridural fibrosis itself is not reduced (20–22). Other forms of purely physical barriers have been explored and tested. These have included mesh forms of Vicril, Dacron weaves, and other synthetic barriers such as Gelfoam sheeting (23). The lack of commercial marketing of these materials as products to reduce fibrosis attests to the fact that none has been found to be effective. Indeed, some, such as Gelfoam sheet, seem actively to promote fibrosis.

Surgical release after fibrosis has formed is not uncommonly attempted but is often unrewarding, providing only temporary benefit in many cases (3). It is suggested that segmental instability in the degenerative spine may promote fibrosis, as may a pseudarthrosis. Certainly, the combination of the two, as seen for example in a failed posterior lumbar interbody fusion, can be associated with awful scarring around the nerve roots and dura. In the more usual situation of clinically significant fibrosis following discectomy, there may perhaps be a role for stabilization of the affected motion segment at the time of any revision procedure, particularly if the patient's symptoms include back pain and there has been progressive disc degeneration. With this exception, surgical release of peridural fibrosis is probably best avoided (13,14).

Commercially available mechanical and biologically active barriers to fibroblastic ingrowth are now becoming available. Preclude is a relatively new addition to the market. It is a synthetic interposition barrier formed from expanded polytetrafluoroethylene. It is designed to be applied as membrane over the exposed nerve roots and dura. It has been tested in the canine model, with favorable results when compared both with free fat grafts and with nonimplanted controls (24). Preliminary studies of Preclude have also been undertaken in a small group of patients undergoing discectomy, with a significant reduction in peridural fibrosis on MRI evaluation when compared with controls (25). However, whether this is reflected in an improved clinical outcome has yet to be demonstrated in clinical studies. Currently, the only mechanical and biologically active barrier preparation to have been tested in controlled, randomized prospective clinical studies is Adcon-L. This product is derived from porcine gelatin, which is composited with a polyglycan ester in buffered saline. The gel is packaged in a syringe delivery system with an applicator to allow deposition of the gel beneath and over the root and dura. *In vivo*, Adcon-L is completely resorbed within 28 days.

Strip assay fibroblast cultures first demonstrated *in vitro* the barrier effect to fibroblastic ingrowth. Fibroblastic cultures on a permissive material showed no ingrowth across strips of the gel, even after 72 hours. Subsequent animal studies, using a rat laminectomy model in one (26) and a canine model in another (27), confirmed that the gel had the potential to significantly reduce peridural fibrosis. In place of the normally found dense fibrosis, surgical sites with Adcon-L were found at blind evaluation to be similar to nonsurgical sites, even after 26 weeks (Fig. 22.2).

As part of these animal studies the effect of blood at the surgical site was evaluated. Mixes of gel and blood in varying proportions were applied. With 50/50 proportions, and even with 75% blood mix, the gel was found to remain effective. This is clearly of importance since a completely bloodless field is a rare luxury, even where great care is taken to achieve hemostasis.

To establish whether this particular gel reduced peridural fibrosis in the surgical situation, and whether this was of clinical relevance, two prospective randomized multicenter studies were undertaken, one in Europe and one in the United States, evaluating patients following discectomy (28). The European study recruited 298 patients and the U.S. study 223. In both studies best current available care was compared with the same but with the added use of the gel at the end of the surgery. Masked MRI evaluation of the extent of fibrosis was performed together with independent and masked clinical assessment. Clinical evaluation was in the form of a visual analog pain scale, together with the Johns Hopkins activity-related pain score and the Roland Morris disability questionnaire. Any adverse events were also documented.

It is probably worth emphasizing initially what the studies *do not* show. The gel does not eliminate peridural fibrosis altogether. Rather, both studies demonstrated a clear

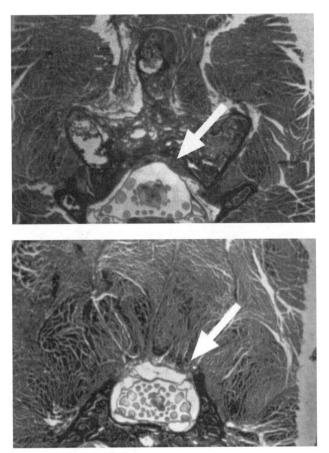

FIG. 22.2. Histologic cross-sections of rat laminectomy sites in a control model **(top)**. The arrow shows dense peridural fibrosis. Histologic cross-sections of rat laminectomy with barrier gel **(bottom)**. The arrow in this case shows a clear plane of separation.

reduction overall in the amount of fibrosis. When plotted graphically this is seen as a shift in the distribution in the treated groups toward less extensive fibrosis (Fig. 22.3). Most importantly, this was reflected in a significant improvement in clinical outcome, both in terms of residual pain and better functional capacity (Fig. 22.4). These effects were sustained between the 6- and 12-month reviews. Furthermore, experience in subsequent surgeries at sites where the gel had been used generally revealed far less scar tissue. This was reflected in shorter surgery times in revision cases, the mean time of 56 minutes for those in the Adcon-L group comparing favorably with 130 minutes for those in the control group.

While the effectiveness of a biologically active and mechanical barrier gel has been established in patients undergoing discectomy, questions remained concerning its use in other lumbar spinal procedures. To address these concerns an additional study has since been undertaken in 401 patients undergoing a range of lumbar spine surgery, including decompression for stenosis, decompression with posterior instrumented fusion, and posterior lumbar interbody fusion (PLIF) (29). Adcon-L was used in 288 patients while a separate 113 patients formed a control group. The gel does not appear to affect fusion

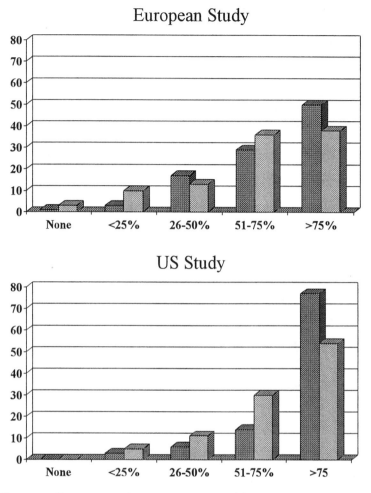

FIG. 22.3. The magnetic resonance image assessment of the extent of peridural fibrosis in the two studies (controls are dark gray; Adcon-L group is light gray). In each study there is a clear and statistically significant shift toward less extensive fibrosis with Adcon-L.

rates, with independent radiologic evaluation of fusion being 91.1% in the control group and 93.1% (no significant difference) in the Adcon-L group. No adverse consequences have been noted. Specifically, while some users have noted occasional pseudomeningocele developing after the gel has been used following spinal decompression, in this study pseudomeningocele was rare (0.7%) and the risk was not significantly greater than in controls. The incidence of peridural fibrosis has again been shown to be reduced in procedures such as spinal decompression and PLIF. In the control group the incidence of late onset sciatica attributed to peridural fibrosis, as shown on Gd-DTPA-enhanced MRI, was 19%. In contrast, in those in whom Adcon-L had been used the incidence was 3.6%, of which nearly half had undergone revision surgery. This difference was highly significant ($P < 0.001$).

Despite all this clinical evidence, the spinal surgeon might still be drawn to conclude that the potential advantages *to the surgeon* of using a barrier gel, in terms of easier revi-

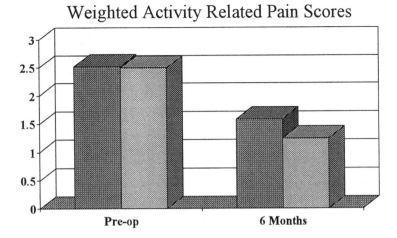

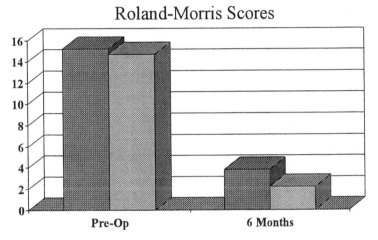

FIG. 22.4. The clinical evaluation of patients at 6 months after surgery without (dark gray) and with (light gray) Adcon-L. In both assessments the percentage of improvement from the preoperative baseline was significantly better in those in whom the gel had been used.

sion surgery, is not warranted in view of the relatively small numbers of patients requiring such surgery. However, this argument ignores the often greatly underestimated financial and human costs of persistent residual symptoms resulting from peridural fibrosis. The costs, in terms of the provision of additional medical care, will include long-term prescription medication, investigations such as MRI scans, and pain clinic procedures such as epidurals and root blocks. Increasingly, providers of medical care must also give consideration to the possibility of litigation. Patients are increasingly well informed and will expect, quite rightly, "state of the art" treatment, including measures to reduce complications, particularly where such measures are supported by sound clinical trials. However, the financial consequences of peridural fibrosis extend beyond the costs of medical care, and must take into account reduced working capacity and the secondary effects that this will have on patients, their families, their employers, and their requirements for benefits and social support services. Cost-benefit analysis undertaken in conjunction with

TABLE 22.1. *Some of the secondary effects of residual symptoms resulting from peridural fibrosis, with clear cost implications, as revealed in the economic survey undertaken in conjunction with the U.S. multicentered study*

	Adcon-L (%)	Control (%)
Considered surgery failure	8	13
Unable to return to work	6	15
Had to change job	6	9
Required prescription medication	12	18
Required additional medical treatment	27	34
Required hospitalization	8	10

the clinical studies of Adcon-L, some of the results of which are shown in Table 22.1, demonstrates convincingly that the additional expense of its use is far outweighed by the benefits of the consequent reduction in peridural fibrosis (30).

REFERENCES

1. Speccia N, Pagnotta A, Toesca A, et al. Fibrosis associated with lumbar disc herniation. Presented at: Second Annual Meeting of the Spine Society of Europe; October 2000.
2. Cooper RG, Freemont AJ, Hoyland JA, et al. Herniated intervertebral disc-associated periradicular fibrosis and vascular abnormalities occur without cell infiltration. *Spine* 1995;20:591–598.
3. Jonsson B, Stromquist B. Repeat decompression of lumbar nerve roots. A prospective two-year evaluation. *J Bone Joint Surg* 1993;75[B]: 894–897.
4. Annertz M, Jonsson B, Stomqvist B, et al. No relationship between epidural fibrosis and sciatica in the lumbar post-discectomy syndrome. A study with contrast enhanced magnetic resonance imaging in symptomatic and asymptomatic patients. *Spine* 1995;20: 449–453.
5. Cervellini P, Curri D, Bernadi L, et al. Computed tomography of epidural fibrosis after discectomy: a comparison between symptomatic and asymptomatic patients. *Neurosurgery* 1988;23:710–713.
6. Quebec Task Force Classification for Spinal Disorders and the Severity, Treatment and Outcomes of Sciatica and Lumbar Spinal Stenosis. *Spine* 1996.
7. Jayson MI. The role of vascular damage and fibrosis in the pathogenesis of nerve root damage. *Clin Orthop* 1992;279:40–48.
8. Ross JS, et al. Association between peridural scar and recurrent radicular pain after lumbar discectomy: MRI evaluation. *Neurosurgery* 1996;38:855–861.
9. Ross JS, Delamarter R, Hueftle MG, et al. Gadolinium-DTPA-enhanced MR imaging of the post-operative lumbar spine: time course and mechanism of enhancement. *Am J Roentgenol* 1989;152:825–834.
10. Ross JS, Obuchowski N, Zepp R. The post-operative lumbar spine: evaluation of epidural scar over a 1-year period. *Am J Neuroradiol* 1998;19:183–186.
11. Fan YF, Chong VF, Tan SK. Failed back surgery syndrome: differentiating epidural fibrosis and recurrent disc prolapse with Gd-DTPA enhanced MRI. *Singapore Med J* 1995;36:153–156.
12. Gundry CR, Fritts HM. Magnetic resonance imaging of the musculoskeletal system: the Spine. *Clin Orthop* 1998;346:262–278.
13. North RB, Campbell JN, James CS, et al. Failed back surgery syndrome: 5-year follow-up in 102 patients undergoing repeated operation. *Neurosurgery* 1991;28:685–691.
14. Gill K, Frymoyer JW. The management of treatment failures after decompressive surgery. In: Frymoyer JW, Ducker TB, et al., eds. *The adult spine: principles and practice*. New York: Raven Press, 1991:1849–1870.
15. Touliatos AS, Soucacos PN, Beris AE. Post-discectomy perineural fibrosis: comparison of conventional versus microsurgical techniques. *Microsurgery* 1992;13:192–194.
16. Hinto JL Jr, Warajcka DJ, Mei Y, et al. Inhibition of epidural scar formation after lumbar laminectomy in the rat. *Spine* 1995;20:564–570.
17. Mayfield FH. Complications of laminectomy. *Clin Neurosurg* 1976;23:435–439.
18. Prusick VR, Lint DS, Bruder WJ. Cauda equina syndrome as a complication of free fat grafting. A report of two cases and a review of the literature. *J Bone Joint Surg* 1988;70A:1256–1258.
19. Mayer PJ, Jacobson FS. Cauda equina syndrome after treatment of lumbar spinal stenosis with application of free autogenous fat graft. A report of two cases. *J Bone Joint Surg* 1989;71A:1090–1093.
20. Bryant MS, Bremer A, Nguyen T. Autogenic fat transplants in the epidural space in routine lumbar spine surgery. *Neurosurgery* 1980;13:367–370.
21. Lee C. Prevention of post-laminectomy scar formation. *Spine* 1984;9:305–312.

22. Martin-Ferrer S. Failure of autologous fat grafts to prevent postoperative epidural fibrosis in surgery of the lumbar spine. *Neurosurgery* 1989;24:718–721.
23. Nussbaum CE, McDonald JV, Baggs RB. Use of Vicril (polyglactin 910) mesh to limit epidural scar formation after laminectomy. *Neurosurgery* 1990;28:692–699.
24. DiFazio FA, Nichols JB, Pope MH, et al. The use of expanded polytetrafluoroethylene as an interpositional membrane after lumbar laminectomy. *Spine* 1995;20:986–991.
25. Mohsenipour I, Daniauz M, Aichner F, et al. Prevention of local scar formation after operative discectomy for lumbar disc herniation. *Acta Neurochir* 1998;140:9–13.
26. Wujek JR, Ahmad S, Harel A, et al. A carbohydrate polymer that effectively prevents epidural fibrosis at laminectomy sites in the rat. *Exp Neurol* 1991;114:237–245.
27. Einhaus SL, Robertson JT, Dohan FC Jr, et al. Reduction of peridural fibrosis after lumbar laminotomy and discectomy in dogs by a resorbable gel (ADCON-L). *Spine* 1997;22:1440–1446.
28. de Tribolet N, Porchet F, Lutz TW, et al. Clinical assessment of a novel antiadhesion barrier gel: Prospective, randomized, multi-center clinical trial of ADCON-L to inhibit post-operative peridural fibrosis and related symptoms after lumbar discectomy. *Am J Orthop* 1998;27:111–120.
29. Boeree NR. Can Adcon-L be used safely and to advantage in all forms of surgery for lumbar degenerative disease? Presented at: Combined Meeting of British Scoliosis Society and Nordic Spinal Deformity Society; April 2000.
30. McKinley D, Shaffer L. Cost effectiveness evaluation of ADCON-L adhesion control gel in lumbar surgery. *Neurolog Res* 1999;21[Suppl]:S67–S71.

New Treatment Modalities and Results

23

Microscopic Surgery Versus Classic Approaches

Björn Rydevik and Bengt Lind

Following the original observations by Mixter and Barr that lumbar disc herniation can cause sciatica and that this condition can be surgically treated, there has been a considerable interest in the management of this condition (11). The standard approach has been an open laminectomy/laminotomy and discectomy, but during the last 10 to 20 years, various alternative surgical techniques have been introduced such as microscopic discectomy, percutaneous nucleotomy, and endoscopic microdiscectomy. This chapter explores whether to use microscopic surgery or classic open discectomy for the treatment of lumbar disc herniation.

ADVANTAGES AND DISADVANTAGES OF THE MICROSCOPE

The surgical microscope has been a well-known tool in neurosurgical management of intracranial tumors and vascular disorders (8). In spine surgery, there has been a gradual introduction of magnification and illumination in terms of using loupes and headlights as well as surgical microscopes. The surgical microscope is superior to loupes for many reasons (Table 23.1). The most important reason is that the surgeon can maintain stereopsis (three-dimensional viewing). Thus, the ability to see the depth in a small wound while maintaining three-dimensional vision requires the use of a microscope.

However, there are some disadvantages in using the microscope. It is also important to point out that the technical advantage of using the microscope may not improve the clinical outcome following lumbar discectomy. Only a small proportion of the surgical success depends on technique; more important is good clinical evaluation leading to proper patient selection for surgery.

One of the limitations when using the microscope is the limited peripheral vision. If the surgical procedure needs to be expanded outside the field of vision, the surgeon has to stop operating and move the microscope. Also, small wounds leave very little room for visualization which requires that the surgeon use instruments which are narrower and longer than standard so that the operating hand can be kept out of the field. Some surgeons believe that the loss of hand–eye coordination creates a problem. As with all surgical techniques, there is a learning curve and the improved vision and the higher resolution will require that the surgeon get accustomed to this new dimension of intraoperative surgical anatomy.

BLEEDING AND INFECTION

Even a small amount of bleeding into the limited operative field under a surgical microscope can interfere with visualization and impair the surgical procedure. Therefore,

TABLE 23.1. *Advantages of the microscope over loupes*

	Loupes	Microscope
Magnification	Fixed and limited in extent	Relatively unlimited and changeable
Illumination	Not parallel to line of vision (paraxial)	Parallel to line of vision (coaxial) and stronger
Deep three-dimensional vision	Limited with less than 65-mm skin incision	Maintained with 25-cm skin incision
Patient size	The larger the patient, the bigger the wound required	Neutralized (every patient is made the same size by the optics)
Teaching	Assistants excluded	Assistants included
Surgeon's neck	Fixed in flexion and requiring repositioning	Spared

(From McCulloch JA. Focus issue on lumbar disc herniation: macro- and microdiscectomy. *Spine* 1996; 21:45S–56S, with permission.)

efforts in preoperative preparation (i.e., stopping nonsteroidal antiinflammatory medication, selection of a spine table, proper patient positioning on the table, and intraoperative control of bleeding) are cornerstones in the surgical management of disc herniation (9,10).

There have been reports of increased rate of disc space infection following microsurgical discectomy, most likely because of the microscope being positioned directly over the surgical wound (16). The microscope is draped with sterile coverage, but there are still some parts that are exposed, for example the eyepieces, which potentially can contribute to wound contamination. The limited operating space between the microscope and the wound can introduce another potential risk in that the surgical technique can be impaired with a risk for wound contamination and infection. Consequently, proper surgical technique and avoidance of contamination of the wound by touching nonsterile parts of the microscope are essential to prevent postoperative infection.

MICROSCOPIC DISC SURGERY: CLINICAL CONSIDERATIONS

McCulloch has stated that "the hidden benefit of the microscope is the more disciplined thinking it forces from the surgeon" (9). When using the microscope the surgeon cannot operate according to the technique of "seek and find;" the pathology to be found and its exact location must be known precisely before the limited skin incision is made.

In microsurgical discectomy a few technical problems are likely to occur and should be identified. When the wound is reduced in length, the surgeon does not have the ability to count the vertebrae from the sacrum for level identification. Thus, there is a risk for exposure at the wrong level in microsurgical discectomy. The use of an image intensifier or a lateral radiograph to localize the correct interspace should therefore be considered. If, during the operation, the surgeon does not find the pathology as seen on computed tomography or magnetic resonance imagine, surgery at the wrong level should be considered and an intraoperative radiograph obtained.

It is imperative to apply proper planning before surgery. As already pointed out, it is very important to recognize the pathology before it is encountered. It is also important to keep in mind that with a deep wound of about 1 inch in length, the use of force on the surgical instruments may create a risk for penetration into a spina bifida with resultant cauda equina damage or through the disc with risk for damage of the anterior vascular structures, the bowel, or the genitourinary system (1,6).

A large number of articles in the literature describe technical aspects of microdiscectomy (2–4,9,15). The patient should preferably be in the kneeling position under general anesthesia. The microscope is usually set up for approximately for 6 to 10 times magnification and an incision of the skin of approximately 2 to 3 cm is made, centered over the interlaminar interval to be exposed, preferably identified by radiographic technique (9). The purpose of the surgical procedure is to leave the nerve root freely mobile. In general, the microsurgical discectomy can be regarded as one type of open discectomy, where the microscope provides good illumination and magnification. Thus, the basic concept of nerve root decompression and disc fragment removal is a common denominator for all surgical types of open discectomy.

RESULTS FOLLOWING MICROSCOPIC DISCECTOMY VERSUS CLASSIC APPROACHES

Only three clinical trials (5,7,13) with data from 219 patients, comparing microscopic discectomy with standard discectomy have been found in the literature (12). The data in these trials regarding outcomes indicate no difference in the clinical results. Use of the microscope lengthened the surgical procedure, but did not appear to make any significant difference regarding perioperative bleeding or other complications, length of inpatient stay, or formation of scar tissue (14). In the study by Tullberg and coworkers, 60 patients were operated on by the same surgeon and randomized to microscopic discectomy or standard discectomy (13). Follow-up was performed by an independent observer at 3 weeks, 2 months, 6 months, and 1 year. The results showed that there was a somewhat longer surgical time with the microscope ($P < 0.01$) but no differences regarding perioperative bleeding, complications, inpatient stay, time lost from work, and clinical results. Tullberg and coworkers conclude that "the decision to use the operating microscope may be left to the surgeon, because it had no effect on the short-term results or those at 1 year" (13).

In a recently published extensive review, using evidence-based medicine technique, Nachemson and Jonsson compiled available data in the literature regarding the scientific evidence of causes, diagnoses, and treatment of neck and back pain (12). Levels of scientific evidence are graded from level A (highest) to level D (lowest). These are reviewed in Table 23.2. In the Nachemson and Jonsson text, Waddell and coworkers conclude that "There is strong evidence (strength of evidence A) that microdiscectomy and standard discectomy give broadly comparable clinical outcomes. In principle, the microscope provides better illumination and possibilities for teaching. These trials suggest that use of the microscope lengthens the operative procedure but despite previous claims, they did not show any significant difference in perioperative bleeding, length of inpatient stay, or the formation of scar tissue (strength of evidence B). However, it is not possible to draw any

TABLE 23.2. *Levels of scientific evidence according to Nachemson and Jonsson, 2000*

A. Support from metaanalysis or systemic review of good quality of two or more studies.
B. Support from one or more randomized controlled trials or good observational studies.
C. Insufficient or inconclusive evidence (no or poor randomized controlled trials or observational studies).
D. No acceptable scientific support from available studies.

(From Nachemson AL, Jonsson E. *Neck and back pain. The scientific evidence of causes, diagnosis and treatment.* Philadelphia: Lippincott, Williams & Wilkins, 2000, with permission.)

firm conclusions about complication rates from these trials (strength of evidence C) (14)."

CONCLUSION

Open discectomy can be performed in different ways in terms of the degree of magnification and illumination. The surgeon may choose to operate with the use of a microscope, with the use of surgical loupes, or without any magnification. All these three types of surgical discectomy should be regarded as different variations of open discectomy. The microsurgical technique may facilitate the procedure but will most likely not improve the overall success rate. Therefore, the choice of surgical technique should be based on the surgeon's preference. Other factors such as careful preoperative patient evaluation/selection and correct indications for surgical intervention are of utmost importance in the management of patients with lumbar disc herniation and sciatica.

REFERENCES

1. Anda S, Aakus S, Skaanes KO, et al. Anterior perforations in lumbar discectomies. *Spine* 1991;16:54–60.
2. Barrios C, Ahmed M, Arrotegui J, et al. Microsurgery versus standard removal of the herniated lumbar disc. *Acta Orthop Scand* 1990;61:399–403.
3. Caspar W, Campbell B, Barbier DD, et al. The Caspar microsurgical discectomy and comparison with a conventional standard lumbar disc procedure. *Neurosurgery* 1991;28:78–87.
4. Delamarter RB, McCulloch JA. Microdiscectomy and microsurgical laminotomies. In: Frymoyer JW, ed. *The adult spine: principles and practice*, 2nd ed. Philadelphia: Lippincott-Raven Publishers, 1996.
5. Henrikson L, Schmidt V, Eskesen V, et al. A controlled study of microsurgical versus standard lumbar discectomy. *Br J Neurosurg* 1996;10:289–293.
6. Kardaun JW, White LR, Shaffer WO. Acute complications in patients with surgical treatment of lumbar herniated disc. *J Spinal Disord* 1990;3:30–38.
7. Lagarrigue J, Chaynes P. Comparative study of disk surgery with or without microscopy: a prospective study of 80 cases [in French]. *Neurochir* 1994;40:116–120.
8. Lang WH, Muchel F. *Zeiss microscopes for microsurgery*. Berlin: Springer-Verlag, 1981.
9. McCulloch JA. Focus issue on lumbar disc herniation: Macro- and microdiscectomy. *Spine* 1996;21:45S–56S.
10. McNulty SE, Weiss J, Azad SS, et al. The effect of prone position on venous pressure and blood loss during lumbar laminectomy. *J Clin Anesth* 1992;4:220–225.
11. Mixter WJ, Barr JS. Rupture of the intervertebral disc with involvement of the spinal canal. *N Engl J Med* 1934;211:210–215.
12. Nachemson AL, Jonsson E. *Neck and back pain. The scientific evidence of causes, diagnosis and treatment*. Philadelphia: Lippincott, Williams & Wilkins, 2000.
13. Tullberg T, Isacson J, Weidenhielm L. Does microscopic removal of lumbar disc herniation lead to better results than the standard procedure? Results of a one-year randomized study. *Spine* 1993;18:24–27.
14. Waddell G, Gibson JNA, Grant I. Surgical treatment of lumbar disc prolapse and degenerative lumbar disc disease. In: Nachemson AL, Jonsson E, eds. *Neck and back pain. The scientific evidence of causes, diagnosis and treatment*. Philadelphia: Lippincott, Williams & Wilkins, 2000.
15. Williams RW. Microlumbar discectomy: a 12-year statistical review. *Spine* 1986;11:851–852.
16. Wilson DH, Harbaugh R. Microsurgical and standard removal of the protruded lumbar disc: a comparative study. *Neurosurgery* 1981;8:422–427.

24

Lumbar Posterior Endoscopic Microdiscectomy: Indications, Technique, and Midterm Results of the First 100 Consecutive Patients

M. Brayda-Bruno

Percutaneous approaches to lumbar discs by a posterolateral entry point date back to 1964, when the use of chymopapain for nucleolysis was first reported (10). In the ensuing years, percutaneous lumbar disc surgery evolved from using manual instruments (7) to the use of automated devices (8) to spinal endoscopy (9) and to that of laser surgery (4), the center of the disc always being approached by a paraforaminal route. None of these methods have proven to be as routinely effective as standard open lumbar disc surgery, especially when a bony or ligamentous pathology is associated to the discopathy, and these are still specific contraindications to percutaneous lumbar discectomy. The real indications for these procedures have generally been limited to contained lumbar disc herniations, and their clinical results are not far indeed from those obtained by any specific and correct conservative treatments.

In the early 1980s, there was a progressive use of the microscope for disc herniation surgery (3), with a less invasive approach and a shorter postoperative recovery of the patient. This technique is still widely used. In the last few years, however, some surgeons matching the microsurgical technique by a midline posterior approach together with modern endoscopic technology developed new systems for endoscopic posterior discectomy, either by a conic "free-hand" working channel (the Endospine by Destandeau) (5) or by a tubular retractor (the MicroEndoscopic Discectomy [MED] system introduced by Foley and Smith in 1996), with preliminary series available at the end of 1997 (6).

The latter technique appears to be very versatile and complete, with a high success rate, and it is still in constant evolution and improvement with the METR'x system. It is a true endoscopic "through-a-tube" surgery that allows for successful removal of disc and/or bony pathology that is compressing the nerve root, similar to open approaches. A small skin incision is made resulting in less disruption of the fascia and the paraspinous muscles which reduces, at a minimum, any postoperative backache. For these reasons, METR'x greatly lowers the average hospital stay for routine lumbar discectomy, and in some conditions it can be an outpatient procedure.

NOTES OF SURGICAL TECHNIQUE

METR'x can be performed under general anesthesia (preferable in the first period of experience), or under epidural anesthesia, which we use periodically to cancel the side effects of general anesthesia (such as postoperative nausea) or in outpatient procedures.

The typical and more common operative position is the "prone" one, with the abdomen free and the spine flexed to open the interlaminar space (i.e., on the Wilson frame), but we prefer a true "genu-pectoral" position, with hip and knee flexed, to maximally reduce the lumbar lordosis. Another position that we often use is the "lateral" decubitus.

The operating room should be equipped with a C-arm fluoroscope, its monitor, and the video equipment for the endoscope. The surgeon stands on the side of the patient ipsilateral to the herniated disc. A flexible arm assembly is attached to the operating table rail; this device holds the tubular retractor with endoscope in a stable position, freeing the surgeon's hands (Fig. 24.1).

The lumbar midline is identified. At 1.0 to 1.5 cm on the side of the herniation, under C-arm control, a spinal needle is inserted, identifying the appropriate disc space.

A small skin incision is made and a guidewire is then advanced through the lumbodorsal fascia, directed toward the inferior edge of the superior lamina. Under fluoroscopic guidance (Fig. 24.2), three or four cannulated, progressive soft tissue dilators are inserted over the guidewire, creating a dilation of the muscular fibers, leaving intact the fascia and the normal muscular attachments to the spinous process and to most of the lamina. The tubular retractor is advanced over the final dilator and down to the lamina, and then connected to the flexible arm assembly to maintain its position. The endoscope is connected to the coupler/camera and the light source, it is then inserted into the tubular retractor and fixed with a ring clamp. This allows the endoscope to be positioned anywhere around the tubular retractor (Fig. 24.3).

Proper image orientation is needed and in the METR'x system this is easily obtained by rotating a small notch that appears on the screen and corresponds to the endoscope position. Standard instruments for microdiscectomy (rongeurs, Kerrison punch, curettes, bipolar forceps) are then used. For bone excision, a high-speed drill (Med-Nex or Midas-Rex) with long, special tips is used, or in absence of this, a thin and long osteotome (4 mm × 200 mm) can be employed.

The inferior edge of the superior lamina is identified using a curette, and residual soft tissues are removed, achieving hemostasis with a modified bipolar forceps. A small

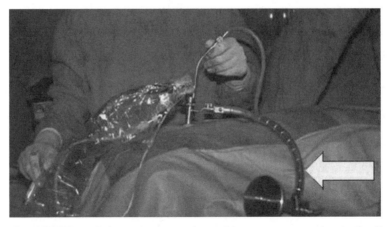

FIG. 24.1. The METR'x technique can be performed by one surgeon due to the flexible arm that holds tube and endoscope (*arrow*).

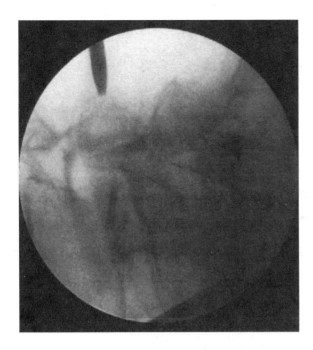

FIG. 24.2. C-arm control of the correct positioning of the dilator on the inferior edge of the L5 lamina, in order to prepare the working tube insertion.

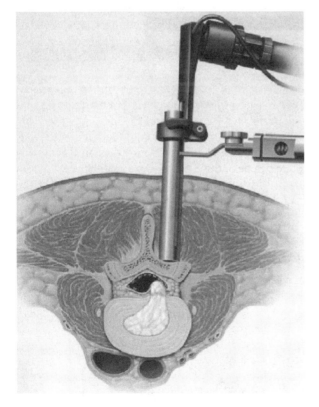

FIG. 24.3. The final position of the working tube with the endoscope, before flavectomy.

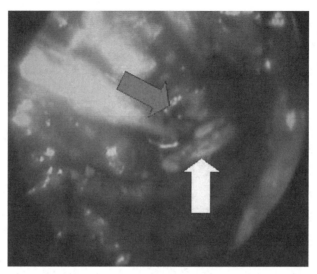

FIG. 24.4. Operative image with suction retractor on the dural sac (*dark arrow*) and the disc herniation (*white arrow*) before removal.

laminotomy and/or minimal facetectomy is performed using a Kerrison punch. In this fashion, adequate bone removal can be obtained to address disc pathology as well as lateral recess and/or foraminal stenosis. Flavectomy is then made, the dural sac exposed, and the nerve root identified. This is explored, retracted medially, and protected with a modified retractor (Fig. 24.4).

The herniated disc is then removed with various pituitary rongeurs in the same fashion of a standard open microdiscectomy. In case of lateral or central stenosis, a wide segmental monolateral laminotomy can be performed ("recalibrage").

By loosening the flexible arm, the tubular retractor can be repositioned in a more convenient way by "wanding" the tube, pivoted within the small skin incision. Using this maneuver, access from pedicle to pedicle can be accomplished through the initial 15-mm skin opening, acting into an inverted cone of work. When the new position is reached, the flexible arm is tightened again, holding the tube in place.

More technical details and techniques can be found in other publications (2,6).

MATERIALS AND METHODS

The first 100 consecutive patients who underwent a MED-METR'x procedure from November 1997 to April 2000 have been studied. The patient population consisted of 56 men and 44 women, between the ages of 21 to 77 years (mean age 40.8), with a mean follow-up of 18 months (minimum 9 months; maximum 35 months).

The disc levels most commonly operated on were L4-L5 (50 patients) or L5-S1 (46), with three cases at L3-L4 and 1 at L2-L3. Most of the disc herniations were intracanalar (11 median, 52 paramedian, 32 lateral), while only five were far lateral or extraforaminal. No significant difference was observed regarding the side: 44 were on the right side and 56 were on the left. More than 40% of these disc herniations were free fragments (Fig. 24.5), while the others were protruded.

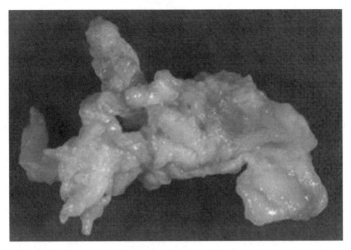

FIG. 24.5. Example of a 3.5-cm free fragment removed through the 1.6-cm working tube of METR'x.

The surgery was performed under general anesthesia in genu-pectoral position in 80 cases. The remaining 20 were done in lateral decubitus with epidural lumbar anesthesia. Mean duration of surgery was less than 1 hour (minimum 35 minutes; maximum100 minutes).

CLINICAL RESULTS

Our clinical results have been very encouraging, similar to those of other previous series (1,6). Among the 100 patients, using modified MacNab criteria and an SF-36 evaluation protocol, good to excellent results have been recorded in 85% of cases, and poor or bad outcomes in only 15%. Of these, 7 patients still experienced some persistent sciatica and eight presented low back pain. However, on a global analysis, 93 patients out of 100 had substantial relief of their radiculopathy.

Especially in the last periods, we have addressed not only true, simple disc herniations, but we have often found some associated spine pathologies. In most of the cases, a concomitant lateral recess and/or central stenosis was present (21 cases), while one patient had a grade 1 spondylolisthesis at the same level and another had a herniation at the first mobile disc, caudal to a spinal fusion.

We have also performed a METR'x technique in some recurrent disc herniations (12 cases), with very good results but some technical difficulties. Three of them were recurrences after MED surgery and the revision was easier than those performed on the hard scar of an open discectomy.

The rate of complications was very low, with five small intraoperative cerebrospinal fluid leaks that did not require any open conversion. We have converted the endoscopic approach in an open microsurgery in four cases (one large L3-L4 central herniation, two very severe central stenoses, and one revision).

We generally discharge patients within 12 to 18 hours after surgery, with prescription of home rest for few days with a lumbar soft brace for 1 week. Because of the negligible muscle disruption significant postoperative low back pain is seldom reported and immediate mobilization of the trunk and lower limbs can be started. Return to work ranges from 6 to 20 days in the noncompensated population (mean: 10 days) and from 14 to 90 days among workers who receive compensation (45% of cases, mean: 42 days).

DISCUSSION AND CONCLUSIONS

METR'x combines standard lumbar microsurgical techniques with endoscopy, and its reliability and versatility has been confirmed, especially in comparison to similar recently proposed systems for a percutaneous approach to the spine. We actually perform 98% of our surgeries for disc pathology by METR'x because it enables the surgeon to successfully address free fragments as well as various posterior lumbar pathologies of the disc, the canal (lateral or segmental stenosis), and bony structures (lamina, facet joint, foramen). With the advantage of a smaller incision and less tissue trauma than standard open microdiscectomy, it is possible to obtain an inverted "cone" of work, moving the tubular retractor with fulcrum on skin and lumbar fascia. The efficacy of all these maneuvers is enhanced by the deep direct observation–magnification and the possible oblique visualization by means of the 25-degree angled endoscope, which can be turned around the tube as needed.

The benefits of this procedure are a very short hospital stay, possibly on an outpatient basis, and a very quick patient recovery due to the minimal muscle and soft tissue disruption, absence of subperiosteal stripping, and negligible blood loss. Last but not least, the very small skin incision generally has an excellent long-term cosmetic outcome.

Among the disadvantages of this technique there are the bi-dimensional vision, as is true with any endoscopic surgery, and a possible longer duration of surgery, particularly at the beginning of the learning curve. For these reasons, we believe that a specific skill in microsurgery and in endoscopic approaches is the best basis from which to begin the experience with METR'x. It is also advisable to start with herniated free fragments in younger patients, and only later on to treat older patients with an associated bony pathology.

In conclusion, METR'x is a unique approach to the surgical management of lumbar disc disease, and it is a comprehensive system for endoscopic posterior spinal microsurgery. The improved micro-instruments (black and glare-resistant, curved bipolar, suction–retraction) and the better image resolution with the new reclavable endoscope allow even easier and safer surgery, as we have experienced in our last 32 cases.

REFERENCES

1. Brayda-Bruno M, Cervellini P, Cinnella P, et al. Microendoscopic posterior lumbar discectomy (MED). Indication and preliminary clinical results of the Italian Multicenter Group Trial. In: Le Huec JC, Husson JL, eds. *Endoscopic and minimal invasive spine surgery*. Montpellier, France: Sauramps Medical, 1999:i–iv.
2. Brayda-Bruno M, Cinnella P. Posterior endoscopic discectomy (and other procedures). *Eur Spine J* 2000;9[Suppl 1]:S24.
3. Caspar W. A new surgical procedure for lumbar disc herniation causing less tissue damage through a microsurgical approach. *Adv Neurosurg* 1977;4:74.
4. Choy DSJ, Case RB, Fielding W, et al. Percutaneous laser nucleolysis of lumbar discs. *N Eng J Med* 1987;317:771.
5. Destandeau J. A special device for endoscopic surgery of lumbar disc herniation. *Neurol Res* 1999;21:39.
6. Foley TK, Smith MM. MicroEndoscopic Discectomy (MED): surgical technique and initial clinical results. Paper presented at: 12th Annual Meeting of the North American Spine Society; October, 1997; New York City.
7. Hijikata S, Yarngislii M, Nakayama T, et al. Percutaneous discectomy: a new treatment method for lumbar disc herniation. *J Toden Hosp* 1975;5:5.
8. Onik G, Helms CA, Ginsberg L, et al. Percutaneous lumbar discectomy using a new aspiration probe. *Am J Roentgenol* 1985;144:1137.
9. Schreiber A, Suezawa Y. Transdiscoscopic percutaneous nucleotomy in disc herniation. *Orthop Rev* 1986;15:75.
10. Smith L. Enzyme dissolution of the nucleus pulposus in humans. *JAMA* 1964;265:137.

25

Sole Discectomy After Lumbar Disc Herniation: Is It Always a Sufficient Treatment? New Aspects by a Dynamic Neutralization System

Dieter Adelt

Unsatisfactory postoperative outcome following nucleotomies are a well-known problem in spine surgery. Grumme states in his textbook *Komplikationen in der Neurochirurgie* (3) that *post*operative instability is the cause of the failed back syndrome in 1% to 3% of all patients undergoing disc surgery and 10% of patients who say they are "not satisfied" after surgical treatment. It is expected that the frequency of *pre*operative existing instability is at least as common. In these cases the disc herniation is just the obvious start of a degeneration of the spine segment, and therefore, the sole nucleotomy cannot be the entire treatment of the disease.

Figure 25.1 depicts the frozen section of the lumbar segment of L4-L5 and L5-S1 in the final state of degeneration in a 70-year-old man (7). This patient had a history of long-standing low back pain, due to the severely degenerated lower lumbar spine. The L4-L5 disc shows loose fragments, complete destruction of the cartilaginous endplates, vacuoles and calcification, and anteriorly projecting osteophytes (spondylosis ridges). The posterior annulus occupies the lower half of the foramen; the upper foramen portion is encroached on by redundant ligamentum flavum. The L4-L5 facet joint is subluxated due to loss of disc height and a pink-colored meniscoid synovial fold is caught in the upper joint space. At L5-S1 the cartilaginous endplates have partially fused, and the outermost annulus projects posteriorly and lies underneath the L5 root.

In the clinical daily routine, practitioners will observe patients in different "pre-stages" of this degenerative disease. Magnetic resonance imaging (MRI) investigations reveal similar conditions as the frozen picture section described in Figure 25.1, but in general, these are seen in younger patients in their fourth or fifth decade. In these patients, it is common to see osteochondrosis with Modic signs, arthrotic joints, and perhaps, arthrotic joints accompanied by space-occupying lesions such as synovial cysts or disc herniations. This occupying lesion is usually the problem to be solved in the short term, but the patient's more pressing problem is the need to repair the complete motion segment. The immediate need is the decompression of nervale structures, but such highly degenerated segments are treated by stabilization after decompression.

In a 3.5-year period from August 1995 to end of 1998, we fused approximately 220 patients with degenerated diseases of the lumbar spine (Table 25.1). Prior to this we used the Dynesys system. Presently, we have stabilized approximately 360 patients.

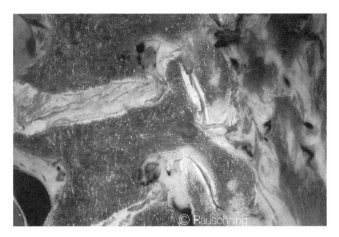

FIG. 25.1. Frozen section of a severely degenerated lower lumbar spine of a 70-year-old old man with a history of long-standing low back pain. (From Rauschning W. Anatomical demonstrations in the lumbosacral junction—a pictorial outline. In: Margulies JY, et al. *Lumbosacral and spinopelvic fixation.* Philadelphia: Lippincott-Raven, 1996, with permission.)

It was very interesting for us to see that 135 patients previously had undergone a disc operation, accounting for 61.4% of all of our fused patients. That means in reverse that the disc operation could not stop the patient's career in nearly two-thirds of the patients to be stabilized.

These findings are surprising when compared to what is reported in the literature concerning long-term follow-ups of disc surgery. Davis (1) examined 984 patients surgically treated for a herniated lumbar disc with a mean follow-up period of 10.8 years. He followed 98% of these patients and found just 30 patients with a pure result. Only three of these patients had any degenerative spine changes. Other causes were worker's compensation, legal claims, radiculopathy, psychological risk, or addiction. The recurrence rate of disc herniation was 6%.

In comparison, Pappas and colleagues (6) report on 655 surgically treated patients, of which a good outcome occurred in 80%. The recurrence rate was 11% among these individuals, but the follow-up period was only 9.7 months.

In 1996, our attention was drawn to the problem of disc recurrences. We often found special constellation beside the herniation, such as severe osteochondrosis, Modic changes at the endplates in MRI (4,5), or hypermobility in radiographs in flexion and extension. At later stages, we found patients with primary disc herniation who had a typical history or complaints, indicative of problems with instability or hypermobility.

TABLE 25.1. *Breakdown of 220 patients fused with degenerated diseases of the lumbar spine*

Diagnoses for spondylodesis (N = 220)	N =	%
Spondylolisthesis	72	32.5
Degenerative instability		
Osteochondrosis without disc herniation	23	10.5
Osteochondrosis after disc operation	85	38.6
Osteochondrosis with acute disc herniation	32	14.5
Spinal canal stenosis with signs of instability	8	3.6

Over a 3-year-period we followed 25 patients with herniations and signs of instability. Of the 25 patients, ten had a first herniation and 11 had recurrent herniations; six had two primary herniations and five had three or more primary herniations. All of these patients had additional signs of a painful segment with a constellation of osteochondrosis, Modic changes in MRI, or hypermobility. The surgeries performed included a discectomy and a fusion of the unstable segment. In 1997, we found that the patients with primary herniations had good results, while patients with recurrent herniations had only fair outcomes.

In recurrent herniations, patients seem to have a higher occurrence of severe degenerated segments than do patients with primary herniations. Osteochondrosis and Modic changes are found more often, giving rise to suspicions that instability is a reason for recurrent herniation. The more sensitive the practitioner is to patients' complaints, the more often primary disc herniation associated with hypermobility as the first sign of instability is found. At this point, it is not sufficient treatment to perform a sole discec-

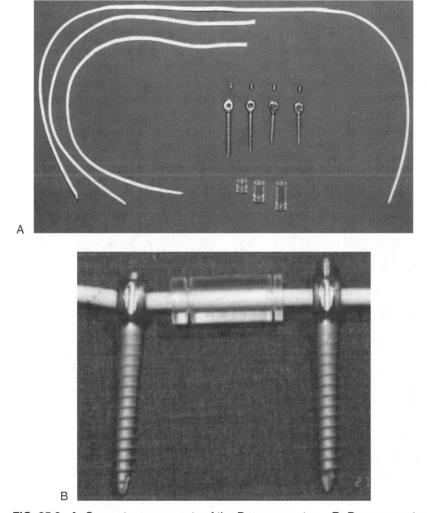

FIG. 25.2. A: Separate components of the Dynesys system. **B:** Dynesys system.

tomy. On the other hand, younger patients need to be treated (mean age in our series was 46.1 years), so one hesitates to do a fusion.

The dynamic neutralization system is a new philosophy for special degenerated spine diseases. It is a dynamic fixation system designed to restabilize motion segments and it allows:

1. A realignment of the posterior disc height and withholding of the posterior ligament and capsular articulation.
2. Realignment of the facets.
3. A controlled range of motion but suppression the discovertebral dyskinesis.

In 1991, Dubois created the idea of the system in France and performed his first surgery using the system in April 1994. The European launch was in 1999. We performed our first surgery with the system in Damp in August 1999 and have subsequently performed approximately 65 more such operations.

The Dynesys system is made up of three different components (Fig. 25.2).

1. Pedicle screws (Protasul-100): These screws anchor the system with the cord fixation. The screws are conical with a soft tip and are available in different sizes.
2. Cord (Sulene-PET): The cord is the connection of the pedicle screw heads, it is fixated with a preload that gives the system a homogeneous rigidity and absorbs tension forces.

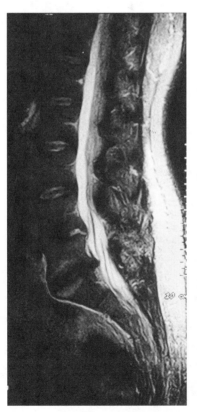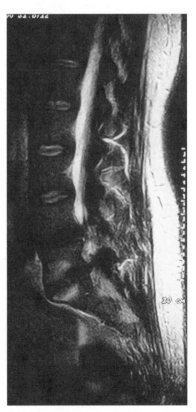

A   B

FIG. 25.3. Magnetic resonance image of a 49-year-old woman with two prior discectomies suffering from sciatica and backache.

3. Modular spacers (Sulene-PCU): The spacers restore the height of the disc space and relieve the facet joints.

An example for the clinical use of the Dynesys system can be found in the history of a 49-year-old woman who had two discectomies. The first was in 1992 at L4-L5 on the right side and the second was in 1999 at L5-S1 on the left side. In January 2000, she had a sciatica S1 on the left side. The MRI revealed scars and protrusions in both levels and also Modic signs in L5-S1. The sciatica was regressive but in only a few weeks the symptoms returned accompanied with severe back pain. In June 2000, we performed a discectomy at L5-S1 on the right side and a Dynesys at L4-L5 and L5-S1 (Fig. 25.3).

In another case, a 56-year-old man suffered more from claudication than from radicular problems. The myelography revealed a disc herniation and a congenital narrow spinal canal, obviously is the hypermobility in function (Fig. 25.4). We performed a decompression of that level and a Dynesys at L3-L4.

In 1999, Dubois published the first results of 57 patients treated with the Dynesys-system (2). None of the patients were lost in follow-up. The follow-up time was 1.5 years. At that time 63% of the patients were free of pain and 30% had only mild lumbago. The remaining 7% complained of serious backache. The intake of analgesics decreased post-

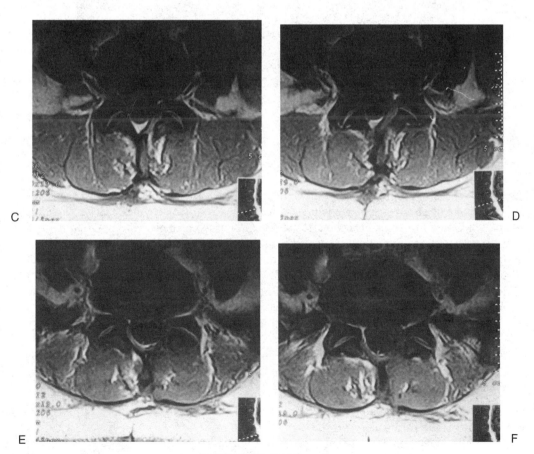

FIG. 25.3. *Continued.*

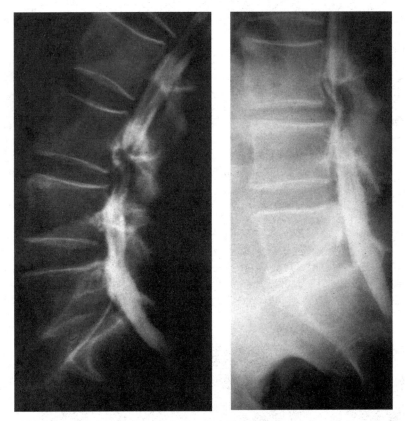

FIG. 25.4. Myelography of a 56-year-old man revealing disc herniation and severe hypermobility.

operatively, more than 85% of the population either do not take analgesics at all or only take them occasionally.

Our results 1 year after surgery are similar to those reported by Dubois. We examined 25 patients of 26 surgeries (one patient moved away from the area and was not included in the follow-up). We had excellent results on 65% of the patients, who reported no pain and had returned to their full work and activity capacity. We had fair results on 35% of the patients, who reported mild pain that did not cause limitations on everyday life, or new mild neurologic symptoms. We found two obvious worker's compensation problems in this group and five patients with sacroiliac joint problems or muscle problems. We found no patients with poor results, such as severe pain or severe neurologic deficits.

The results are promising but a longer follow-up period is mandatory. The early success of the surgery is associated with a decompression of the compressed nervale structures and that is no service of the system. The success is the loss of backache for a long period and the Dynesys system has to prove this problem. The advantages of the Dynesys system are:

1. It is not a destructive management procedure.
2. It treats the adjacent levels with care.
3. It allows later on every surgical procedure which is needed.
4. It provides physiologic support for the spine.

REFERENCES

1. Davis RA. A long-term outcome analysis of 984 surgically treated herniated lumbar discs. *J Neurosurg* 1994;80: 415–421.
2. Dubois G, de Germay B, Schaerer NS, et al. Dynamic neutralization: a new concept for restabilization of the spine. In: Szpalski M, Gunzburg R, Pope MH, eds. *Lumbar segmental instability.* Philadelphia: Lippincott Williams & Wilkins, 1999:233–240.
3. Grumme T, Kolodziecjzyk D. *Komplikationen in der neurochirurgie, wirbelsäulen-, schmerz- und nervenchirurgie,* vol 1. Berlin: Blackwell Wissenschafts-Verlag, 1994.
4. Modic M, Pavlicek W, Weinstein M, et al. Magnetic resonance imaging of intervertebral disk disease. *Radiology* 1984;152:103–111.
5. Modic M, Ross J. Magnetic resonance imaging in the evaluation of low back pain. *Orthop Clin North Am* 1991; 22:283–301.
6. Pappas CTE, Harrington T, Sonntag VKH. Outcome analysis in 654 surgically treated lumbar disc herniations. *Neurosurgery* 1992;30:862–866.
7. Rauschning W. Anatomical demonstrations in the lumbosacral junction—a pictorial outline. In: Margulies JY, et al. *Lumbosacral and spinopelvic fixation.* Philadelphia: Lippincott-Raven, 1996.

26

Soft Hardware for the Spine: OptiMesh— A Preview of Some Novel Tools and Methods for Manipulating and Stabilizing Bone Graft and Bone Graft Substitutes

Stephen D. Kuslich

This chapter introduces a new and promising technology for manipulating and stabilizing bone graft and bone graft substitutes. The basic innovations involve methods and tools to prepare cavities and to inject, contain, and retain bone graft or bone graft substitutes within a porous balloon. Utilizing certain physical characteristics of granular mechanical systems, the resulting balloon-graft construct then performs the stabilization functions normally carried out by more invasive hardware systems. The term, "soft hardware for the spine" has been coined to best convey the essence of our system.

This technology is the product of a 20-year program of research and development that sought to understand the nature of lumbar degenerative pain syndromes and their treatment by mechanical stabilization. Our methodology may be a useful strategy for several indications in spinal surgery, including interbody fusion and stabilization of vertebral compression fractures. Our goal was to develop a technology that would prove capable of effectively treating certain orthopedic and spinal conditions in a manner that was faster, easier, and safer than existing forms of management.

BACKGROUND

The diagnosis and treatment of low back pain is a complex subject. The symptoms may be caused by a variety of organic and nonorganic pathologies. No one possesses a complete knowledge of its origin, pathophysiology, natural history, or methods of cure. On the other hand, a nihilistic declaration of complete ignorance would be incompatible with the facts and disregard the substantial progress that has been made in the past few decades. Experienced spinal professionals know that, in spite of our lack of a complete understanding of the entire subject, we are usually able to arrive at a defensible diagnosis, and we are often able to provide effective treatment of symptoms, even if a complete cure remains out of our reach (Fig. 26.1).

A substantial body of evidence has convinced most practicing spinal surgeons that the degenerative disc is the most common causative agent. Evidence for the discogenic hypothesis is derived from multiple lines of investigation. The evidence includes:

• The common association of advanced disc degeneration with clinical symptoms.
• The presence of nociceptive nerve components in the annulus of degenerative discs.

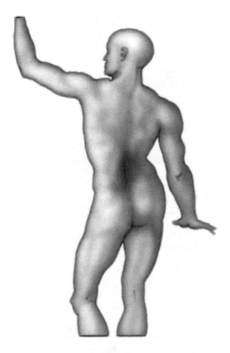

FIG. 26.1. Mechanical low back pain is one of the most common and most challenging conditions treated by spinal surgeons. The past decade has produced several new promising treatments. The most noteworthy of these has been the interbody fusion cages. Future advances are likely to be achieved in the arenas of prevention, disc replacement (either artificial or biological), or perhaps, less invasive methods of stabilization. This chapter deals with a novel approach that might prove effective for stabilization and/or perhaps, biological replacement.

- The ingrowth of new afferents into certain degenerating discs.
- The production of typical symptoms when the annulus is mechanically stimulated during surgery under local anesthesia.
- The elimination of symptoms when the disc tissue is blocked with local anesthesia.
- The elimination of symptoms when the motion segment is successfully stabilized by a variety of surgical techniques, even when that stabilization is less than absolutely rigid (Fig. 26.2).

The author and his collaborators, and many colleagues and competitors have developed a variety of methods for mechanically stabilizing the intervertebral disc. Various forms of surgical fusion are known to produce an amelioration of symptoms in appropri-

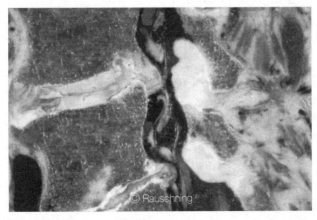

FIG. 26.2. Multiple lines of evidence implicate the degenerative disc as the primary source of mechanical low back pain.

ately selected cases. The use of bone graft, with and without instrumentation, is probably the most commonly employed technique. Recently, interbody fusion cages have been extensively employed for that purpose. The BAK (developed by Bagby and Kuslich) interbody fusion cage, and many other fusion cages, have been in wide use for more than 8 years. Short-, medium-, and long-term studies, involving hundreds of patients in carefully performed multicenter trials, proved their effectiveness. Success of the BAK, the Ray, and the Brantigan cages spawned a large number of other cage designs. While the results of these newer designs are less completely documented, and therefore less convincing, the author believes that they will prove to be similarly effective. It is now abundantly clear that success in this field of surgery depends more on careful case selection and surgical expertise, and less on the brand of cage used. Progress in the future will likely consist of faster, easier, and safer technologies, rather than the "invention" of different geometric shapes, different materials, or different surface features on "new" cages.

COMPONENTS OF OUR PROPOSED SOLUTION

During the mid-1980s, our research group began experimenting with a variety of methods for stabilizing and "fusing" the interbody space. Most of our attempts involved the development of a variety of rigid interbody cages. Time and space do not allow an exhaustive display of our prototypes and procedures, but in summary, we designed and tested a number of rigid or semi-rigid containers (in addition to the BAK) for interbody bone graft or bone graft substitutes. After several years and many dead ends as well as some substantial successes, our group realized that the geometric shape and material of the container of the graft might be less important than the nature of the graft itself (e.g., the graft shape, porosity, chemical and biological composition, and the degree to which it fills the cavity created by the removal of the degenerated disc). The rigidity and strength of the cage might also be less important than the "minimalness" of the exposure required for implantation, and the preservation of normal anatomic stabilizing structures.

Rather than attempting to answer the following questions:

• What is the strongest and largest possible container for interbody graft?
• What is most rigid possible construct?

We began to consider other questions:

• What is smallest, thinnest, least bulky, and least obtrusive device that might be used to contain and retain interbody graft?
• What procedure would produce the least collateral damage (e.g., the smallest exposure, the least destruction of anatomic biological stabilizers, the least amount of bleeding, the shortest operating time, the least postoperative swelling)?
• What procedure would lead to the fastest recovery?

Our answers to the latter set of questions constitute the discoveries and inventions that comprise the "OptiMesh system."

WHAT IS THE OPTIMESH SYSTEM?

The OptiMesh system consists of a series of new devices, new tools, and new methods for containing and/or retaining tissue graft or tissue graft substitutes within a defined space. That space may be any cavity existing in, or created in, any bone or joint or other bodily structure. The OptiMesh system, as outlined in several issued patents and pending patent applications, teaches the use of certain mesh containers, geometrically structured to hold the graft material within the confines of a three-dimensional space. One unique characteristic of our system is the ability to fill the mesh containers *within* the body cavity by first placing the unfilled mesh container into the cavity. This feature allows the surgeon to insert the mesh and its fill materials through very small entrance portals, thus limiting the surgical exposure and its resultant collateral damage.

The OptiMesh system includes several novel instruments for creating and filling cavities. The first instrument is an expanding reamer that allows the surgeon to create a cylindric, elliptic, or spheric cavity deep within a hard tissue structure—a cavity that is larger (up to 2.5 times larger) than the entrance hole through which the tool is placed. For instance, we are now able to enter the intervertebral disc through an 8- to 10-mm hole and then easily and rapidly create a cavity having a diameter of 22 to 25 mm within the disc. This capability was impossible before the invention of our reamer (Figs. 26.3 and 26.4).

The second novel instrument is our circumferential or peripheral resecting, reciprocating reamer that allows the surgeon to evacuate a toriodal-shaped (tire-shaped) cavity in bone or joint tissue. When this instrument is used in the disc space, after first evacuating the nuclear space with the expanding reamer, the resultant cavity will have a Saturn-like shape—a sphere with a tire around it. A cavity of this shape results when the surgeon removes the degenerated nucleus and the inner annulus and a millimeter or two of endplate, leaving the outer annulus. Such a shape would be ideal for creating an interbody fusion cavity.

The third novel instruments are our filling tubes. These tubes are long (10 to 25 cm) metal cylinders with thin rigid walls. They have a highly polished internal wall surface constructed with the appropriate internal diameters that permit graft material to be easily forced (by means of a piston) into the cavity at its distal end. After experimenting with various lengths and diameters, we settled on certain lengths and diameters that optimize the flow of graft material. In addition to straight tubes, we have a patent-pending design that permits the surgeon to direct fill material 90 degrees away from the main axis of the tube. This feature gives the surgeon the capability to direct the graft material in the direction required for intervertebral distraction, or to reduce the kyphosis produced by a compression fracture.

The forth novel instrument is our injection tube-loading tool. This tool allows the surgeon or their assistant to easily and quickly fill injection tubes with graft or graft substitutes.

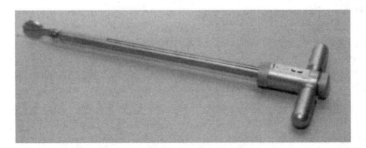

FIG. 26.3. The Spineology Group's expandable reamer provides the surgeon with the capability to remove the central portion of the disc and adjacent endplate through a very small entrance portal.

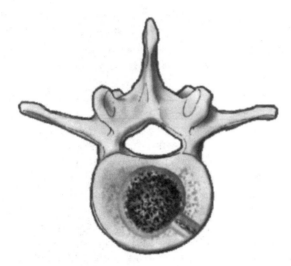

FIG. 26.4. The expandable reamer removes the central disc and overlying endplate. The resulting cavity can be up to 2.5 times the diameter of the entrance portal. The tool can be employed by any commonly used approach; anterior, anterolateral, lateral, posterolateral (TLIF), or direct posterior (laminotomy).

THE SCIENTIFIC BASIS FOR OPTIMESH SYSTEM TECHNOLOGY

A subspecialty of physics known as granular mechanics deals with the unique physical characteristics of granular materials. Granular materials consist of finely ground or morselized compounds such as sand, gravel, cereal grains, or bone graft particles. These materials exhibit certain unique physical characteristics. One especially useful characteristic of granular materials is their ability to change phase from liquid-like to solid-like. For instance, they sometimes "act" like solids (i.e., they can be rigid and "nonflowable"). On the other hand, they may "act" like liquids (i.e., they can be made to flow through tubes and through openings). The mode of behavior of granular materials is governed by several ambient circumstances including the size and shape and consistency of the granules, the degree of wetness of the granular pack, the pressure applied to the granular pack and the timing sequence of pressure application, and other factors.

The unique characteristics of granular materials can be useful to the spinal surgeon who is attempting to transport graft material into spinal cavities for the purpose of interbody fusion. For instance, if the proper tools and conditions are present, a surgeon is able to transport a volume of morselized bone graft through a small portal and into the interdiscal space. Once that space is filled, the further application of pressure can cause the morselized bone granular pack to change phase from a flowable liquid to a solid structure that is capable of withstanding compression loading without flowing back through the injection portal. The capabilities described earlier, when combined with our unique technology for creating large cavities through small portals, allows the surgeon to fill and stabilize the interbody space—in a manner similar to a rigid cage—but with much less surgical exposure and therefore less damage to nearby anatomy. We label our technology a "system" because it includes all of the tools and procedures necessary to fully utilize the unique and beneficial characteristics of granular materials: flowability, porosity, and eventual stability.

OptiMesh itself can be any porous balloon whose porosity restricts the passage or leakage of graft material while permitting the passage of liquids, ions, and cells, as well as the ingrowth and through-growth of blood vessels and trabecular bone (Figs. 26.5, 26.6, and 26.7). Thus far, we have developed mesh constructed from polymeric fibers

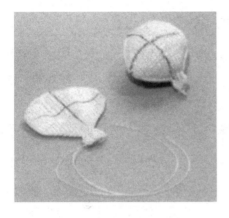

FIG. 26.5. The OptiMesh container is a hollow, porous container and retainer of bone graft or bone graft substitutes. This version consists of a woven polyester fabric. We have also patented, developed, and built containers by injection molding and weaving. We have tested several different materials including absorbable fibers and metal fibers.

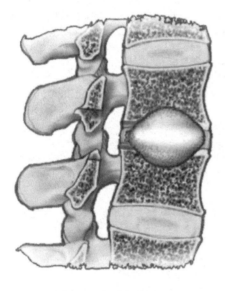

FIG. 26.6. When the OptiMesh container is inflated with graft material using sufficient pressure—a procedure that requires special proprietary instrumentation—the graft material changes phase from liquid to solid, but retains porosity. This expansion places tension on the annulus, and thereby develops improved segmental stability. Depending on the nature of the injected material, the motion segment might be stimulated to fuse by bony union, or a new fibrocartilaginous "biological disc replacement" could result.

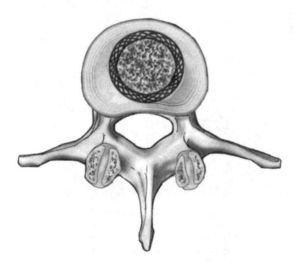

FIG. 26.7. A transverse section through a disc with a filled mesh in place. The OptiMesh does not function like a fusion cage (i.e., it does not hold the vertebral bones apart). Rather, it retains and contains the graft material, preventing flow out of the cavity and causes the graft to shift phase from liquid-like slurry to solid. The graft pack itself then performs the mechanical load-bearing function. That, together with the concomitant stretching of the annulus, provides a remarkable degree of segmental stability.

(absorbable and nonabsorbable) and metal fibers; and we have created containers by injection molding plastics.

MECHANICAL AND BIOLOGICAL TESTING

When we tested the OptiMesh system's ability to stabilize the motion segment, we found that while the graft-filled container was somewhat less rigid than a metal interbody cage, the annulus did tighten substantially, and the motion segment was therefore stabilized compared to the intact segment. The application of additional posterior stabilization in the form of pedicle fixation systems, trans-facet screws, or posterior tension bands would likely further improve stability.

Using a validated rabbit tibial defect model, we showed that our polymeric woven BAK did not create an inflammatory response, and it allows unimpeded bony union around and through the OptiMesh (Fig. 26.8).

Last year, we began an animal trial using the OptiMesh system for interbody fusion in the sheep model. Early results indicate that the system is capable of inducing stability and bony fusion at 6 months. We are currently studying the effects of various fill material within the containers including autograft, allograft, autogenous growth factor, BMP, marrow blood, and certain proprietary bioceramic granules.

We are currently testing the ability of our system to reduce and stabilize vertebral compression fractures by filling the OptiMesh with bone graft, bone graft substitutes, or bone cement. Early results are encouraging.

Finally, we are testing the utility of the OptiMesh system in the treatment of several common orthopedic conditions and problems such as tibial plateau fractures, avascular necrosis of the femoral head, cruciate ligament anchorage, and nonspinal joint arthrodesis.

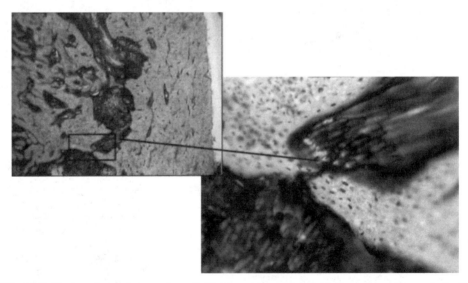

FIG. 26.8. These photomicrographs—**(left)** low power, **(right)** high power—demonstrate the unimpaired bony through-growth during this rabbit tibial osteotomy experiment. The dark filaments are the fibers of the OptiMesh container. Note that bone is growing through the porosities of the fabric. There is no apparent inflammatory or fibrous reaction to these polyester fibers.

THE FUTURE

After more than 3 years of intensive research and development, our system is almost ready for human use. We plan a careful introduction of the technology, starting with small numbers of patients treated by a group of experienced spinal surgeons. Interested surgeons should contact the author.

27

Prosthetic Disc Nucleus Implants: An Update

Charles D. Ray, Barton L. Sachs, Britt K. Norton,
Elizabeth Smith Mikkelsen, and Nan Clausen

Spinal surgeons continue to focus their attention on new directions and solutions for back pain caused by degenerative disc disease (DDD). Natural aging phenomena of the spine, or trauma, can produce physiologic deterioration of the disc leading to relative segmental spinal instability and subsequent anatomic structural changes and functional abnormality. As degeneration causes a loss in disc height, stabilizing spinal structures become lax, enabling relatively excessive, abnormal motion. Loss of disc height also leads to facet joint impingement on the nerve root foramen, and stretching of small nerves innervating the disc annulus. A bulge or herniation through the compromised annulus may also contribute to the patient's painful clinical symptoms. Further degeneration, as described by William W. Kirkaldy-Willis in *The Degenerative Cascade*, stabilizes, even fixates the segment, effectively stopping all practical motion and pain.

Contemporary medical or surgical treatment has yet to find the means to halt or reverse degenerative processes in the spine. The standard of care for many patients today involves fusing the spine to eliminate motion in the painful spinal segment. To accomplish fusion, devices or grafted bone permanently implanted in the spine maintain fixation of the spinal elements. Although normal spinal function is sacrificed, fusion is considered to be clinically successful when abnormal, painful motion is eliminated.

For many patients, a more acceptable surgical treatment solution would provide biomechanical stability and pain relief while preserving normal segmental spinal motion. The spinal disc provides flexibility while constraining motion to protect the adjacent spinal structures. The ideal treatment would have as its goal maintenance and augmentation of the natural spinal segment, its functions, and its structures while relieving pain to restore the patient's near-normal activities of daily living.

To offer surgical treatment options that better preserve spinal integrity, much research has focused on development of a prosthetic spinal disc that would serve to replace functions lost through degeneration and alleviate disabling pain. After many years of analysis, research, design, development, and testing, under direction of the senior author of this chapter (C.D.R.), the Raymedica prosthetic disc nucleus (PDN) was developed for use in cases of DDD in the human lumbar spine that fail to respond to conservative care. The intended role of the device is to replace the functions of the native nucleus pulposus. These functions include: separating and cushioning adjacent vertebrae; enabling appropriate deformation of the disc in spinal flexion and extension; responding to gravitational force with cyclic, diurnal volumetric changes that theoretically maintain the health of the disc through the supply of nutrients; and removal of waste byproducts. Designed with these natural functions in mind to restore spinal stability and preserve segmental motion, the PDN device offers a unique and novel solution to a costly, widespread, and debilitating health problem.

Implanted in pairs, each PDN device comprises a structural polymeric hydrogel constrained in a woven, high-strength polyethylene jacket. The two implants are tethered together and positioned transversely, side by side in the enucleated disc space. The dehydrated and mechanically compressed state of the hydrogel core of the implant at implantation, and the placement of two separate implants, reduces the volume and profile required to pass through the opening in the annulus. Once in the body, the hydrogel swells and absorbs fluid, restoring more normal biomechanics to the motion segment and surrounding structures. The fully hydrated implants provide resistance to deformation similar to that of an intact disc.

ANATOMY OF THE DISC

The intervertebral disc structure is a force-operated system, which is reflected in its structure viewed in cross-section. Much like the structure of an automobile tire, the outer annulus of the disc is made up of multiple plies or laminations. In the normal disc, there may be as many as 20 plies or circumferential layers, with the fibers inserted into the vertebral bodies above and below at roughly a 30- to 40-degree angle in both directions, binding the adjacent vertebrae together. This arrangement particularly resists dislocation and torsion (8,10).

Strong and flexible, but inelastic, type I collagen fibers make up the bulk of the annulus. Based on their material properties, these structures must be separated by another material that is both elastic and conformable—a gel, the same as that found in the disc nucleus. This gel, as the nucleus pulposus, is comprised of complex polysaccharide (sugar) and aminoglycans (protein) plus short collagen fibers. The nucleus pulposus serves the function of the air in the automobile tire analogy; that is, it keeps the annulus in tension and redistributes the considerable forces within the disc.

Primarily serving as a cushion, the intervertebral disc permits controlled motions between the vertebrae of the axial skeleton. Flexibility of surrounding soft tissues and ligaments, disc tissue, and facet joints plays the largest role in range of motion. Segments of the lumbar spine are most flexible in flexion–extension (approximately 11 degrees), have limited lateral bending (approximately 3 to 5 degrees), and are quite restricted in rotation (approximately 1 degree). Excessive rotation would pose the biggest structural threat to the spinal segment integrity (1,4,5,6).

Sources of Pain

Other than nerve pressure/tensions from disc herniation or stenoses, root entrapment in spondylolisthesis or facet arthralgia, fractures, or tumors, structural changes of the spine in and of themselves seldom produce symptomatic problems (12). In nearly all cases, it is the pain resulting from such changes that drives the spine–related disability in vulnerable patients. Aging, disease, or disorder can alter any of the body's tissues because they all have viscoelastic components (1,7,8,14,16,24). The degenerative process that ends in painful symptoms usually follows a pattern: as the nucleus loses its ability to retain water and loses disc height, the annulus buckles (1,14). Torsional delamination of the concentric plies begins and radial tears may occur. Normal biomechanics are compromised and the downward spiral of loss of function and pain is set in motion.

The central part of the disc comes under extreme pressure during exertion. Normal resting pressure in the nucleus at L5-S1 has been measured at about 0.5 MPa (about 75 psi); the pressure is more than tripled by exertion, especially hyperextension (8). The pressure is perhaps 50% higher still in discs that are degenerating, with loss of hydration and annular stiffening (1,8). This internal pressure prohibits vascularity of the inner annulus and nucleus, rendering their meager metabolism anaerobic. The pressure around the outer margin of the annulus, especially the outer six layers, is sufficiently low to allow for small arterioles and free nerve endings. These nerve endings are polymodal, meaning that they can be stimulated by stretch, thermal changes, or chemical events. Therefore, a progressive delamination of layers, separating as the result of degeneration, will apply traction to the free nerve endings and cause pain.

Many of the byproducts produced by anaerobic metabolism, as is the case inside the disc nucleus, are toxic to the aerobic structures. If a break or tear occurs in the annulus, the byproducts may reach the free nerve ending and cause severe pain. The pH (normally about 7.2) inside the degenerative nucleus is considerably more acid, perhaps as low as pH 6.8 (15). If this pH falls to 6.2, regeneration of the gel and inner annulus stops.

Mechanical irritation to free nerve endings of the outer annulus may also cause pain. Disc sensations, exclusively pain and pressure, are detected by small somatic nerves that encircle the annulus and penetrate the annular layers for a short distance (6 to 8 mm) (6). Pain may be initiated by shearing motions of a torn annulus, across which tiny nerve fibers must pass on their inward path, or by the escape of anaerobic metabolites of the nucleus to reach the polymodal, free-nerve endings or the nearby emerging root ganglion.

DISC REPLACEMENT CONSIDERATIONS

Functionality and biocompatibility place rigorous demands on device design and materials for a spinal disc replacement. Over the average human lifespan, the spine is subjected to an estimated 100 million cycles of motion, including minor ones such as in walking or breathing (9,11,13,24). The optimal lifetime for spinal implants is considered to be approximately 30 million cycles where 10 million is the fully loaded test minimum (11). These requirements present quite a challenge for implanted mechanical devices, since the elastic behavior of most elastomeric polymers will degrade, metals will wear, etch or be otherwise attacked, constant motion and stress will lead to metal fatigue, and wearing out cannot be repaired or replaced as can natural tissues (18).

Artificial disc devices have principally been designed by surgeons and most have had the sole purpose of replacing lost biomechanics. Early inventors largely took a pragmatic approach using "generic" construction concepts, whether or not the appropriate tested materials and fabrication methods were available at that time. Those designs were premised upon stopping all, or nearly all, of the six reciprocal degrees of motion of the spinal segment. Based on the idea that motion of the spine had to be dramatically decreased, hardware was developed. Early designs were more conceptual, to be reduced to any material (metal or polymer) with flexibility, and to any rubber material or metal spring. Considerably larger problems have been glossed over in many designs (e.g., attachment to bone, resistance to expulsion, tissue compatibility, mechanical failure modes, or longevity).

Many inventor/authors have not described in their patents the particular disc functions to be replaced or imitated. The lead author of this chapter (CDR) was one of the first to indicate the potentiality of a prosthetic nucleus, to restore nuclear function and to promote healing of the annulus (19–23). When he began development of an artificial disc, Dr. Ray decided that the device would not be attached at any point within the nucleus cavity, neither to the annulus nor to the bone, which could lead to fusion formation and was therefore not an option. His goal was to elevate the disc and tighten the annulus to restore functional stability to the spinal segment. Also, he planned that the device would swell and shrink by approximately 20% at each level, elevating the disc space 1 to 1.5 mm under the diurnal loading cycle to mimic the natural function of the disc.

The Raymedica prosthetic disc nucleus has shown a reasonable ability to imitate the structure and functions of the normal disc nucleus, but requires several compromises to reach full clinical utility. The fluctuating hygroscopic-related behavior of the normal disc nucleus (in the diurnal cyclic loading with resultant change in disc height) proved easier to replicate than the apparent rheology of the nucleus tissue. The semi-flexible hygroscopic gel material of the implant pellet showed excellent biocompatibility and could reasonably replicate the function of the natural nucleus.

DEVICE DESIGN

The PDN device currently in use reflects 16 years of experience with early device design and surgical technique. Tethered together after insertion into the enucleated disc space, to function as a composite construct, the pair of implants is positioned transversely (Fig. 27.1). The devices are dehydrated before packaging to minimize their profile, facilitate their placement in the disc space, and allow the surgeon to minimize the perforated annular access. Once implanted, the hydrogel core absorbs moisture from the surrounding tissue and expands. When fully hydrated, the PDN devices swell, increasing disc height by approximately 1 to 3 mm, restoring tension in the surrounding annulus, as would a normal disc nucleus (Fig. 27.2). As such, disc height and proper biomechanical

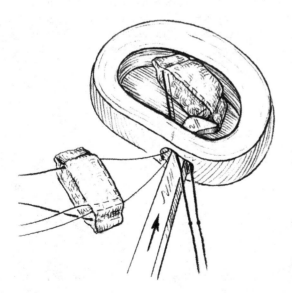

FIG. 27.1. Tethered prosthetic nucleus device implants.

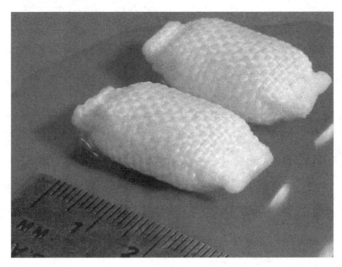

FIG. 27.2. Fully hydrated prosthetic nucleus devices.

function are restored to the affected area of the spine, the patient's pain is reduced, and the segment then exhibits the normal range of motion.

The hydrogel core (Hypan) of the PDN implant is a polyacrylonitrile–polyacrylamide multiblock copolymer with memory capability (Fig. 27.3). This material, depending on the grade used, will absorb 50% to 90% of its dry weight in water when fully hydrated. The high-strength woven polyethylene jacket provides dimensional control of the fabricated pellet. The strands of the jacket, made of a highly oriented, ultrahigh molecular weight polyethylene (UHMWPE) fiber similar to that used in bulletproof vests, are woven in a tubular pattern that maximizes strength and minimizes circumferential elastic stretch. After completely removing the disc nucleus, the surgeon selects implants from a range of sizes and shapes to accommodate patient anatomy based upon preoperative disc measurements and other intraoperative sizing observations. As intended, the implants remain in place in the disc nucleus without fixation (Fig. 27.4).

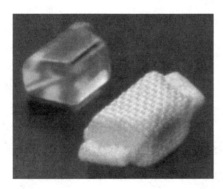

FIG. 27.3 Hydrogel core and finished prosthetic nucleus device.

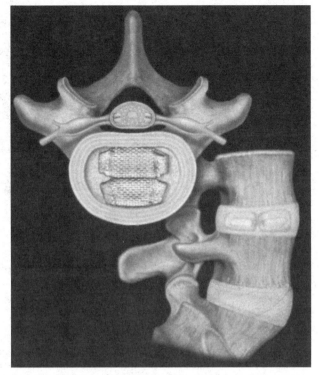

FIG. 27.4. Prosthetic nucleus devices *in situ*.

DEVICE TESTING

The PDN device has been thoroughly evaluated with regard to biological safety, durability, and performance characteristics. These tests indicate that the device is safe for long-term implant, is durable over the expected life of the implanted device, and restores the stability of the degenerated disc.

Biological Safety

The biological safety of the device was tested in accordance with U.S. Food and Drug Administration/ISO 10996 guidelines. The device was also tested for possible mutagenic and genotoxic effects. The individual tests are listed in Table 27.1. In addition to these tests, the Hypan hydrogel core material was subjected to a carcinogenicity assay in the transgenic mouse model (p53-knockout strain). The study design included sham surgery controls, positive and negative implant controls, positive controls via chemical ingestion, and positive and negative controls in the wild-type (nongenetically modified strain) mouse. Two grades of the Hypan hydrogel core material were tested and proved to be as inert as other recognized noncarcinogenic implant materials such as polyethylene and silicone.

The PDN device was evaluated in a long-term implant study in the dog model. Appropriately sized PDN device prototypes were implanted in three dogs. In each dog, one intact device was implanted in a single intervertebral disc, samples of jackets or gel were

TABLE 27.1. *Mutagenic and genotoxic testing of prosthetic disc nucleus device*

Test	Result
Hemolysis	Nonhemolytic
Cytotoxicity (in L-929 mouse cells)	Noncytotoxic
Material-mediated pyrogenicity (rabbit)	Nonpyrogenic
Sensitization (guinea pig)	Nonsensitizing
Intracutaneous reactivity (rabbit, 72 hrs)	Nonirritating, nontoxic
Acute systemic toxicity (mouse, 72 hrs)	Nontoxic
Chronic systemic toxicity (rat, 13 wks)	Nontoxic
Muscle implant (rabbit, 26 wks)	Slight irritant
Genotoxicity (hamster cells, chromosomal aberration)	Nongenotoxic
Genotoxicity (Ames test, *Salmonella typhimurium*)	Nonmutagenic
Genotoxicity (mouse, bone marrow micronucleus)	Nongenotoxic

implanted alone at other levels in the same animals as controls, and a sham surgery was performed in a disc at least two levels away from the implant site. No local or systemic tissue toxic effects were found from any implants after 12 months.

Durability

PDN devices installed in mechanical testing blocks surrounded by saline have been evaluated for the production of Hypan hydrogel polymer degradation, polyethylene particle generation, and maintenance of mechanical performance characteristics following accelerated fatigue testing. Hydrated PDN devices were cycled between compressive forces of 200 N and 800 N four times per second (4 Hz) for 50 million cycles at 37°C. Fifty million cycles presumably represent 200 to 500 years of life for a typical person. Following completion of 50 million cycles, the test fluid (sterile saline) was microfiltered and visually scanned for particles using polarized light microscopy. No particulate matter of biological significance was found (such as those with size and shape reportedly associated with bone necrosis seen in some solid UHMWPE acetabular cups for prosthetic hip implants).

The fatigue test fluid was also evaluated for theoretical Hypan hydrogel breakdown byproducts. Because the hydrogel material is a poly-block (acrylonitrile–acrylamide) copolymer, the test fluid was analyzed for acrylonitrile and acrylamide monomers using high-performance liquid chromatography. The test results indicated monomer levels at, or below, the detectable limits of 95 ppb (parts per billion) and 25 ppb, respectively.

The test-fatigued devices were visually inspected and subjected to performance testing that included dimensional analysis, load-deflection testing to 2,200 N, and severe load testing to 6,000 N. At this load, which represents the ability of the device to separate, the vertebrae was unchanged after 50 million cycles.

PERFORMANCE CHARACTERISTICS

The goal of a PDN is to restore the biomechanical performance of the degenerated disc as closely as possible to approximate that of the healthy disc. It should match the energy absorption and possess the same viscoelastic properties as the undamaged disc. It should also restore the dynamic stability of the spine as measured in spinal segment flexion–extension, lateral bending, and rotational motion.

TABLE 27.2. *Energy absorption testing of prosthetic disc nucleus device*

Device nominal size	Work to 400 N (N-mm)	
	Mean ($N = 6$)	Standard deviation
7 mm	200.0	8.0
9 mm	232.3	5.3
Target work value from cadaver testing	143.9–278.1 N-mm	

Since the intervertebral disc, as with all body tissues containing water, is viscoelastic, the stiffness of the joint increases with a higher loading rate. The hydrogel-based PDN device is viscoelastic, and this characteristic was evaluated, as well as the compressive energy absorption of intact and enucleated cadaveric lumbar spinal segments, calculated as work. These studies were conducted at the Orthopedics Research Department at Emory University in Atlanta, Georgia (2,17). The viscoelastic properties of the cadaveric lumbar spinal segment were evaluated in intact specimens. The stiffness and compressive energy absorption of the spinal segments, before and after enucleation, were evaluated at varying loading rates, and compared with the same properties of hydrated PDN tested at the same loading rates (Table 27.2). The PDN device exhibited energy absorption and viscoelastic properties matching those of the human intervertebral disc.

Restoration of dynamic stability of the spinal segment has been demonstrated by two different biomechanical studies in the cadaver spine. At the Institute for Biomechanics at the University of Ulm in Germany (25), a flexibility study evaluated the neutral zone and range of motion in cadaveric lumbar spines in the intact state, postnucleotomy, and following implantation of the PDN device. Motions included flexion–extension, lateral bending, and rotation during application of a 200-N preload. Following the nucleotomy, the neutral zone and range of motion in all axes of load application increased. Implantation of the PDN device restored the values for the neutral zone and range of motion to that of the intact state.

Further study at Emory University evaluated the stiffness and energy absorption in intact cadaveric lumbar spines, postnucleotomy, immediately following implant of the PDN device, and after 96 hours of hydration (3). This evaluation included compression, flexion–extension, and lateral bending while applying a 700-N preload. As in the flexibility study, the enucleated spinal segment exhibited decreased stability, but implanting the PDN device restored much of the stiffness (stability) to the spinal segment; the stiffness was nearly identical to that of the intact spine, following hydration of the devices.

These tests indicate that the device is safe for long-term implant, is durable over the expected life of the implanted device, and acts to restore the stability of the degenerated, lax disc.

PATIENT SELECTION

Appropriate patient selection and preoperative planning are essential to the successful outcomes for the PDN device. The patients selected for the PDN prosthesis must be between 18 and 65 years of age with DDD with or without herniation, generally confirmed by MRI. Conservative (nonoperative) treatment for 6 months or longer must have failed to relieve the patient's symptoms of severe low back pain, with or without leg pain. This low back pain must be of such magnitude and/or frequency that it has seriously affected the patient's lifestyle and ability to function in normal daily activities. Along with this pain, patients may present with frank spinal instability, abnormal neurologic findings, diminished range of segmental motion, muscle spasms, spinal deformities, or bony changes associated with the vertebrae.

EARLY RESULTS

The PDN device has demonstrated both efficacious results and an acceptable safety profile for use in treating DDD. When efficacy is compared to preoperative baseline results, the postoperative 6-month outcome from two clinical trials has shown that patients see a 64% improvement in their ability to function as measured by the Oswestry Scale, and a 63% improvement of their perceived pain as estimated by the 11-Point Box Visual Pain Scale. When evaluated at 6 months, medial disc height for these patients increased by 22% (average 2 mm) over their preoperative measurement. An analysis of patients' 6-month postoperative follow-up showed 85% device success as measured by no additional surgical intervention. While these results are preliminary, they show significant promise for the treatment of DDD by the presently available PDN device and method of implantation.

EARLY FEASIBILITY STUDIES

In 1996, Raymedica began a feasibility trial with Professor Robert Schoenmayr at the Horst-Schmidt Clinic in Wiesbaden, Germany. In this trial, which was completed in two phases, 16 patients were implanted with the original PDN device design, using the surgical technique for that study protocol. Over the next 2 years, an additional 57 patients were enrolled in feasibility studies and implanted with the device at sites in Sweden, Saudi Arabia, Egypt, and the United States.

When designing each of these trials, new technique or device modifications from its predecessors were carefully examined and incorporated as dictated by experience. These early trials proved valuable learning experiences; their data exhibited an overall device movement rate of 37.3%, reflecting an expected early learning curve and the need for device and technique modification. Device movement was the single most important safety consideration in these trials. All other observed and reported postsurgical complications and presentation of symptoms were transitory and expected postspinal surgery occurrences; nevertheless, no patient was adversely affected in this study.

The device efficacy variables all yielded very positive improvements from baseline. Variables were measured, as indicated previously using the Oswestry Low Back Pain Disability Scale, the Prolo Economic Functioning Scale, the 11-Point Box Visual Pain Scale, and medial disc height measurements. At 6 months, efficacy improved 40% to 70% according to functional and pain variables, and averaged a 14% increase in medial disc height.

REVISIONS IN DEVICE DESIGN AND OTHER FACTORS

In early 1999, a significant redesign and revisions of the PDN device geometry, the preoperative patient selection and device selection, surgical technique, and postoperative patient rehabilitation were implemented. These features had all been identified as key variables in the successful placement of the PDN device and the positive patient outcomes, even though the population was small. During early exposure and learning, surgical success declined predictably at times, which affected overall product performance measures (Fig. 27.5). The surgical success curve rose as study experiences were applied to improve product design, patient selection, and surgical technique.

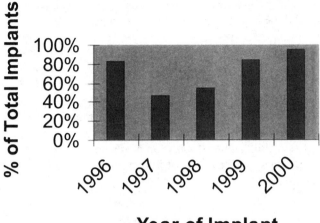

Year of Implant

FIG. 27.5. Surgical success rate: total patients with secondary surgical intervention/total patients implanted.

ADDITIONAL FEASIBILITY TRIALS

In 1999, two new feasibility trials under EN 540 regulations were initiated: a single site trial in Sweden and a multicenter trial in Germany. In addition to the new feasibility evaluations in Europe, the redesigned product and application features were approved for placement of the CE (European conformity) mark, with open marketing and sale of the

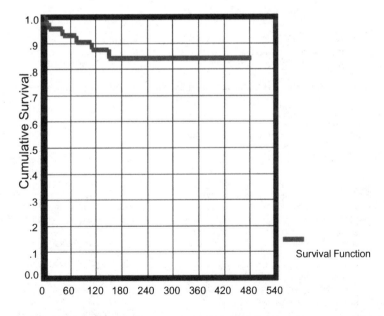

Time after Implant (days)

FIG. 27.6. Freedom from device movement for patients implanted with a prosthetic disc nucleus device between 1999 and 2000.

device in the European Economic Area (EEA) beginning in August 1999. Several product and market evaluations were concurrently undertaken in other countries with the CE marked product.

The data from the new 1999–2000 EN 540 trials have shown that there has been a dramatic reduction in the incidence of movement of the device after placement, as well as continued good efficacy results. In the cohort of 47 patients enrolled and implanted in 1999–2000, incidence of device movement dropped from the previous 25 of 67 patients to 6 of 46 patients. When device movement did occur, it was within the first 6 months postimplantation, with most occurring earlier than 4 months. Movement of the devices in patients in the early feasibility studies was evaluated using Kaplan-Meier actuarial analysis (Fig. 27.6) to evaluate the incidence of a given outcome as it relates to duration of device implantation.

CONCLUSION

The PDN device offers a novel and unique solution for providing spinal stability while preserving segmental spinal motion and reducing discogenic segmental pain. It is the only disc nucleus prosthetic device available for insertion through a relatively less invasive surgical approach from the dorsal or lateral aspect of the spine. It is anticipated that a percutaneous implantation method will be developed, potentially permitting an outpatient surgical procedure. Preclinical biomechanical and laboratory animal testing has demonstrated an acceptable safety profile that supports proceeding with clinical use in human subjects. The early clinical experience has provided very positive efficacy results. Based on a clinical need and demonstrable data, the PDN device presently serves as an important contribution to the treatment of back pain.

REFERENCES

1. Adams MA, Hutton WC. Gradual disc prolapse. *Spine* 1985;10:524–531.
2. Bain AC, Sherman T, Norton BK, et al. A comparison between the viscoelastic properties of a prosthetic disc nucleus and the intervertebral disc. Paper presented at: The 2000 IITS Annual Conference; June 2000; Williamsburg, VA.
3. Bain AC, Sherman T, Norton BK, et al. A biomechanical evaluation of a prosthetic disc nucleus. Paper presented at: The 2000 NASS Annual Conference; October 2000; New Orleans.
4. Berry JL, Moran JM, Berg WS, et al. A morphometric study of human lumbar and selected thoracic vertebrae. *Spine* 1987;12:362–367.
5. Biondi J, Greenberg BJ. Redecompression and fusion in failed back syndrome patients. *J Spinal Disord* 1990;3: 362–369.
6. Bogduk N, Tynan W, Wilson AS. The nerve supply to the human lumbar intervertebral discs. *J Anat* 1981;132: 39–56.
7. Fung YC. *Biomechanics: Mechanical properties of living tissues.* New York: Springer-Verlag, 1981.
8. Ghosh P. *The biology of the intervertebral disc*, vols I and II. Boca Raton, FL: CRC Press, 1988.
9. Hedman TP, Kostuik JP, Fernie GR, et al. Artificial spinal disc. US patent 4,759,769, June 12, 1988.
10. Keller TS, Hansson TH, Holm SH, et al. In vivo creep behavior of the normal and degenerated porcine intervertebral disk: A preliminary report. *J Spinal Disord* 1989;4:267–278.
11. Kostuik JP, Hedman T, Hellier W, et al. Design of an intervertebral disc prosthesis. *Spine* 1991;16[Suppl]: S256–S260.
12. Lee CK. Clinical biomechanics of lumbar spine surgery. In: White AH, Rothman RH, Ray CD, eds. *Lumbar spine surgery: Techniques and complications.* St. Louis: Mosby, 1987.
13. Lee CK, Langrana NA, Alexander H, et al. Fiber-reinforced functional disc prosthesis. Abstract presented at: Orthopaedic Research Society Annual Meeting, 1989.
14. Miller JAA, Schmatz C, Schultz AB. Lumbar disc degeneration: correlation with age, sex and spine level in 600 autopsy specimens. *Spine* 1988;13:173–178.
15. Mooney V. A perspective on the future of low back research. In: Guyer RD, ed. *Spine: state of the art reviews*, vol 3. Philadelphia: Hanley and Belfus, 1989:173–183.

16. Nachemson A. Some mechanical properties of the lumbar intervertebral discs. *Bull Hosp Jt Dis (NY)* 1962;23: 130–132.

17. Norton BK, Kavanagh S, Bauer L, et al. Mechanical evaluation of a structural hydrogel for use as a spinal disc nucleus. Paper presented at Biomaterials 2000 conference.

18. Ray CD, ed. *Medical engineering*. Chicago: Year Book, 1974.

19. Ray CD. Artificial disc [abst]. Challenge of the lumbar spine. Proceedings of the Annual Meeting, 1988:67.

20. Ray CD, Corbin T. Prosthetic disc and method of implanting. US patent 4, 772, 287, September 20, 1988.

21. Ray CD. Prosthetic nucleus as an artificial disc. Proceedings of the North American Spine Society Annual Meeting; June 30, 1989 [poster and abstract].

22. Ray CD, Corbin TP. Prosthetic disc containing therapeutic material. US patent 4,904,260, February 27, 1990.

23. Ray CD. Lumbar interbody threaded prostheses. Flexible, for an artificial disc and rigid, for a fusion. In: Broch M, Mayer HM, Weigel K, eds. *The artificial disc*. Heidelberg: Springer-Verlag, 1991:53–67.

24. White AA, Panjabi MM. The basic kinematics of the human spine. *Spine* 1978;3:12–20.

25. Wilke HJ, Kavanagh S, Neller S, et al. Prosthetic disc restores the flexibility and height of a disc after nucleotomy. Paper presented at: The 6th World Biomaterials Congress; May 2000; Kamuela, HI.

28

Indications for Disc Replacement Following Lumbar Discectomy

Thierry David

In some patients with chronic low back pain, a new posterior surgery for recurrent hernia may induce bad results and future failed back syndrome. A second surgery by anterior approach with a lumbar disc prosthesis, however, may offer improved results.

This chapter discusses a study of 15 cases of disc replacement for recurrent hernia, reviewed with a minimum of 1-year follow-up.

MATERIALS AND METHODS

Fifteen patients with recurrent and severe sciatica had a disc replacement between September 1997 and September 1999. All cases were reviewed in 2000. All of the patients had undergone surgery previously had been by a posterior approach for a disc hernia; eight in L5-S1 and seven in L4-L5.

The patients had a fair result after the first surgery in terms of chronic low back pain but had a good resolution of their sciatica. At some point, each of them presented with a new acute sciatica at the same level.

Diagnosis was made by magnetic resonance imaging (MRI) with gadolinium. In five cases we observed Modic I inflammatory signs around the disc.

An anterior approach was possible in only one case of contained hernia sub or completely extruded and migrated (therefore only accessible by posterior approach). To be certain, all patients had discography and computed tomography (CT) in order to fulfill these conditions (Fig. 28.1).

The disc replacement was made by an anterior left extraperitoneal approach, and the prosthesis was always a LINK SB CHARITE III.

It is mandatory not to put the patient in hyperlordotic position before excision of the hernia to avoid migration and neurologic complication.

RESULTS

No major complications were noticed immediately following surgery. There was one epidural vein hemorrhage that was easily stopped. Among Stauffer-Coventry classification modified by Cauchoix in four grades with an average follow-up of 25 months, we had only excellent (eight patients) and good results (seven patients) and no residual sci-

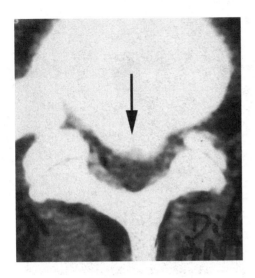

FIG. 28.1. Computed tomography image showing a subligamentous herniated disc, reachable only by an anterior approach.

atica. Ten of the 15 patients returned to work. Seven of these individuals returned to jobs that included heavy physical labor.

One patient required another surgery for a secondary disc hernia L5-S1 below the L4-L5 disc prosthesis.

All of the prostheses were in place at the follow-up point with no migration.

The average mobility was in flexion extension 11 degrees for L5-S1 and 13 degrees for L4-L5. The mobility in bending left and right was, respectively, 5 degrees for L5-S1 and 6 degrees for UL5 (Figs. 28.2 and 28.3).

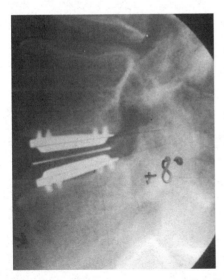
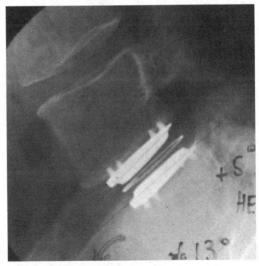

FIG. 28.2. L4-L5 prosthesis implanted after recurrence of herniated disc previously operated on by classic posterior approach and laminectomy. At 3 months after implantation, this sagittal view demonstrates a good 13-degree mobility in the sagittal plane (flexion–extension).

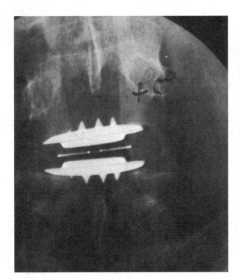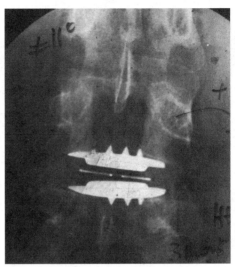

FIG. 28.3. Anteroposterior view of the same patient as in Fig. 28-2, showing a good mobility of 11 degrees in the frontal plane (lateral flexion).

CONCLUSION

The disc replacement by anterior approach for patients with chronic low back pain and acute sciatica with a recurrent hernia has many advantages in comparison with a repeated posterior surgery with or without fusion.

The procedure completely treats the problem of sciatica and low back pain with conservation of the mobility, it limits scar tissue formation and the risk of root deterioration. These first results from 15 patients are very encouraging.

29

What Is Failed Back Surgery? How Do We Treat?

Gordon Waddell

There are many case series, discussions, and even books on failed back surgery and repeat back surgery, which mostly focus on the technical details of why the primary procedure failed, how to assess and investigate the present situation, and alternative techniques for revision procedures. This chapter will not repeat these technical details, but will focus instead on some fundamental, if more philosophical, principles about how we should approach the patient with persistent pain and disability after spinal surgery. These concerns include:

- Indications for surgery and diagnosis of a surgically treatable lesion.
- Patient selection and psychological overlay.
- Not relying excessively on images to make a diagnosis.
- Is it really "failed back surgery" or rather patients with persistent or recurrent pain and disability after back surgery?
- The fact that there may or may not be any surgical answer.
- Are the problems persistent ones, or new ones?
- Is there currently a surgically treatable lesion?
- Is this patient likely to be helped by further surgery or might surgery make them worse?
- Is a surgeon the right person to continue looking after this patient?

Disc surgery has withstood the test of time for more than half a century because it is one of the most successful orthopedic and neurosurgical procedures ever devised, with a success rate of 80% to 90% in carefully selected patients. The major proviso, of course, is in carefully selected patients. Every analysis of failed back surgery emphasizes that the most common reason for failure is inadequate diagnosis of a surgically treatable lesion which is likely to respond to surgical treatment. Too often, the indications for disc surgery are severity of symptoms, failure to respond to conservative treatment, distress, desperation, and a desire to help. Unfortunately, these common selection criteria have very little to do with diagnosing a surgically treatable lesion or predicting a successful outcome. As one of the nineteenth-century pioneers of abdominal surgery recognized: "He who operates for pain rarely finds it." Many studies show that the outcome of disc surgery depends on completely different issues of the accuracy of the diagnosis of a surgically treatable lesion, efficient uncomplicated surgery, and good postoperative rehabilitation. Yet spinal surgeons seem to have difficulty separating the patient's needs and demands for help and their own natural and laudable desires to provide help—from rational, objective indications for surgery. A good analogy may be made with carcinoma, where surgeons, even spinal surgeons, have no such difficulty recognizing whether or not there is a surgical answer, and accepting the need for detached and rational decisions without being unduly swayed by emotional issues. We must recognize that the first spinal operation is always the best and often the last chance to get things right. If ever there is a need for detached, rational decision making, it is in the initial decision to perform the first surgical invasion of a patient's back. There is no such procedure, or there should be no such procedure, as "exploration of the spine."

I alluded briefly to the need for careful patient selection, which raises issues of psychological overlay, nonorganic findings, and illness behavior. Many patients with severe back pain and sciatica become distressed and if pain and disability become chronic they may become angry or depressed, and even show signs of illness behavior. This is all a natural and an entirely secondary effect of their entirely genuine physical problem: it does not tell us anything about the original cause of their pain, and it does not mean their pain is psychogenic. It is not a question of whether the pain is organic or nonorganic: many patients have both physical and psychological components to their clinical presentation, and it is important that we recognize and treat *both*. The presence of overt distress, nonorganic signs, and behavioral responses to examination therefore does not preclude a surgically treatable lesion and should not rule out patients from disc surgery. However, we must recognize that such patients may need more careful assessment, and additional support and help in their postoperative recovery and rehabilitation, and even then the clinical outcome and success rate may not be quite as good.

When it comes to repeat spinal surgery, however, psychological overlay and nonorganic features become much more important, and that was the context in which they were first recognized. Unfortunately, in practice, they add greatly to the pressure on the surgeon to "do something" but at the same time often confuse clinical assessment and diagnosis. So they tend to increase the surgeon's belief that there may be something they can operate upon and that they should perhaps "give the patient the chance." Contrary to such wishful thinking, the reality is that psychological and nonorganic findings usually indicate a greatly reduced chance of a successful clinical outcome from repeat back surgery. Instead of being used as argument that this patient is in greater need of help and therefore lowering the decision threshold to operate, the surgeon should actually increase that threshold. If psychological overlay and nonorganic features are marked, there is even greater need to demand objective and unequivocal evidence of a surgically treatable lesion before embarking on repeat spinal surgery.

It may be pertinent at this point to remind readers of the dangers of relying too much on imaging studies such as computed tomography (CT) and magnetic resonance imaging (MRI). The high false-positive rate of these sensitive investigations is now well known and all surgical texts emphasize the need to match them against the clinical findings. Unfortunately, too many spinal surgeons seem to have difficulty remembering this and continue to either find CT and MR images dangerously seductive, or perhaps find it intellectually easier to use the illusion of concrete anatomic images for surgical decision making rather than the much more difficult and demanding need to assess the patient. It is even more important not to rely heavily on imaging studies when considering repeat spinal surgery. When a spine has already been operated upon, CT and MRI changes are almost universal (though there are no published series of imaging studies in asymptomatic patients with successful previous spinal surgery, which would be an original and useful research project). Therefore, it is absolutely essential to base the decision to perform a subsequent surgery on clinical indications, and only to use the images as a tool to plan the technical details, not to influence the decision.

If disc surgery has an 80% to 90% success rate, that implies about 15% are failures. One author has calculated this means that several hundred thousand patients each year throughout the world have "failed back surgery." Various large, population-based series show that 5% to 15% of all patients undergoing disc surgery sooner or later come to repeat surgery. However, there is no such thing as "failed back surgery" and I strongly object to that term because it implies a blinkered professional focus on the technical problem. It loses sight of the reality that what we must deal with are patients who have persistent or recurrent pain and disability after our failed spinal surgery. As one of the pioneers of disc surgery wrote 30 years ago: "No operation in any field of surgery leaves in its wake more human wreckage than surgery on the lumbar discs." Spinal surgery demands a much more holistic approach to each individual patient, with careful assessment of all the biomedical and biopsychosocial aspects of their problem. If you are not prepared or equipped to address these issues, you are not fit to be doing repeat spinal surgery. Above all, back pain demands recognition that there may not be any surgical solution, that the answer may lie elsewhere, and that we must be prepared to recognize and admit that we do have any surgical answer. This may be a particularly difficult admission for the surgeon who is responsible for the original failed surgery, which is an argument for demanding an independent second opinion in this situation before embarking on repeat surgery.

There is a major difference between patients who have a good clinical outcome from their spinal surgery and then later develop recurrent problems and patients who never get relief or who have rapid recurrence of symptoms after a brief placebo response (and surgery is probably the most powerful placebo known). Patients who have at least 6 to 12 months' good outcome and then develop clear-cut and objective findings of a recurrent disc prolapse generally have clear indications for surgery and do reasonably well from a repeat operation. Patients who have persistent pain and disability after their first disc operation are very different. The usual reason for failure in that case is that the first operation was performed for the wrong reasons and some post hoc analyses have suggested that in one-third to one-half of patients there was never any good indication for surgery. There is usually then no good indication for reoperation. You cannot "re-operate on an operation" and there is no place for "exploring the back" or "giving the patient one last chance." Now, above all, severity of symptoms, failure to respond to conservative treatment, distress, desperation, and the desire to help are totally insufficient indications for repeat spinal surgery. Now, above all, there is a need for detached, rational decisions based on clear, objective evidence of a surgical treatable lesion which is likely to respond to repeat surgery.

I will not consider failed disc surgery because of technical error or complication in detail and would refer the reader to the appropriate surgical texts. However, despite claims by some senior spinal surgeons that they are able to diagnose such technical explanations in most cases (even when no one else can), I am totally convinced that clearly defined and objectively demonstrable technical causes of failure actually only account for a small proportion of failed disc operations. The only specific point I would add is that wound infection is commonly associated with chronic back pain and disability and is then an almost complete contraindication to further surgery for pain (this is, of course, quite different from dealing with any residual infection).

We then must make and give to the patient an honest assessment of the likely success rate of repeat surgery, which can never be as high as for a primary procedure. If the success rate for primary disc surgery is 80% to 90%, that of a second procedure is probably about 60% to 80%, and that of a third or later procedure is probably 50% or less. What few spinal surgeons seem to recognize is that spinal surgery can also make pain and disability worse. We all recognize and accept that surgical complications may lead to lasting problems, although these are fortunately rare. However, much more commonly, patients complain of increased pain and disability after spinal surgery without any overt complications. That is increasingly important after repeat surgery. With each successive operation the chances of good relief of pain and disability become less, but, conversely, the chances of increased pain and disability become greater. One study estimated that by the fourth operation, repeat spinal surgery was more likely to make the patient's pain and disability worse rather than better. Surgeons and patients embarking on repeat spinal surgery must recognize and acknowledge that possibility. It is totally wrong to suggest that "this patient's pain and disability are so severe that I cannot make them any worse, so I might as well give him or her a chance, however small." As one well-known spinal surgeon puts it: "They're no-hopers—but you give them another scratch." Unfortunately, the reality is that you can *always* make their pain and disability even worse.

Regrettably, for most patients with "failed back surgery," we must recognize that there is no surgical answer and increasingly desperate attempts by patient and surgeon to "try, try, and try again" are not commendable efforts to help but sheer stupidity. It is difficult and painful for surgeons and patients faced with this desperate situation for which we often share responsibility to admit openly that we do not have any easy solution, but that may be the essential first step to dealing with the problem. Once both surgeon and patient confront this reality, the logical implication is that a surgeon is no longer the best person to go on looking after this patient. The danger is that if such a patient does remain under the care of surgeons, one will sooner or later yield to pressure and temptation and stick a knife into the patient's back. Our professional duty to the patient with failed disc surgery is to recognize when it would be better for the patient to move to a different kind of specialist and stay well away from surgeons.

Economic and Ethical Considerations in the Management of Spinal Stenosis

30

Principles of Quality Assessment

Christian Mélot

改善　方針

Kaizen	Houshin
A continual improvement process involving everyone in a personal quest for excellence. It consists of doing things better, little by little.	*Orientation defined by a plan or a policy. Improvement following a main idea or a general direction.*

Of the many issues now confronting medical professionals, none seems more perplexing than the debate about the quality of care. In the past, physicians could be confident that they alone had a social mandate to judge and manage the quality of care. Now that mandate is contested by those taking part in the process of care, as well as the patient. The language about the quality of care leaves many physicians uncomprehending: observed and expected mortality, outcome and process measures, SF-36 (36 item short-form questionnaire for quality of life), case-mix and case severity adjustments, HEDIS (Health Plan Employer Data and Information Set) measures, CONQUEST (Computerized Needs-Oriented Quality Measurement Evaluation System) system, control charts, continuous quality improvement, total quality management. Few of the terms seem, at first glance, to be related with the day-to-day realities of providing care for individual patients. Moreover, none of these terms were taught to most of the physicians now in practice.

DEFINITION OF QUALITY OF HEALTH CARE

Experts have debated for decades to formulate a concise, meaningful, and generally applicable definition of quality of health care. In 1980, Donabedian defined high-quality care as "that kind of care which is expected to maximize an inclusive measure of patient welfare, after one has taken account of the balance of expected gains and losses that attend the process of care in all its parts" (7). In 1986, the American Medical Association defined high-quality care as care "which consistently contributes to the improvement or maintenance of quality and/or duration of life" (1). One of the most widely cited recent definitions, formulated by the Institute of Medicine in 1990, holds that quality consists of the "degree to which health services for individuals and populations increase the likelihood of desired health outcomes and are consistent with current professional knowledge" (20). The Joint Commission on Accreditation of Healthcare Organizations (JCAHO) defined quality as "the degree to which patient care services increase the probability of undesired patient outcomes and reduce the probability of undesired outcomes given the current state of knowledge."

Health care professionals tend to define quality in terms of the attributes and results of care provided by practitioners and received by patients. Although the perspective of health care professionals is important, other perspectives on quality have been emphasized in recent years. The most important change has been a growing recognition of the preferences and values of the consumers of health care services as they have been introduced in economic evaluation (3,21). Other perspectives on the quality of care that have recently become more influential are those of health care plans and organizations as well as those of organized purchasers of health care services: employers, unions, and consumer cooperatives.

FACETS OF QUALITY ASSESSMENT

Donabedian identifies three key categories within quality assessment and monitoring: structure, process, and outcome variables (Table 30.1) (7,8).

Structure represents the stable attributes of the settings in which care occurs. This includes the attributes of material resources (facilities, equipment, etc.), of human resources (the number and qualification of personnel), and of organizational structure (medical staff organization, methods of peer review, methods of reimbursement).

Process includes the interventions performed by the health care team and involves how skillfully these interventions are executed. Process denotes what is actually done in giving and receiving care. It includes the patient's activities in seeking care and carrying it out as well as the practitioner's activities in making a diagnosis and recommending and implementing treatment.

Outcome denotes the effects of care on health status of patients and populations. Improvements in the patient's behavior as well as the patient's satisfaction with care are included under the definition of health status.

This three-step approach to quality assessment implies a relationship between structure, process, and outcome.

TABLE 30.1. *Definitions and nonexhaustive examples of each type of measure in quality assessment*

	Structure	Process	Outcome
Definition	The inputs or elements that facilitate care	Functions of the care providers	Results of care
Examples	Resources Equipment Numbers of staff Qualification of staff	Assessment Planning Treatment Timeliness	Short-term results Complications Adverse events Satisfaction Long-term results Changes in health status

THE MANAGEMENT OF QUALITY

Total Quality Management

Total quality management (TQM) (Fig. 30.1) is an industrial model developed in the United States and successfully implemented in Japan following World War II. The TQM philosophy provides a managerial approach encompassing meeting the customers' requirements, error-free performance (doing it right the first time), and the concept of continuous quality improvement (known in Japan as *kaizen*) using a series of problem-solving tools and techniques related to statistical process control (quality control).

TQM requires a commitment to an organized, systematic, collaborative, and pervasive quality program with dedicated resources. It requires rigorous process flow and techniques for statistical analysis, evaluation of all ongoing activities, methods for managing large data sets, and recognition and application of underlying psychosocial principles affecting individuals and groups within an organization. TQM assumes that most problems are not the result of administrative or clinical professionals' errors, but the inability of the structure (system) to perform adequately. The focus of TQM is on process, not individuals.

Quality Assurance

Traditionally, quality assurance (QA) has been perceived as a fragmented, oversight mechanism to enhance public accountability through various monitoring and evaluation reviews (Fig. 30.1). QA is concerned by the characteristics that determine the value or degree of excellence and by the mechanisms to efficiently and effectively monitor and improve patient care provided by competent professionals with appropriate resources. QA is the quantitative and qualitative measurement of the quality of existing processes and systems. QA is driven by accreditation and regulatory requirements. QA aims to protect and preserve the actual quality level. While quality improvement and quality assurance are not synonymous, they do have a symbiotic relationship.

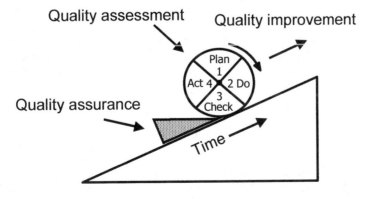

FIG. 30.1. The management of quality.

Quality Assessment

Quality assessment (Fig. 30.1) is the measurement of the level of quality at some point in time. It consists in monitoring in data collection, and in making a judgment regarding adequacy with no effort to change or improve. Quality assessment is *not* synonymous with quality assurance.

Continuous Quality Improvement

Continuous quality improvement (CQI) (Fig. 30.1) is the relentless drive for improvement based on: assessing (a) structure, including the competence of professionals practicing in a resource-relevant culture; (b) process, including the activities and behaviors employed; and (c) acceptable clinical outcomes. Based on a comprehensive, integrated, and coordinated quality improvement program, CQI acknowledges the humanity and complexity of health care organizations. CQI consists of a wide array of clinical, managerial, and organizational activities designed to remove waste and unpredictability, and to achieve previously unprecedented levels of performance. CQI focuses on "process" rather than the individual. Outcomes are measured in terms of the needs and expectations of customers, who are the recipients of the processes. CQI implies that a process and its service/outcome are never optimized (core of TQM philosophy). CQI and quality assurance (QA) are *not* synonymous.

Benchmarking

Benchmarking is the continuous process of comparing products, services, and practices with internal or external competitors recognized as leaders in the field. Benchmarking can be comparative in nature or process-oriented. In comparative benchmarking, an organization compares its performance with the performance of others by using performance measures and indicators. Process benchmarking may start as a comparison of data but evolves into the evaluation of processes. The evaluation of processes is necessary to recognize and identify the best practices. Health care organizations usually benchmark critical processes such as flow through an operating room (24,27).

Reengineering

Reengineering is the fundamental rethinking and radical redesign of business processes to achieve dramatic improvement in performance in areas such as cost, quality, service, and speed. Reengineering involves finding new and improved ways to accomplish work (13).

Kaizen and *Houshin*

Kaizen is a Japanese concept of a continual improvement process involving every member of a work team in a personal quest for excellence. It consists of doing things better, little by little, all the time. *Kaizen* is similar to the concept of CQI. *Houshin*, on the other hand, means improvement of process following a main idea, a general direction, or an orientation defined by a plan or a policy.

MODELS FOR QUALITY IMPROVEMENT

Evaluation models typically found in health care include the Plan-Do-Check-Act (PDCA) cycle, the FOCUS-PDCA, and the Cycle for Improving Performance. These quality improvement models are used by work groups for continuous improvement.

The Plan-Do-Check-Act (PDCA) Cycle

The PDCA cycle (Fig. 30.1), developed by Walter Shewhart and widely taught by W. Edwards Deming (6), is useful in planning, testing, assessing, and implementing improvement actions. The PDCA cycle, which is a variation of the input-processing-output model is defined as follows:

Plan: determine how an issue or potential improvement will be studied (what data will be collected to answer a defined question).
Do: implement the plan on a small scale.
Check: check the data or information gathered to analyze the effect of the action under study.
Act: implement the action or improvement and continue the process for further improvement.

The FOCUS Procedure

FOCUS, as outlined in *An Integrated Approach to Medical Staff Performance Improvement* by the JCAHO (17), means:

*F*ind a process for improvement
*O*rganize a team that knows the process
*C*larify current knowledge of the process
*U*nderstand causes of process variation, and
*S*elect the process improvement

The FOCUS procedure immediately precedes implementation of the PDCA cycle. Both the PDCA model and the FOCUS-PDCA are examples of the influence of quality improvement concepts on the evaluation process. Characteristics of quality improvement that have affected the evaluation process are: (a) inclusion of those affected or involved in the evaluation process; (b) emphasis on work groups and group evaluation activities; (c) inclusion of tools such as fishbone diagrams, control charts, flowcharts, histograms, and Pareto charts to enhance an understanding of processes (16); and (d) emphasis on continual change as compared with a snapshot or one-time assessment of a program or evaluation.

The Cycle for Improving Performance

The JCAHO developed a flowchart to illustrate the cycle for improving performance and outcomes (Fig. 30.2) (18). The JCAHO cycle for improving performance and outcomes is ongoing and is designed to consider the external and internal environments of a health care organization. A health care organization can use the cycle in multiple improvement efforts, for example, designing a new program or service, creating a flow-

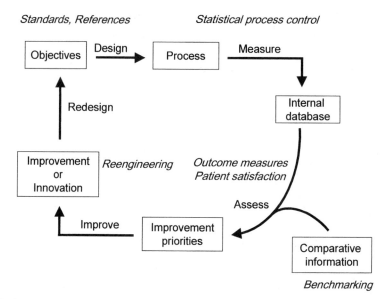

FIG. 30.2. Improving organization performance function. (From JCAHO 2001©, adapted and reprinted with permission.)

chart of a clinical process, measuring patient outcomes, comparing its performance to other organizations, establishing quality improvement priorities, or piloting innovations. The cycle can be entered at any stage but is described in this chapter as being initiated in the design stage.

Design Stage

In the design stage, the staff have clearly identified the process or outcome they wish to improve. They address the relationship of the process to the organization's mission, vision, values, and priorities. The needs and expectations of the customers or patients affected by the process must be determined and influence the design phase. The staff need to develop clear objectives to guide the process improvement. State-of-the-art knowledge about the process must be researched and considered in the proposed design. Baseline performance expectations are established to guide the next two stages: measurement and assessment.

Measurement Stage

Measurement is the foundation for all improvement activities. The leaders for the improvement of performance should delineate the measures that will be necessary to assess the process initially, support the changes, and evaluate the improved process and outcomes. Potential measurements include outcomes, process parameters, customer or patient satisfaction, and costs associated with the process improvement and outcomes. The leaders and staff of an organization must determine the scope, focus, and priorities for measurement activities. Then the organization must organize the measurement activities into a systematic approach, determine the frequency and intensity of each measure, and incorporate the measurements into daily work processes. This data collection may be periodic and ongoing or more intensive. A balanced approach to measurement includes both outcomes and process measures. Outcomes are measured to understand results and processes are measured to understand the causes of results.

Assessment Stage

The assessment stage may now be initiated and should be systematic and interdisciplinary. Assessment is supported by a variety of methodologies including the use of statistical analysis tools, graphic tools, cause-and-effect diagrams, peer review, and comparative information. Cause-and-effect (fishbone) diagrams and flowcharts are often used early in the assessment phase. Comparative information includes assessing the organization's own performance and comparing it with others. A control chart is an example of internal performance, and benchmarking is a method of comparing with others. A health care organization may use a variety of assessment frameworks, for example, internal comparisons over time, comparison with practice guidelines or parameters, comparison with reference databases, or benchmarking.

Improvement and Design/Redesign Stages

In the improvement stage an improvement process model should be used. An organization can improve its processes and outcomes by designing new processes or redesigning current processes (reengineering). The leaders and staff identify the potential improvement, test or pilot an improvement strategy or innovation, assess data to determine if the improvement produced the desired results, and implement the improvement systemwide if the improvement is effective. Ongoing measurement and assessment are needed to verify that the improvement is maintained. The staff who have implemented an improvement may determine, through ongoing measurement and assessment, that the design/redesign stage may be indicated again. The JCAHO cycle for improvement supports a philosophy of continuous improvement (TQM).

HEALTH-RELATED QUALITY OF LIFE

Recent advances in quality assessment have been especially impressive for measures that elicit information directly from users of the health care system. These measures include questions that ask patients what they experienced during a particular clinical episode (process measures) or about a patient's health-related quality of life (HRQoL) before and/or after treatment (outcome measures).

The term "health-related quality of life" is often used because widely valued aspects of life exist that are not generally considered as "health" (e.g., income, freedom, quality of the environment, etc.) (12). HRQoL is important for measuring the impact of chronic disease. Physiologic measures provide information to clinicians but are of limited interest to patients. They correlate poorly with functional capacity and well being, the areas in which patients are most interested and familiar.

Two basic approaches to HRQoL measurement are available: generic instruments that provide a summary of HRQoL; and specific instruments that focus on problems associated with single disease states, patient groups, or areas of function. Generic instruments include health profiles and instruments that generate health utilities. Both approaches are not mutually exclusive.

Most commonly, HRQoL instruments are questionnaires made up of a number of items or questions. These items are added up in a number of domains (also called dimensions). A domain or dimension refers to the area of behavior or experience that we are trying to measure. Domains might include mobility and self-care (sometimes aggregated into a physical function domain), or depression, anxiety, and well being (sometimes aggregated into an emotional function domain).

The types of HRQoL measures for generic instruments consist of health profiles and utility measures. Health profiles are instruments that attempt to measure all important aspects of HRQoL. The Sickness Impact Profile (SIP) is an example of a health profile and includes a physical dimension, a psychosocial dimension, and five independent categories including eating, work, home management, sleep and rest, as well as recreation and pastimes. Major advantages of health profiles include dealing with a variety of areas and use in any population, regardless of the underlying condition. Because generic instruments apply to a variety of populations, they allow for broad comparisons of the relative impact of various health care programs. Generic profiles may, however, be unresponsive to changes in specific conditions. Utility measures of quality of life are based on decision theory and are widely used in cost–utility analyses (22). They reflect the preferences of patients for treatment process and outcome. The key elements of utility measures are that they incorporate preference measurements and relate health states to death, i.e., quality with quantity of life. In utility measures, HRQoL is summarized as a single number along a continuum that usually extends from death (score: 0) to perfect health (score: 1). Utility scores reflect both the health status and the value of that health status to the patient. Utility measures are useful for determining if patients are, overall, better off, but they do not show the domains in which improvement or deterioration occurs.

The rationale for the specific instrument approach lies in the potential for increased responsiveness that may result from including only important aspects of HRQoL that are relevant to the patients being studied. The instrument may be specific to the disease (i.e., heart failure or asthma), to a population of patients (i.e., older people), to a certain function (i.e., sleep or sexual function), or to a problem (i.e., pain).

OUTCOME MEASURES: ARE MORTALITY INDICATORS GOOD INDICATORS OF HEALTH CARE QUALITY?

Consumers and payers increasingly demand data with which to evaluate health care providers. While publication of risk-adjusted, hospital-specific death rates is one response, debate continues over whether higher than predicted mortality is warning about quality of care or rather a reflection of a hospital's atypical patient population.

Mortality rates for certain interventions or disease states have been used over the last decade as indicators of the quality of care provided by a given hospital, unit, or medical team. If published, these rates would be a useful tool for decision makers in the process of fund allocations, for public information, and for promoting improved care in hospitals or units with low classifications.

It is difficult to adjust an indicator of mortality to disease-related risk factors and any modification of this adjustment can have major consequences on the validity of subsequent comparisons (11,14,15). The differences in mortality observed between hospitals and physicians can reflect not only differences in quality of care but also differences in approaches to disease-related risk factors, therapeutic choices, or coding practices (2). The lack of statistical power is a major limiting factor in interpreting differences in mortality rates. To evidence a statistical significant difference in mortality between two hospitals whose rates are respectively 0.5% and 1% (e.g., in total hip replacement patients) it would be necessary to include 4,673 patients, a number that would correspond to 20 years of data for a hospital performing 230 interventions per year. Consequently, the number of interventions performed in the most active hospitals would not be sufficient to make such comparisons.

Some studies have demonstrated that the publication of mortality rates does not have a major influence on patients' decisions nor on physicians' choice of a referral hospital (25). It would have no effect on improving health care quality of the institutions cited. On the contrary, some perverse effects have been observed: modification in patient recruitment and higher-risk patients being referred to hospitals with unpublished mortality rates (23). For many authors, procedure indicators are more pertinent than outcome indicators for detecting differences in health care quality between different care structures.

ASSESSMENT OF QUALITY IN CLINICAL TRIALS

In clinical trials, HRQoL measures are used increasingly as primary or secondary endpoints. Initially, when studying a new therapy (such as a new drug), investigators rely on disease-specific measures. Disease-specific measures are clinically sensible in that patients and clinicians intuitively find the items directly relevant. A study by the Canadian Erythropoietin Study Group (19) used a questionnaire designed specifically for patients with chronic renal failure and showed that erythropoietin-induced increases in hemoglobin levels improved HRQoL in renal failure patients.

A number of specific measures can be used together in a battery of trials to obtain a comprehensive picture of the impact of different interventions on HRQoL. A variety of instruments, including measures of well being, physical function, emotional function, sleep, sexual function, and side effects, were used to show that antihypertensive agents have a differential impact on many aspects of HRQoL (5).

A number of situations exist in which generic measures are highly appropriate for clinical trials. Utility measures are particularly relevant if the economic implications of an intervention are a major focus of investigation. In one randomized trial, investigators (26) showed that a compliance-enhancing maneuver for patients with chronic lung disease involved in exercise rehabilitation improved HRQoL, and the cost was approximately $25,000 per quality-adjusted life-year (QALY) gained.

Investigators must utilize appropriate methods for incorporating HRQoL information when comparing treatment options in clinical trials. Such methods are especially useful when there is a trade-off between increased treatment toxicity and improved response. For example, a new therapeutic regimen may significantly delay disease recurrence or progression, but may also have undesirable side effects compared with a standard treatment. It is important that the evaluation of HRQoL is made within the context of clinical outcomes related to the disease and its treatment.

The *Quality-adjusted Time Without Symptoms* of disease and *Toxicity* of treatment (Q-TWiST) methodology focuses on the integration of both quality and quantity of life into a single analysis to be used for treatment comparisons (4,9). The Q-TWiST method makes treatment comparisons in terms of survival time without symptoms of disease or toxicity of treatment (i.e., the survival time remaining after subtracting periods of time with symptoms or toxicity from the overall survival time). The Q-TWiST method allows a portion of the time spent with toxicity, relapse, or other clinical health states to be included in the comparison, as these health states often have some HRQoL value for patients. Q-TWiST was originally designed to compare therapies in cancer settings, but the methodology has been applied in other disease. The Q-TWiST method makes treatment comparisons in terms of quality and quantity of life by penalizing treatments that have negative HRQoL effects and rewarding those that increase survival and have other positive HRQoL effects. As in an ordinary survival analysis, the focus of the method is on time, but rather than evaluating a single end-point such as overall survival or disease-free survival, multiple outcomes corresponding to changes in HRQoL are considered. The multiple outcomes partition the overall survival time into clinical health states that may differ in HRQoL. These clinical health states are selected to be relevant to the clinician and patients. Each clinical health state is assigned a weight (utility score) that corresponds to its value in terms of HRQoL relative to a state of best possible health. A utility score of 0 indicates that the health state is as bad as death, and a score of 1 indicates perfect health (Fig. 30.3). Utilities can be computed using standard gamble or time trade-off techniques (22).

The first step in the analysis is to define quality of life-oriented health states that are appropriate for the disease setting under study. For example, we can define a period of toxicity of the treatment, a period free of symptoms (TWiST), and a period of relapse of the disease process. The utility score for the TWiST period is usually assumed to be unity because it characterizes a period of relatively perfect health. In some treatment comparisons TWiST might be assigned a value of less than unity, such as when one therapeutic regimen might return patients to a better state than another. The other clinical health states (toxicity, relapse) are generally associated with diminished HRQoL (Fig. 30.3). Patients progress through the health states chronologically, possibly skipping one or more states, but never backtracking. This allows for a patient dying prematurely or not experiencing treatment toxicity.

In the second step, Kaplan-Meier curves for the times to events that signal transitions between the clinical health states are used to partition the area under the overall survival curves separately for each treatment. As a useful visual display, the survival curves corresponding to the multiple outcomes that define transitions between health states for the treatment under evaluation can be plotted on the same graph. These are called partitioned survival plots (Fig. 30.4) (4).

The third step is to compare the treatment regimens using the weighted sum of the mean duration of each clinical health state as calculated in step 2. For example, in a disease setting involving TWiST and two other clinical health states (toxicity of treatment and relapse of the disease)

Mean Q-TWiST = 0.5 × Time with toxicity + 1.0 × TWiST + 0.5 × Time with relapse

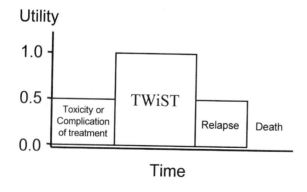

FIG. 30.3. Utility assigned to different health states.

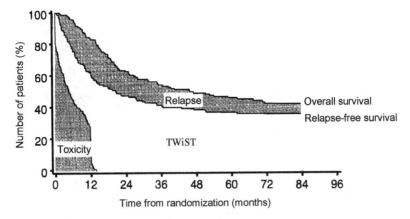

FIG. 30.4. Partitioned Kaplan-Meier survival plots for Eastern Cooperative Oncology Group (ECOG) study of patients with malignant melanoma treated with interferon-α. Survival curves are plotted for overall survival, relapse-free survival, and treatment toxicity. Area between curves represents mean time spent with toxicity, with relapse, and without symptoms of relapse or toxicity (TWiST). (Redrawn from reference 26, with permission.)

Where *time with toxicity, TWiST,* and *time with relapse* represent the average amounts of time spent in each state, and *0.5, 1.0,* and *0.5* represent the utility scores. Treatment effects are compared by computing these differences in mean Q-TWiST. This quality-adjusted survival comparison offers the opportunity to include the utility weights to reflect the relative value to the patient of the different clinical health states. Treatment comparisons are made using a sensitivity analysis, called threshold utility analysis, which displays the treatment comparison for varying values of the utility scores (10).

Several extensions of the basic Q-TWiST methodology have been proposed which incorporated patient-derived preferences by examining longitudinal utility scores in each patient and prognostic factors using proportional hazard regression.

CONCLUSION

Quality management methods have a rich heritage from the history of traditional quality assurance and assessment. They have been enhanced and expanded by quality improvement and reengineering initiatives leading to the TQM concept. As quality management evolves, there will be continuing challenges to develop performance measurement and reporting systems that meet the external demands for accountability in addition to the internal demands.

ACKNOWLEDGMENT

The author thanks Dr. Arino Yaguchi for her help in the translation of Japanese concepts of *Kaizen* and *Houshin*.

REFERENCES

1. American Medical Association, Council of Medical Service. Quality of care. *JAMA* 1986;256:1032–1034.
2. Chassin MR, Hannan EL, DeBuono BA. Benefits and hazards of reporting medical outcomes publicly. *N Engl J Med* 1996;334:394–398.

3. Cleary PD, Edgman-Levitan S. Health care quality. Incorporating consumer perspectives. *JAMA* 1997;278: 1608–1612.

4. Cole BF, Gelber RD, Kirkwood JM, et al. Quality-of-life adjusted survival analysis of interferon alpha-2b adjuvant treatment of high-risk resected cutaneous melanoma: an Eastern Cooperative Oncology Group (ECOG) study. *J Clin Oncol* 1996;14:2666–2673.

5. Croog SH, Levine S, Testa MA, et al. The effects of antihypertensive therapy on the quality of life. *N Engl J Med* 1986;314:1657–1664.

6. Deming WE. *Out of control*. Cambridge, MA: Massachusetts Institute of Technology Press, 1986.

7. Donabedian A. Explorations in quality assessment and monitoring. In: *The definition of quality and approaches to its assessment*, vol. 1. Ann Arbor, MI: Health Administration Press, 1980.

8. Donabedian A. The quality of care. How can it be assessed? *JAMA* 1988;260:1743–1748.

9. Gelber RD, Goldhirsch A. A new endpoint for the assessment of adjuvant therapy in postmenopausal women with operable breast cancer. *J Clin Oncol* 1986;4:1772–1779.

10. Glasziou PP, Simes RJ, Geler RD. Quality adjusted survival analysis. *Stat Med* 1990;9:1259–1276.

11. Green J, Passman LJ, Wintfeld N. Analyzing hospital mortality. The consequences of diversity in patient mix. *JAMA* 1991;265:1849–1853.

12. Guyatt GH, Feeny DH, Patrick DL. Measuring health-related quality of life. *Ann Intern Med* 1993;118:622–629.

13. Hammer M. Reengineering work: don't automate, obliterate. *Harvard Business Review* 1990;July–August: 104–112.

14. Iezzoni LI, Ash AS, Shwartz M, et al. Predicting who dies depends on how severity is measured: implications for evaluating patient outcomes. *Ann Intern Med* 1995;123:763–770.

15. Iezzoni LI. The risks of risk adjustment. *JAMA* 1997;278:1600–1607.

16. Ishikawa K. *Guide to quality control*. White Plains, NY: Kraus International Publications, 1987.

17. Joint Commission on Accreditation of Healthcare Organizations. *An integrated approach to medical staff performance improvement*. Oakbrook Terrace, IL: The Joint Commission on Accreditation of Healthcare Organizations, 1996.

18. Joint Commission on Accreditation of Healthcare Organizations. *Comprehensive accreditation manual for hospitals*. Oakbrook Terrace, IL: The Joint Commission on Accreditation of Healthcare Organizations, 2001.

19. Laupacis A. Changes in quality of life and functional capacity in hemodialysis patients treated with recombinant human erythropoietin. The Canadian Erythropoietin Study Group. *Semin Nephrol* 1990;10(2)[Suppl 1]:11–19.

20. Lohr KN. *Medicare: a strategy for quality assurance*. Washington, DC: Institute of Medicine, National Academy Press, 1990.

21. Mélot C. Economic evaluation in health care. In: Gunzburg R, Szpalski M, eds. *Lumbar spinal stenosis*. Philadelphia: Lippincott Williams & Wilkins 2000:357–365.

22. Mélot C. Principles of cost–benefit analysis. In: Szpalski M, Gunzburg R, Pope MH, eds. *Lumbar segmental instability*. Philadelphia: Lippincott Williams & Wilkins 1999:259–273.

23. Omoigui NA, Miller DP, Brown KJ, et al. Outmigration for coronary bypass surgery in an area of public dissemination of clinical outcomes. *Circulation* 1996;93:27–33.

24. Patrick M, Alba T. Health care benchmarking: a team approach. *Qual Mgmt Health Care* 1994;2:38–47.

25. Schneider EC, Epstein AM. Influence of cardiac-surgery performance reports on referral practices and access to care. *N Engl J Med* 1996;335:251–256.

26. Toevs CD, Kaplan RM, Atkins CJ. The costs and effects of behavioral programs in chronic obstructive pulmonary disease. *Med Care* 1984;22:1088–1100.

27. Weissman NW, Allison JJ, Kiefe CI, et al. Achievable benchmarks of care: the ABCs of benchmarking. *J Eval Clin Pract* 1999;5:269–281.

31

Prediction of Results in Lumbar Disc Herniation

Federico Balagué, Ali Sheikhzadeh, and Margareta Nordin

The term "sciatica" describes pain and possibly paresthesias radiating down the leg with dermatomal distribution. These are the signs and symptoms for nerve compromise and a possible intervertebral disc herniation (DH). Pain radiating below the knee is documented as a robust sign for a DH and nerve compromise (13). Sciatica prevalence in an adult population has been estimated at 1.6% for symptoms lasting more than 2 weeks (13) and 3% of patients reporting lower back pain (LBP) (52). Annual incidence rates range from 1% to 10% (15,28,44). Risk factors for lumbar DH have been associated with occupational, biomechanical, and/or lifestyle characteristics (13). The cause–effect relationship of DH and pain remains unclear, and recently the value of clinical assessment has been questioned (1,34).

A minority of patients with sciatica will require surgery (13). While some indications for surgical referral are generally accepted, the large geographic variations in the rates of lumbar surgery performed in the United States widely suggest differing practice styles among physicians (13). The only absolute indication for surgery is the presence of the cauda equina syndrome according to Svartzman and colleagues (45). Inappropriate patient selection has been suggested as the most common cause of failure after lumbar laminectomy (22). A Swiss retrospective study of 196 subjects surgically treated for DH concludes that 23% of indications were inappropriate, 29% were equivocal, and 48% were appropriate (39). These figures support Weber's statement that "approximately 60% of the operated patients may have been submitted to an unnecessary surgical procedure" (50). Different authors state that the option to undergo surgical or conservative management should remain with the patient (45,51).

Long-term outcome after surgical or conservative management of patients with sciatica remains controversial. Since November 1993, we have conducted a prospective study on patients with acute severe sciatica in Fribourg (Switzerland). The results of baseline evaluation and evolution during 1-year follow-up have been previously published (3).

Our aim for this chapter regarding this study is: (a) to describe overall recovery during 1 year in terms of well being; (b) to identify acute phase predictors strongly associated with recovery at 1 year; and (c) to report on overall evolution after 3 to 6.5 years of follow-up.

MATERIALS AND METHODS

A prospective cohort of patients with severe acute sciatica due to the involvement of a single nerve root (L5 or S1) was evaluated by means of a standardized protocol, and followed prospectively for 1 year.

Subjects

Consecutive patients were hospitalized in the Cantonal Hospital of Fribourg for treatment of severe sciatica and were evaluated for inclusion in the study. Medically necessary reasons for hospitalizations were intensive pain management (including bed rest, epidural injections, medications, and other treatements), neurologic deficit, and residing too far from the hospital for ambulatory treatment (10). The inpatient program included bed rest (less than 1 week), medication (narcotic analgesics, nonsteroidal antiinflammatories, sedatives), physical medicine modalities, transcutaneous electrical nerve stimulation (TENS), exercise in a swimming pool, instruction, and other exercises. The average duration of hospitalization was 3 weeks. Cauda equina syndrome and progressive motor deficit (manual motor test less than 3) were indications for immediate surgery. Surgery was elective for intolerable pain refractory to aggressive drug therapy, or for lack of improvement after 2 to 3 weeks of hospitalization (22,51).

Inclusion Criteria

All the patients were admitted to the Department of Rheumatology, Physical Medicine, and Rehabilitation for conservative management of sciatica and were considered potentially eligible for inclusion in the study. Inclusion and exclusion criteria were similar to those used in the literature, and have been described in detail elsewhere (3).

Informed Consent

The ethical committee of the Cantonal Hospital of Fribourg approved the project. The study started in November 1993 and the follow-up of the last patient was conducted in November 1998. A survey was performed to evaluate the rate of inclusions and exclusions among the overall sciatica admissions to the Department of Rheumatology. With this purpose, each admission was dated and recorded together with the preliminary diagnosis.

Process

Short-Term (1-Year) Follow-Up

All the subjects were evaluated five times: at admission and discharge from the hospital, and then at 3, 6, and 12 months after discharge (visits 1 to 5). The first evaluation (visit 1) was performed within the first 24 hours of admission, and the second evaluation took place during the last 2 to 3 days of hospitalization. The treating physician performed clinical evaluation at admission (visit 1) and at discharge (visit 2). Follow-up (visits 3 to 5) was performed by an independent physician. The evaluations were standardized according to an agreement between the physicians reached during the pilot study. An inter-observer study was performed with ten patients for the straight leg raising (SLR) test and spinal mobility ($R = 0.88$ to 0.98; $P < 0.05$).

Long-Term Follow-Up

A subgroup of 33 patients underwent a sixth evaluation by an independent physician 3 to 6.5 years after visit 1.

Data Collection

Data collected at admission included demographics, clinical examination, self- administered questionnaires on function, pain, and quality of life, electrodiagnostics (electromyography), imaging (computed tomography scans or magnetic resonance imaging), and blood specimens. At discharge and follow-up visits a clinical examination was performed and questionnaire data were collected.

Imaging

Computed tomography (CT) scans or magnetic resonance imaging (MRI) of the L4-L5 and L5-S1 levels was done. The imaging was evaluated by an experienced radiologist blinded to the origin of the images (12). We developed a scoring system to standardize the reading of the imaging. A subsample of ten files was selected at random to evaluate the intra-observer agreement, which was at least 65% (range 65% to 80%). A subset of 15 patients treated conservatively underwent a second CT scan limited to the level identified at the first imaging on average 46.3 months after the first evaluation.

Electrodiagnostics

Electrodiagnostic tests were performed on patients with leg pain duration longer than 3 weeks. Electromyography (EMG) was evaluated by an independent neurologist and focused on nerve root impairment, localization of lesion, acute or chronic lesion, and presence of signs of polyneuritis. Results were classified as abnormal or normal.

Blood Samples

Within 24 hours of admission, a 10-mL fasting blood sample was taken from 68 of 82 patients. The sample was centrifuged; plasma was divided into 1-mL aliquots, frozen at $-60°$, and shipped frozen to the Department of Neurochemistry at Sahlgrenska University Hospital in Molndal, Sweden, for assays. Specimens were analyzed for the presence of autoantibodies against a number of glycosphingolipids, most of which have been previously discussed as potential autoantigens in other neuropathies to investigate whether production of autoantibodies to the glycosphingolipids occurs in patients with sciatica. Since these antibodies may be present at low titers in normal individuals (35) and there is no clear limit for pathologic levels in serum, we used pooled serum from blood donors as a negative reference.

Antiglycosphingolipid antibodies were assayed by a microtiter–enzyme-linked immunosorbent assay (ELISA) method (17,18).

A second blood sample was obtained and the same tests performed on a sample of 23 patients at the last follow-up visit (6).

Self-Administered Questionnaires

The self-administered questionnaires and standardized clinical evaluations were adapted from the protocol of the Model Clinic of the Occupational and Industrial Orthopedic Center in New York City (8,37).

The intake protocol included a questionnaire eliciting age, work activities, gender, previous medical history, previous sciatica, marital status, duration of symptoms of current episode, cause of injury, smoking, and country of birth.

The questionnaire also ascertained pain related to functional disability by Oswestry (16). The last item of the original Oswestry questionnaire, concerning sexual life, was not included due to low acceptance rate of the question from the patients. Therefore, our scores ranged from 0 to 45 and were then recoded to 100%.

Pain was ascertained by visual analog scale (VAS) (where 0 is no pain and 100 is the worst pain imaginable), and a pain drawing divided into five categories: low back, buttock, thigh, below the knee, and foot.

Clinical Examination

Clinical examination included functional spinal mobility evaluation (modified Schober test and finger-to-floor distance in centimeters) and SLR test. The SLR test was entered as a dichotomous variable. Greater than 60 degrees of SLR was coded as normal. SLR of less than 60 degrees and/or enhanced SLR by dorsiflexion of the ankle, internal rotation of the hip, and/or flexion of the cervical spine were considered positive tests.

Light touch was tested by the examiners touching the different dermatomes with their fingers. Both sides were tested simultaneously, and the results compared. The findings were graded as normal or abnormal sensitivity using a dichotomous variable to determine normal or abnormal sensitivity.

Manual muscle power was tested according to the description of Kendall and colleagues (27). The great toe extensor and other dorsiflexors of the foot as well as plantar flexors of the foot were tested (13). For each leg, the lowest score was recorded for the L5 and S1 muscle group. The score was entered as a dichotomous variable where less than 4 is "abnormal" and greater than or equal to 4 is "normal."

Statistical Test

For baseline and follow-up data, descriptive statistics were computed, as appropriate for categorical and continuous variables. Contingency table methods were employed for evaluating associations between the clinical and the imaging tests and biomarkers at admission. Fisher's exact probability was computed for statistical hypothesis testing. Recovery was summarized as an index determined as perceived disability (Oswestry score less than 20), pain intensity (VAS score less than 15), and no pain below the knee. Factors associated with surgery and factors associated with recovery at 1 year were evaluated by contingency table methods if categorical and by comparison of means if continuous. Fisher's exact probability was computed for contingency tables and Wilcoxon's rank sum statistic was computed for continuous variables. For all hypotheses testing, alpha was set at 0.05.

RESULTS

During the study period, 1,239 patients were admitted to the Department of Rheumatology. Sciatica patients represented 25% ($N = 315$) of the total admissions; and 25% ($N = 82$) of the cases with sciatica were included in the study. The reasons for exclusion have been reported (3).

Nine patients (11%) discontinued the study within the first follow-up year, either because they moved away from the area ($N = 1$) or did not wish to continue ($N = 8$). These figures compare favorably with a study by Patrick and colleagues (38). Patients characteristics and the results of the overall evolution during the first 12 months have been published elsewhere (3).

Clinical Evolution of Recovery

Table 31.1 describes the clinical evolution with respect to clinical tests and perceived patient outcomes.

At 1-year follow-up, 30% of patients reported that they had no residual pain at all (VAS: 0/100). The same percentage reported a perfectly normal function as assessed by an Oswestry index of 0/100. We also used a composite index including little pain (VAS less than 15/100), an acceptable function (Oswestry less than 20/100), and normal muscle function (M5). With this definition, recovery occurred in about one-third of our cohort.

At long-term follow-up, 16 of 33 patients reported no LBP at all (48.5%) and 25 of 33 no leg pain at all (75.8%). However, only 17% had a perfectly normal score (0/100) on the Oswestry disability inventory.

None of the patients who underwent a second CT scan at visit 6 showed any increase in the amount of nucleus pulposus visible into the lumbar spinal canal. There was either a radiologic reduction or stability of the herniation.

We compared the patients at first visit for successful recovery at 1 year, using the recovery index (Oswestry less than 20, VAS score less than 15, and no pain below the knee). Patients who met the recovery index criteria were compared to patients who did not meet the criteria for recovery. Only the duration of pain was different at visit 1. Patients with good outcome had a duration of pain of 17 ($\pm$13) days compared to 42 ($\pm$46) days ($P = 0.012$) among patients not meeting the recovery index.

Factors Associated with Recovery at 1 Year

We examined univariate associations of age, gender, duration of pain, severity of pain, history of smoking, previous episodes of sciatica, EMG, Body Mass Index (BMI), Swiss

TABLE 31.1. *Summary of the evolution of some clinical tests and patient-reported outcomes*

Variables	Visit 1 (N = 82)	Visit 5 (12 months) (N = 72)	Visit 6 (52 months) (N = 33)
Age (yrs)	43		
Female:Male	34%:66%	30%:70%	30%:70%
Oswestry (%)	55	16	15.1
Trunk list (yes)	22%	1%	3%
Limp (yes)	38%	5%	3%
Modified Schober index (cm)	18.8	20.3	21.3
Finger–floor distance (cm)	36.4	17.0	15.5
LBP on palpation (yes)	85%	28%	42%
LBP on trunk flexion (yes)	52%	23%	30%
Leg pain on trunk flexion (yes)	73%	20%	21%
Motor deficit (yes)	21%	1%	3%
Sensory deficit (yes)	48%	20%	27%
Achilles reflex (missing)	46%	24%	12%
SLR ipsilateral (≤60°)	78%	32%	15%
SLR contralateral (≤60°)	20%	3%	none

LBP, lower back pain; SLR, straight leg raising.

TABLE 31.2. *Three models of recovery from lumbar disc herniation*

Definition of recovery at 1 year	Prevalence	Predictors	O.R. (C.I.)
VAS <15 Osw <20 No distal pain[a]	40%	Duration of pain†	4.8 (1.2–18.7)
VAS <15 Osw <20 Normal muscle strength	50%	Neurotot[c] Smoking	4.3 (1.4–13.3) 0.33 (0.1–0.99)
VAS <15 Osw <20	54%	Antibodies anti-GD1a	3.7 (1.01–13.7)

Osw, Oswestry questionnaire; VAS, visual analog scale
[a]No distal pain means that the pain drawing at 1 year did not contain any leg pain below the knee.
†Defined as duration of sciatica >30 days at admission.
[c]Neurotot was defined as any kind of neurologic deficit at visit 1.

birth, quality of life, Oswestry, pain (VAS), imaging results, neurologic tests (Neurotot), SLR, and antibody test results with recovery at 1 year as expressed by the composite variable (Table 31.2). Only duration of pain was significantly associated with recovery (i.e., the longer the pain duration the less recovery). The analysis was repeated using a little broader definition of recovery including only pain intensity (VAS less than 15) and self-reported functional capacity (Oswestry less than 20).

At long-term follow-up, the variables collected at visit 1 were examined with regard to their predictive value for disability pension application.

DISCUSSION

This study describes the characteristics, admission diagnostics, and recovery of otherwise healthy patients with severe sciatica. The patients were enrolled at admission to hospital and followed prospectively for 1 year. The cohort was restricted to patients without comorbidities, systemic or other orthopedic bases for sciatica, or prior history of surgery. A subgroup was followed up to 6.5 years.

The majority of patients in this study were male (male:female ratio 1.93:1). This is consistent with other reports that have male:female ratios ranging from 2.6:1 to 1.3:1 (2, 7,9,19,22,24,29,50,53). Men opted slightly more for surgery than did women in this study, which supports the findings from Hurme and coworkers and Matray (23,32).

Our patients have a similar age range to reports in the literature. Mean ages vary from 38 to 48 years (2,5,7,9,22–24,29,32,51).

As in other reports, a large proportion of patients could not identify a precipitating event for their sciatica (13,51). Among the 280 patients described by Weber (50), the sciatica "began insidiously."

A large proportion of patients (57%) in our study had a history of cigarette smoking. Smokers are in less good health than nonsmokers (4,20,55). In our study, smoking was not associated with outcome.

Imaging

In a recent study by means of MRI, the intra-observer variability at 2-month interval was 0.86 (composite index: 0.65, 1.00) (40). Our intra-observer agreement was 65% or 80%. The best agreement was found at the L4-L5 level.

In Carragee and Kim's study, morphometric features of disc herniation and the spinal canal (by MRI) were predictors of surgical outcome (9). Different methods have been described to evaluate the size of disc herniations (7,11,14,31,33,36,47).

Radiologic evolution over time was not the purpose of our research; rather, we wanted to know whether imaging at admission could help predict neurologic and/or functional outcome or the choice of surgical treatment. Our method was a modification of those mainly used by Ninomiya and Muro (36) and Maigne and coworkers (31). We used nerve roots as anatomic landmarks both in the frontal and sagittal planes.

No correlation was found by Thelander and associates either between SLR and the size or position of the hernia or between the decrease in hernia size over time and the improvement in SLR (46). In our study, the percentage of positive agreement was 74% between positive SLR at visit 1 and positive CT scan, defined as the herniation grade 2 or 3 at the proximity of the nerve root.

Factors Associated with Recovery at 1 Year

A substantial percentage of patients with acute severe sciatica had not recovered by 1 year after discharge in our study. The same has been reported by others (41,54). Overall, only 21 patients recovered on our composite index. Only 21 (29%) of the patients were totally free of pain and 22 patients perceived no disability (Oswestry less than 5) regardless of treatment. Twelve percent still reported radiating pain into the foot. A recent study performed in France, where subjects with acute sciatica were treated as inpatients in rheumatology departments, showed several similarities with our results mainly in terms of need for surgery, lack of predictive value of some clinical parameters, and so forth (5). Our figures are lower than those reported by Vroomen and colleagues who found more than 85% of patients improved after 12 weeks (48).

Our finding that major recovery occurs within the first 3 months is in agreement with the results reported by Woertgen and associates (54).

Only duration of pain at admission was associated with recovery at 1 year. The lack of other strongly associated demographic, clinical, and paraclinical factors suggests that as with nonspecific low back pain, the biopsychosocial model (49) may be more appropriate for the treatment of sciatica patients than the purely medical or surgical model. This is consistent with Hasenbring and coworkers' statement that some predictors of chronicity in nonspecific LBP, are also predictors of outcome among patients with radicular pain (21).

Patients who underwent surgery reported significantly greater pain intensity at admission than patients who did not go on to surgery. There were no differences in findings on the clinical and imaging examinations. This confirms that surgery is an option chosen more for patient perception reasons than for objectively demonstrated pathoanatomic findings. Patients who had surgery did not have significantly different outcomes than patients who did not have surgery. Given that patients undergoing surgery reported borderline greater pain at admission, the lack of a difference in composite recovery at 1 year is consistent with a reduction in self-reported pain intensity without affecting pain below the knee, functional disability, quality of life, or muscle function. Evaluating the efficacy of surgery compared to medical treatment was not the purpose of this study (21,25, 26,30).

Nevertheless, these results are consistent with other reports (7,42,43,50). Only randomized controlled trials can determine the efficacy of different treatments.

Limitations of the Study

Hospital treatment for severe sciatica is not a universal practice. It is possible that the hospitalization of the patients as practiced in Switzerland reinforces the sick role and perceived seriousness of the condition. Thus perceived, recovery may have been delayed in these patients. While the homogeneous nature of the cohort permitted focus on this subgroup of sciatica patients, the results of this study may not be able to be generalized for patients who have already experienced spine surgery, or to patients with comorbidities.

CONCLUSIONS

The primary purposes of this study were to describe the presentation and recovery of severe sciatica and to examine the value of commonly used tools as well as some new tools for the prediction of recovery. The study shows that a large proportion of patients with acute severe sciatica have positive imaging or EMG tests. Perceived pain and disability measures do not correlate with clinical findings or imaging results in these acute severe patients. Thus, the severity of pain and functional disability is not explained by structural derangement or by disturbed nerve function alone.

Autoantibodies to 3'LM1 were associated with positive neurologic tests, perhaps indicating an immune response leading to neurologic deficit. This may be a biomarker of neurologic damage and may identify patients in need of targeted interventions.

Recovery in severe sciatica, in terms of an overall index of pain, disability, quality of life, and muscle function, is not as good as might be expected based on reports of surgical outcomes. The lack of predictors of 1-year recovery in this group of patients is interesting and should be further explored. As in nonspecific LBP, patients' coping mechanisms, beliefs about back pain, social circumstances, and other psychosocial factors may have an important role in recovery.

There is very little recovery after 3 months' postdischarge. Thus, further interventions may be introduced for patients who have not recovered by this time.

Educating patients to understand that total recovery occurs in about one-third of cases regardless of whether surgery is performed may result in more realistic patient expectations.

REFERENCES

1. Albeck MJ. A critical assessment of clinical diagnosis of disc herniation in patients with monoradicular sciatica. *Acta Neurochir (Wien)* 1996;138:40–44.
2. Atlas SJ, Deyo RA, Keller RB, et al. The Maine lumbar spine study, part II. 1-year outcomes of surgical and nonsurgical management of sciatica. *Spine* 1996;21:1777–1786.
3. Balagué F, Nordin M, Sheikhzadeh A, et al. Recovery of severe sciatica. *Spine* 1999;24:2516–2524.
4. Bartecchi CE, MacKenzie TD, Schrier RW. The human costs of tobacco use. *N Engl J Med* 1994;330:907–912.
5. Berthelot J, Rodet D, Guillot P, et al. Is it possible to predict the efficacy at discharge of inhospital rheumatology department management of disk-related sciatica? A study in 150 patients. *Rev Rhum (Br)* 1999;66:207–213.
6. Brisby H. *Nerve tissue injury markers, inflammatory mechanisms and immunologic factors in lumbar disc herniation* [dissertation]. Göteborg University (Sweden); 2000.
7. Bush K, Cowan N, Katz DE, et al. The natural history of sciatica associated with disc pathology. A prospective study with clinical and independent radiologic follow-up. *Spine* 1992;17:1205–1212.
8. Campello M, Weiser S, van Doorn J, et al. Approaches to improve the outcome of patients with delayed recovery. In: Nordin M, Cedraschi C, Vischer T, eds. *New approaches to the low back patient.* London: BailliÈre's Clinical Rheumatology, International Practice and Research, Harcourt Brace Jovanovich Ltd, 1998:93–113.
9. Carragué EJ, Kim DH. A prospective analysis of magnetic resonance imaging findings in patients with sciatica and lumbar disc herniation. *Spine* 1997;22:1650–1660.
10. Cherkin DC, Deyo RA. Nonsurgical hospitalization for low-back pain. Is it necessary? *Spine* 1993;18: 1728–1735.

11. Delauche-Cavallier M-C, Budet C, Laredo J-D, et al. Lumbar disc herniation. computed tomography scan changes after conservative treatment of nerve root compression. *Spine* 1992;17:927–933.

12. Deyo RA, Andersson G, Bombardier C, et al. Outcome measures for studying patients with low back pain. *Spine* 1994;19:2032S–2036S.

13. Deyo RA, Loeser JD, Bigos SJ. Herniated lumbar intervertebral disk. *Ann Intern Med* 1990;112:598–603.

14. Ellenberg MR, Ross ML, Honet JC, et al. Prospective evaluation of the course of disc herniations in patients with proven radiculopathy. *Arch Phys Med Rehabil* 1993;74:3–8.

15. Errico TJ, Fardon DF, Lowell TD. Contemporary concepts in spine care. Open discectomy as treatment for herniated nucleus pulposus of the lumbar spine. *Spine* 1995;20:1829–1833.

16. Fairbank JCT, Couper J, Davies JB, et al. The Oswestry low back pain disability questionnaire. *Physiotherapy* 1980;66:271–273.

17. Fredman P. The role of anti-glycolipid antibodies in neurological diseases. *New York Acad Sci* 1998;845: 341–352.

18. Fredman P, Lycke J, Andersen O, et al. Peripheral neuropathy associated with monoclonal IgM antibody to glycolipids with a terminal glycoronyl-3-sulfate epitope. *J Neurol* 1993;240:381–387.

19. Hakelius A. Prognosis in sciatica. A clinical follow-up of surgical and non-surgical treatment. *Acta Orthop Scand* 1970;1–76.

20. Hanrahan JP, Sherman CB, Bresnitz EA, et al. Cigarette smoking and health. *Am J Respir Crit Care Med* 1996;153:861–865.

21. Hasenbring M, Marienfeld G, Kuhlendahl D, et al. Risk factors of chronicity in lumbar disc patients. A prospective investigation of biologic, psychologic, and social predictors of therapy outcome. *Spine* 1994;19:2759–2765.

22. Herron LD, Turner J. Patient selection for lumbar laminectomy and discectomy with a revised objective rating system. *Clin Orthop* 1985;199:145–152.

23. Hurme M, Alaranta H, Einola S, et al. A prospective study of patients with sciatica. A comparison between conservatively treated patients and patients who have undergone operation, part I: Patient characteristics and differences between groups. *Spine* 1990;15:1340–1344.

24. Jönsson B, Strömqvist B. Neurologic signs in lumbar disc herniation. Preoperative affliction and postoperative recovery in 150 cases. *Acta Orthop Scand* 1996;67:466–469.

25. Junge A, Dvorak J, Ahrens S. Predictors of bad and good outcome of lumbar disc surgery: a prospective clinical study resulting in recommendations for screening to avoid bad outcome. *Spine* 1994;20:460–468.

26. Junge A, Fröhlich M, Ahrens S, et al. Predictors of bad and good outcome of lumbar spine surgery: a prospective clinical study with 2 years' follow-up. *Spine* 1996;21:1056–1065.

27. Kendall HO, Kendall FP, Wadsworth GE. *Les muscles, bilan et Ètude fonctionnelle.* Paris: Maloine S.A., 1974.

28. Lawrence RC, Helmick CG, Arnett FC, et al. Estimates of the prevalence of arthritis and selected musculoskeletal disorders in the united states. *Arthritis Rheumatism* 1998;41:778–799.

29. Leclaire R, Blier F, Fortin L, et al. A cross-sectional study comparing the Oswestry and Roland-Morris functional disability scales in two populations of patients with low back pain of different levels of severity. *Spine* 1997;22:68–71.

30. Little DG, MacDonald D. The use of the percentage change in Oswestry disability index score as an outcome measure in lumbar spinal surgery. *Spine* 1994;19:2139–2143.

31. Maigne J-Y, Rime B, Deligne B. Computed tomographic follow-up study of forty-eight cases of nonoperatively treated lumbar disc herniation. *Spine* 1992;17:1071–1074.

32. Matray L. *Etude sur les facteurs pronostiques des lombo-sciatalgies à 5 ans* [dissertation]. Lausanne: Faculté de Médecine de Lausanne (Switzerland), 1994.

33. Matsubara Y, Kato F, Mimatsu K, et al. Serial changes on MRI in lumbar disc herniations treated conservatively. *Neuroradiology* 1995;37:378–383.

34. Michel A, Kohlmann T, Raspe H. The association between clinical findings on physical examination and self-reported severity in back pain. *Spine* 1997;22:296–304.

35. Mizutamari RK, Wiegant H, Nores GA. Characterization of anti-ganglioside antibodies present in normal human plasma. *J Neuroimmunol* 1994;50:215–220.

36. Ninomiya M, Muro T. Pathoanatomy of lumbar disc herniation as demonstrated by computed tomography/discography. *Spine* 1992;17:1316–1322.

37. Nordin M, Skovron M, Hiebert R, et al. Early predictors of delayed return to work in patients with low back pain. *J Musculoskeletal Pain* 1997;5:5–27.

38. Patrick DL, Deyo RA, Atlas SJ, et al. Assessing health-related quality of life in patients with sciatica. *Spine* 1995;20:1899–1909.

39. Porchet F, Vader JP, Larequi-Lauber T, et al. The assessment of appropriate indications for laminectomy. *J Bone Joint Surg (Br)* 1999;81:234–239.

40. Rankine JJ, Fortune DG, Hutchinson CE, et al. Pain drawings in the assessment of nerve root compression: A comparative study with lumbar spine magnetic resonance imaging. *Spine* 1998;23:1668–1676.

41. Rompe J, Eysel P, Zöllner J, et al. Prognostic criteria for work resumption after standard lumbar discectomy. *Eur Spine J* 1999;8:132–137.

42. Saal JA. Natural history and nonoperative treatment of lumbar disc herniation. *Spine* 1996;21:2S–9S.

43. Saal JA, Saal JS. Nonoperative treatment of herniated lumbar intervertebral disc with radiculopathy. An outcome study. *Spine* 1989;14:431–437.

44. Savettieri G, Rocca WA, Slemi G. Prevalence of lumbosacral spondylitic radiculopathy (LSR): a door-to-door survey in two Sicilian municipalities. *Neurology* 1992;42:355(abst).
45. Shvartzman LEW, Sherry H, Levin S, et al. Cost–effectiveness analysis of extended conservative therapy versus surgical intervention in the management of herniated lumbar intervertebral disc. *Spine* 1992;17:176–182.
46. Thelander U, Fagerlund M, Friberg S, et al. Describing the size of lumbar disc herniations using computed tomography. A comparison of different size index calculations and their relation to sciatica. *Spine* 1994;19: 1979–1984.
47. Thelander U, Fagerlund M, Friberg S, et al. Straight leg raising test versus radiologic size, shape, and position of lumbar disc hernias. *Spine* 1992;17:395–399.
48. Vroomen P, De Krom M, Wilmink J, et al. Lack of effectiveness of bed rest for sciatica. *N Engl J Med* 1999;340:418–423.
49. Waddell G. Biopsychosocial analysis of low back pain. In: Vischer NM, Vischer T, eds. *Common low back pain: prevention of chronicity*. London: Baillière's Clinical Rheumatology, International Practice and Research, Harcourt Brace Jovanovich Ltd, 1992:523–557.
50. Weber H. Lumbar disc herniation. A controlled, prospective study with ten years of observation. *Spine* 1983;8: 131–140.
51. Weber H. Spine update. The natural history of disc herniation and the influence of intervention. *Spine* 1994;19: 2234–2238.
52. Wipf JE, Deyo RA. Low back pain. *Med Clin North Am* 1995;79:231–246.
53. Woertgen C, Holzschuh M, Rothoerl RD, et al. Clinical signs in patients with brachialgia and sciatica: A comparative study. *Surg Neurol* 1998;49:210–214.
54. Woertgen C, Rothoerl R, Breme K, et al. Variability of outcome after lumbar disc surgery. *Spine* 1999;24: 807–811.
55. Wyser C, Bolliger CT. Smoking-related disorders. In: Bolliger CT, Fagerström KO, eds. *The tobacco epidemic*. Basel: Karger, 1997:78–106.

32

Epidemiology, Fitness for Work, and Costs

Marc Du Bois and Peter Donceel

In the United States, surgical decompression for a prolapsed or herniated lumbar intervertebral disc is the most frequently performed spinal intervention and one of the most commonly performed surgical procedures with approximately 200,000 cases being reported each year (1,10). A common operation worldwide, disc herniation surgery puts an important social and economic burden on society since the end results are inconsistent. Reported results of surgical discectomy have shown success rates that vary between 50% to 95% (4,10,13). In the case of surgery for low back pain, return to work and the value of time lost from work is of major significance to patients, employers, and the entire economy and should be an important element in its evaluation. In an era of increasingly limited health care resources it seems prudent to consider the cost and effectiveness of discectomy before making treatment recommendations for patients (5,6,12). It is likely that direct medical costs alone exceed 5 to 6 billion dollars for the more than 200,000 lumbar discectomies performed in the United States each year.

The present study was undertaken to investigate the trends in surgery rates for cervical and lumbar disc herniation and to assess return to work rates 1 year after surgery. An additional objective was to identify factors associated with the return to work and to delineate costs related to disc herniation surgery.

METHODS

This study was based on the administrative patient record files from the largest Belgian Sickness Fund. It covers approximately 45% of the Belgian population, where sickness insurance is legally mandated. All claim files of the Christian Sickness Fund that were related to a surgical intervention for cervical or lumbar disc herniation performed in 1998 were reviewed according to the Belgian procedure code for medical and surgical procedures. The procedure code is a numerically encoded system that refers to the official description of a surgical intervention for financial reimbursement purposes. The surgeon has to register every intervention for disc herniation in line with this procedure code. Between January 1998 and January 1999, 203 enrollees in the Christian Sickness Fund underwent surgical intervention for cervical disc herniation whereas 2,105 underwent surgery for lumbar disc herniation. Patient records were followed until 1 year after surgical intervention. Five interventions were studied: standard surgery for disc herniation of the cervical spine, standard surgery for disc herniation of the lumbar spine, combined discectomy and fusion of the lumbar spine, and percutaneous nucleotomy and chemonucleolysis of the lumbar spine. Details about medical condition, clinical or radiologic signs were not included in the database. Since these data are used primarily for reimbursement purposes, they may be vulnerable to erroneous and biased coding.

Trends in Surgery Rates

Surgery rates were based on the data of the Official Authority of Sickness and Invalidity Insurance in Belgium. Since sickness insurance is mandatory, these figures cover the entire Belgian population. Surgery rates were calculated by dividing the number of treated patients by the year-specific total sickness fund enrollees for 1989 to 1999. Rates were not adjusted for sex or age.

Fitness for Work

Patients were evaluated by social security medical advisers. Individual medical evaluations took place regularly from about 1 month after surgical intervention until patients were judged fit for resuming work according to the legal criteria in the sickness and invalidity insurance. In the first 6 months of work incapacity, the medical adviser evaluated fitness for work with regard to the patient's most recently held job. After an incapacity period of 6 months, the criteria were extended to all occupations the patient may have access to, according to jobs performed in the past, present career, and education. The return to work rate after surgery for cervical or lumbar disc herniation was determined from claim files of patients belonging to the working population who were operated on in 1998. There were 1,499 men and 809 women in the study. The available preoperative features were gender, occupation, and work incapacity period prior to surgery. This information is obtained through a review of the individual files of the claimants and is depicted in Table 32.1. Patients who returned to work within 1 year after surgery for disc herniation were classified as good outcomes.

Analysis of Costs

In Belgium, health care and sickness benefits are insured by a social security system that is financed by contributions from both employees and employers. In the health care insurance tariff, agreements are made between health care providers, the government, and sickness funds. In this system each medical procedure or intervention is valued at a fixed

TABLE 32.1. *Worker's compensation population characteristics (N = 2.308)*

Characteristic	% (Mean)
Gender	
Male	65
Female	35
Occupation	
Self-employed	6
Blue-collar worker	62
White-collar worker	32
Surgery	
Standard discectomy C-spine	8
Standard discectomy L-spine	80.5
Fusion L-spine	9
Chemonucleolysis L-spine	1
Percutaneous nucleotomy L-spine	1.5
Age	40.5 yrs
Work incapacity period	5 months

price. A day lump sum is provided for hospitals to finance medical equipment, nursing, lodging, and administration. Patients belonging to the working population are compensated during the recovery period until fitness for work is determined. They receive a daily compensation in accordance with their previous salary level. The expenditures for medical procedures, work incapacity compensation, hospital nursing, lodging, and administration add up to the social insurance costs.

The cost–assessment phase of the study determined the social insurance cost for a follow-up of 1 postoperative year. In view of the retrospective design of the present study, we were not able to rule out medical care costs unrelated to surgery for lumbar or cervical disc herniation.

The individual files were broken down into the following cost items: office visits, kinesitherapy, anesthesia, surgery, radiology, implants, nursing, and lodging. Daily sickness fund payments compensating for work time lost after 1 month of work incapacity were calculated for the working population. No information about compensation payments during the first month of sick leave was available. (In the Belgian social security system this is paid by the employer.) Cost items were retrieved from the Christian Sickness Fund data warehouse via the Oracle 8i database management system. All costs are expressed in 1999 U.S. dollars.

Statistics

The data were analyzed using distinct statistical analyses. The relationship between outcome and the various associated factors were investigated employing parametric univariate analysis. Kruskal-Wallis one-way analysis of variance was used to identify continuous factors related to ability to work postoperatively. Logistic regression was performed to identify factors independently associated with return to work status 1 year after intervention. Forward stepwise logistic regression was conducted to discover the combinations of variables that might be associated with return to work 1 year after surgery. The variables tested were duration of work incapacity before surgery, gender, age, and professional status. The appropriate statistical procedures and Kaplan-Meier curves were performed using Statistical Package for the Social Sciences (SPSS) 10.0. Costs were analyzed and trend figures were drawn using Excel 7.0 for Windows. For all tests a 5% significance level was used.

RESULTS

Trends in Surgery Rates

From 1989 to 1999, 7,725 surgical interventions for cervical disc herniation were performed in Belgium. In the same period there were 88,512 operations for standard lumbar disc herniation, 8,107 combined lumbar discectomy and fusion operations, 4,359 chemonucleolysis procedures, and 3,566 percutaneous nucleotomies (Fig. 32.1). The 1999 annual rate of standard surgery for cervical disc herniation was 10.04 per 100.000 inhabitants. There was a steady increase over the 1-year period with approximately 12%. We found a steady state of approximately 95 operations per 100,000 inhabitants for standard lumbar disc herniation surgery. For combined lumbar discectomy and fusion there was an increase of 124% over the studied period. This trend goes along with the substantial decrease in percutaneous nucleotomy or chemonucleolysis. The decrease of percutaneous nucleotomy is about 40% over the 11-year period.

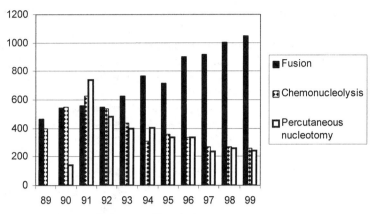

FIG. 32.1. Trends in surgery rates.

Fitness for Work

There were 1,499 men and 809 women in the working population who had an intervention for lumbar or cervical disc herniation in 1998. One year after combined lumbar disc herniation and fusion 194 patients (41.2%) were still unable to resume work (Table 32.2). Return to work rates 1 year after standard surgery for cervical or lumbar disc herniation were 76.8% and 80.9%, respectively. For percutaneous nucleotomy and chemonucleolysis, the number of cases were too small to make valid conclusions.

Comparison of the features among the bad and good outcome groups showed that there was a significant statistical difference in working capacity with respect to gender. About 25% of the women had an unsatisfactory result with only 19% of the men reporting an unfavorable outcome.

The period of work incapacity before surgical intervention affected postoperative work capacity. Of the patients who were out of work for more than 6 months at the time of surgery, 79.7% were still unable to return to work after 1 year. For patients out of work less than 1 month prior to surgery, only 9% were unable to work 12 months later (Fig. 32.2). Age was significantly associated with return to work. Of the patients younger than 30 years, 86% resumed work within 1 year postsurgery in contrast with 64% of patients older than 50 years.

Professional category had an effect on postoperative working capacity: 12 months after surgery for lumbar disc herniation 23% of the blue-collar workers were still unable to resume work. For white-collar workers this figure was just 13% (Fig. 32.3).

In the regression analysis, the duration of work incapacity before surgery was significantly ($P < 0.001$) associated with a return to work within 1 year after surgery. This vari-

TABLE 32.2. *Percentage of patients unable to resume work after surgery for disc herniation*

Surgical intervention	% unable to resume work (N)
Standard discectomy C-spine	23.2% (203)
Standard discectomy L-spine	19.1% (1862)
Fusion L-spine	41.2% (194)
Chemonucleolysis L-spine	29.0% (31)
Percutaneous nucleotomy L-spine	22.2% (18)

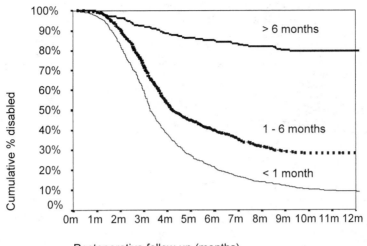

FIG. 32.2. The period of work incapacity before surgical intervention and how it affected postoperative work capacity.

able explained substantially the variance in return to work (partial correlation coefficient = 0.27).

Analysis of Costs

The administrative database also provides information on costs (Table 32.3). The mean social security cost of standard surgery for cervical disc herniation in the year after operation was $4,525 per case. For combined lumbar discectomy and fusion, the costs add up to $7,563. Each record file can be broken down into the following cost items: office vis-

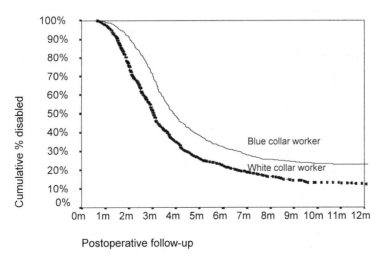

FIG. 32.3. Professional category and its effect on postoperative working capacity for blue-collar workers and white-collar workers.

TABLE 32.3. *Mean Social Security cost per case (USD)*
during a 1-year period after surgery for disc herniation
(Mean Social Security cost for standard surgery of the lumbar spine = 100%)

	Mean cost	Index (%)
Standard surgery-CS	$4,525	140
Standard surgery-LS	$3,239	100
Fusion-LS	$7,563	233
Chemonucleolysis-LS	$6,048	187
Percutaneous nucleotomy-LS	$5,102	158

its, kinesitherapy, anesthesia, surgery, radiology, implants, nursing, and lodging. Costs of implants are very important in the total social security costs of combined lumbar discectomy and fusion: they add up to 26% of the total costs. Costs for surgery are relatively less important for chemonucleolysis. For chemonucleolysis nursing and lodging constitutes the highest relative part (40%) of the social security costs.

DISCUSSION

Our study has strengths and weaknesses. First, the evaluation of fitness for work was performed by social security medical advisers. They are independent observers of return to work capacity. Second, since the Christian Sickness Fund covers more than 45% of the mandatory insured population in Belgium, this study concerns all Belgian centers where spinal surgery is performed. Third, valid conclusions can be drawn on a sufficient sample since more than 2,300 patients were involved. Nonetheless, the study was retrospective in nature and as such suffers from the shortcomings of retrospective design (4). It was therefore impossible to provide information concerning preoperative symptoms, coexisting diseases, and imaging.

We found an annual rate of 95 standard operations for lumber disc herniation per 100,000 inhabitants. According to literature, incidence of disc surgery varies tenfold among industrialized countries, differences that cannot be explained by biological factors alone. Rather, secondary gain, health care organization, social insurance, availability of medical resources, and local traditions seem to be important. For Belgium, we found a tremendous increase in surgery rates for combined discectomy and fusion operations. This may be due to the growing quality of implants as well as to the better reimbursement for that type of surgery in contrast with less invasive procedures like percutaneous nucleotomy or chemonucleolysis (14).

The study demonstrates a high percentage of unsatisfactory results in patients who had standard surgery for lumbar or cervical disc herniation. At a follow-up of 1 year, 19.1% to 23.2% of the patients were still unable to resume work. A meaningful comparison of these results to those of other studies is rather difficult. This is due to the fact that outcome measures are different. Short-term studies with less than a 2-year follow-up tend to give an optimistic success rate that exceeds 90%. It is generally known that objective outcome measures tend to give less favorable results than objective outcome measures. But the trend toward a less favorable return to work after combined discectomy and fusion is consistent with the results of other studies.

Despite advancements in diagnostic imaging and refinement of surgical technique, the results after lumbar disc surgery do not seem to have improved during recent decades (11,13,15). Some 15% to 20% of patients do not recover and a few have severe chronic pain syndromes. The end results of such treatment have been inconsistent. The most likely factors leading to variable results are patient selection, varying follow-up intervals, and differences in analyzing outcomes (4).

In this as in many other disc herniation studies, women were associated with a poor outcome (4,15). In general, women also appear to be more prone to chronic pain syndrome than men. It is assumed that cultural, social, and biological factors work in concert to make middle-aged women particularly vulnerable.

The results of the study indicate that employment status is correlated with the working incapacity period after surgery for disc herniation. Jobs requiring significant physical strenuousness predispose to an unfavorable outcome (10). Blue-collar workers are especially vulnerable since they are most often involved in the heaviest manual work with most back strain (4,9,15). Additionally, they have less possibility of changing their working conditions than does a patient with a light occupational activity. Only 13% of the white-collar workers had unsatisfactory results, compared with 23% of the blue-collar workers. Some studies do not support this finding. This may be due to difficulties in classifying the strenuousness of work from traditional job descriptions. It could be hypothesized that because of the unsatisfactory work conditions the patient uses his restriction in daily activities as an excuse to not return to work. It is assumed that patients with stressful work conditions do not tend to return to work even if the discectomy was successful from a surgical point of view. Improvements in working conditions particularly from the psychological point of view, could play a significant role in the rehabilitation of a patient after discectomy. However, the exact mechanisms thus far remain unclear and deserve further attention and evaluation.

Patients who were older showed significantly negative association with return to work This is in line with the fact that prognosis after lumbar disc surgery is known to deteriorate with age at referral (3). However, if multivariate analysis is controlled for preoperative period of work incapacity no significant effect is revealed.

Return to work is very important both from the social and economic perspective. It is apparent from our data that a high rate of patients were still unable to return to work after surgery for disc herniation. A major finding of this study was that the preoperative period of work incapacity was significantly associated with return to work. The importance of the work incapacity prior to surgery should be taken more into account in further research. It also implies that our attention should be drawn to the determination of the indication and the timing of surgery (7,8). It is also generally assumed that prolonged waiting among patients with sequestrated herniations is meaningless and only causes unnecessary suffering (15). The best surgical results occur when surgery is performed before 3 months have elapsed since the onset of symptoms.

The general conclusion that can be drawn from the cost–assessment phase is that the social security costs of combined discectomy and fusion for lumbar disc herniation are 2.3 times higher than for the standard procedure. With regard to the high direct and indirect costs of surgery for disc herniation, reliable and valid screening instruments that allow a more comprehensive patient evaluation for surgery with emphasis on the length of work incapacity before surgery must be developed on the basis of further research (2,4,8).

REFERENCES

1. Andersson GB, Weinstein JN. Disc herniation. *Spine* 1996;21:1S.
2. Andersson GBJ, Brown MD, Dvorak J, et al. Consensus summary on the diagnosis and treatment of lumbar disc herniation. *Spine* 1996;21:75S–78S.
3. Chen TY. The clinical presentation of uppermost cervical disc protrusion. *Spine* 2000;25:439–442.

4. Loupasis GA, Stamos K, Katonis PG. Seven- to 20-year outcome of lumbar discectomy. *Spine* 1999;24: 2313–2317.
5. Malter AD, Weinstein J. Cost-effectiveness of lumbar discectomy. *Spine* 1996;21:69S–74S.
6. Maniadakis N, Gray A. Health economics and orthopedics. *J Bone Joint Surg* 2000;82-B:2–7.
7. McCulloch JA. Focus issue on lumbar disc herniation: macro- and microdiscectomy. *Spine* 1996;2145S–21456S.
8. Rasmussen C. Lumbar disc herniation: favourable outcome associated with intake of wine. *Eur Spine J* 1998;7: 24–28.
9. Rasmussen C. Lumbar disc herniation: social and demographic factors determining duration of disease. *Eur Spine J* 1996;5:225–228.
10. Shade V, Semmer N, Main CJ. The impact of clinical, morphological, psychological and work-related factors on the outcome of lumbar discectomy. *Pain* 1999;80:239–249.
11. Sonntag VKH, Klara P. Controversy in spine care. Is fusion necessary after anterior cervical discectomy? *Spine* 1996;21:1111–1113.
12. Stevenson RC, McCabe CJ, Findlay AM. An economic evaluation of a clinical trial to compare automated percutaneous lumbar discectomy with microdiscectomy in the treatment of contained lumbar disc herniation. *Spine* 1995;20:739–742.
13. Takeshima T, Kambara K, Mijata S. Clinical and radiographic evaluation of disc excision for lumbar disc herniation with and without posterolateral fusion. *Spine* 2000;25:450–456.
14. Van de Belt H, Deutman R. Repeat chemonucleolysis is safe and effective. *Clin Orthop* 1999;363:121–125.
15. Vucetic N, Astrand P, Güntner P, et al. Diagnosis and prognosis in lumbar disc herniation. *Clin Orthop* 1999;361: 116–122.

33

The Technique of Local and Regional Anesthesia for Lumbar Disc Surgery

Stephen D. Kuslich

The most commonly used anesthetic technique for lumbar spine surgery is undoubtedly general endotracheal anesthesia, and for good reasons. The method is generally safe, comfortable for the patient, and convenient for the surgical team. However, general anesthesia for spinal surgery does have some drawbacks:

- The unconscious patient's down-turned face is not easily visible or accessible.
- Positioning errors can result in pressure areas, some of which (e.g., the eyes) can cause serious long-term complications.
- Positive pressure ventilation is not normal ventilation. It results in elevated intrathoracic pressures during inspiration. These elevated pressures cause elevated pressures in the entire venous system, including the inferior vena cava, Batson's vein complex, and hence, the epidural veins. Elevated epidural vein pressure can result in bleeding, decreased surgical visibility, longer operations, and probably higher rates of epidural fibrosis and other complications.

While the author did not invent or originate the use of local and regional anesthesia for lumbar surgery, he probably has more experience with the technique (about 4,000 cases) than most spinal surgeons (3). This chapter will acquaint the reader with the details of this technique, and the benefits and drawbacks of local and regional anesthesia as applied to lumbar spinal surgery.

The author learned the technique of operating with local anesthesia in 1966 while studying general surgery with a gifted Minneapolis surgeon, Dr. Daniel Moos. Dr. Moos performed all of his cholecystectomies and inguinal hernia repairs with local anesthesia. Later, the author became aware of the literature concerning the use of local anesthesia for lumbar spinal surgery by studying the publications of Falconer and colleagues (1), Murphy (4), Spurling and Granthum (7), and Wiberg (8), and Smith and Wright (6). In 1991, the author published his large experience with local anesthesia for spinal surgery (2). More recently, Nystrom confirmed his observations (5).

The following summary provides details of the author's preferred technique. Other techniques and agents may also be effective, but in the author's hands, the following procedure has been exceedingly safe and effective. After more than 20 years of use, without changing the sequence, technique, or medications, the author is convinced that it will prove to be safe and effective in the hands of others as well.

PREOPERATIVE PREPARATION

Informed consent is obtained by telling the patient of the reasons for the anesthetic choice and describing the technique. Apprehension is greatly relieved by explaining to

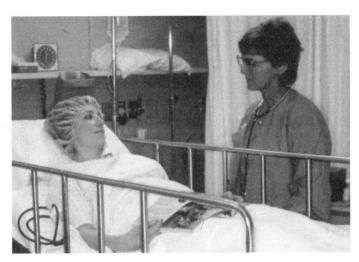

FIG. 33.1. The proper use of local and/or regional anesthesia begins in the office visit and continues during the preoperative visit. It is remarkable how simple it is to get patients to agree to this form of anesthesia once they understand the benefits, including the safety features of the technique. Intravenous sedation is given before the patient enters the operating theater.

the patient the advantages in terms of safety, and the fact that no tube will have to be placed in the throat. Finally, informing the patient that the intravenous and local medications will relieve any immediate preoperative and postoperative discomfort usually results in their consent (Fig. 33.1).

INTRAVENOUS PHARMACOLOGIC AGENTS

We use an intravenous injection of a short-acting narcotic (fentanyl) and a short-acting sedative (Versed) before and during the procedure. The dose is titrated to alleviate appre-

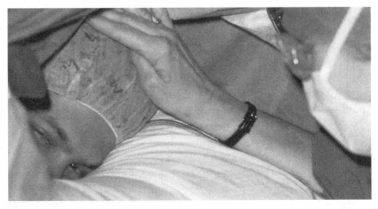

FIG. 33.2. Intravenous sedation and analgesia are given by titration as necessary. Ideally, the patient is sedate and not anxious, but cooperative and capable of answering questions and following instructions. "Verbal anesthesia" (i.e., talking to the patient) is part of the experience. Patients enjoy being part of the therapeutic team and knowing what is going on, rather than awakening from general anesthesia and wondering: "What really happened?"

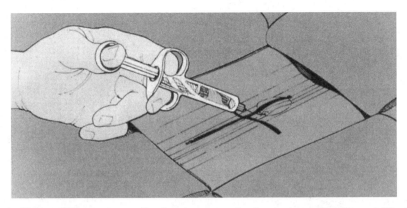

FIG. 33.3. Using a 25-gauge needle, the dermis and subcutaneous tissue are infiltrated with 1% Xylocaine with 1:100,000 epinephrine.

hension, while keeping the patient sufficiently conscious to cooperate with the surgical team. When properly performed, the patient is sedate but is able to carry on a conversation and move enough to protect anatomic sites from damage (Fig. 33.2).

Local Injection Technique

We infiltrate the skin and subcutaneous region using a few cc's of Xylocaine (lidocaine), 1% with 1:100,000 epinephrine (Fig. 34.3).

Then, we inject 2 to 3 cc at two to three sites at the base of the paravertebral muscles, just posterior to the posterior elements, to block the posterior primary ramus (Fig. 33.4).

Careful retraction of the muscle laterally exposes the interlaminar space. The laminar bone and ligamentum flavum are not sensitive, so no anesthetic agent is needed in these tissues (Fig. 33.5).

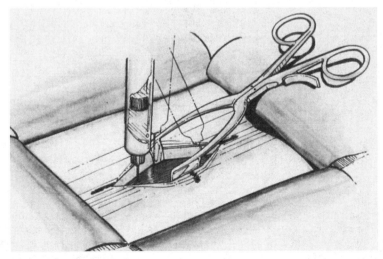

FIG. 33.4. Using a 22-gauge, 3.5-inch needle, the deeper tissues are infiltrated with 1% Xylocaine at the base of the musculature at the level of the lamina.

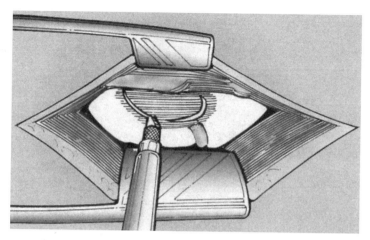

FIG. 33.5. The ligamentum flavum and laminar bone require no anesthesia, but great care must be taken to be gentle when approaching the spinal canal. The operating microscope is essential during this phase of the surgery when using local or regional anesthesia.

Tissues within the spinal canal space will likely be very tender in cases of nerve root compression, therefore, after careful removal of the ligamentum flavum using microsurgical instruments, proper illumination, and magnification, the nerve root may be injected using a 30-gauge needle just proximal to the site of compression. Only 0.5 cc of Xylocaine is necessary (Fig. 33.6).

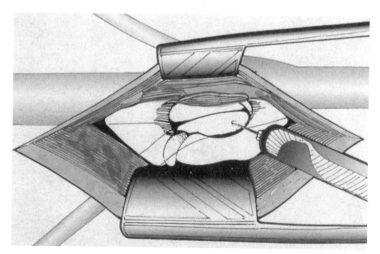

FIG. 33.6. After very carefully removing the ligamentum flavum and sufficient laminar bone, 0.5 cc of 1% Xylocaine is gently injected beneath the sleeve of the nerve root, proximal to the area of compression. This produces a very brief re-creation of the patient's sciatica for a few seconds, but all rootlet pain is immediately relieved for the remainder of the procedure. If all compression is then removed—by excision of the offending disc fragment and stenosing bone, etc.—the sciatic relief will be permanent. If a very small diameter syringe is used, visibility is enhanced. The use of the operating microscope is essential for this step.

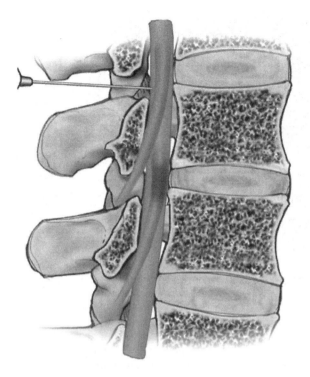

FIG. 33.7. Complete sensory analgesia at and below the target level can be acheived by performing a subarachnoid injection one level above the target level. A 25-gauge, 3.5-inch spinal needle is inserted blindly (by feel) through the ligamentum flavum one level above. The author recommends using 3 to 5 cc of 1% plain (unpreserved, sterile) Xylocaine. This produces a block of the unmyelinated sensory fibers, but leaves the myelinated motor fibers unblocked; therefore the patient can continue to contract leg muscles. By these means, complete, bilateral, multilevel spinal stenosis decompressions may be performed.

Alternatively, the subarachnoid space may be blocked by blindly inserting a 25-gauge spinal needle one level above the target level, and installing 3 to 5 cc of plain Xylocaine 1%. This subarachnoid injection allows the surgeon to perform extensive decompressions, and even interbody fusions at any level below the injected segment. The block affects the unmyelinated fibers of the sensory afferents only, leaving the myelinated motor fibers functional. Therefore, the patient is able to contract the leg musculature even though he or she is unable to feel the result. Such movement is beneficial in preserving venous blood flow. This injection, however, does not completely block the autonomic innervation of the disc, so care must be taken to avoid vagal symptoms by gentle manipulation of the disc (see treatment of complications below) (Fig. 33.7).

If the disc annulus is tender, as it is in about one-half to two-thirds of cases, the disc should be infiltrated with 2 to 3 cc of Xylocaine before fenestration.

We use the kneeling–sitting position provided by the Andrew's table, but other positioning devises also work (Fig. 33.8).

Handling Intraoperative Problems

Using local or regional anesthesia requires patience on the part of the surgeon. It takes a little more time than general anesthesia—about 15 minutes longer—but the benefits in terms of safety and postoperative comfort far outweigh this minor disadvantage. The technique "forces" the surgeon to be gentle when manipulating tissues. Such gentleness is rewarded by minimal bleeding and less postoperative pain and swelling.

Most cases proceed uneventfully as long as the surgeon is patient and careful. Because the disc is innervated by the autonomic nervous system, vagal type symptoms arise in a small percentage of patients in the form of nausea, hypotension, and bradycardia. These symptoms

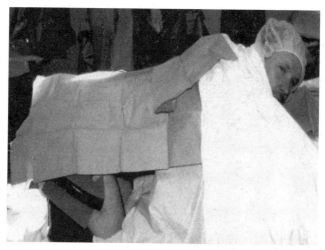

FIG. 33.8. Any standard spinal surgery positioning device may be used, but the Andrew's frame is preferred because it is inexpensive, easy to set up, comfortable, and allows complete decompression of the abdominal contents, thereby leading to relief of venous compression.

and signs can be quickly relieved by a 0.4- to 0.8-mg intravenous injection of atropine. In more than 3,000 cases, the author has never had to convert to general anesthesia.

Advantages of Local and Regional Anesthesia in Spinal Surgery

Safety

The operation is safer because the likelihood of stasis and pressure-point phenomena are greatly reduced. Endotracheal tube-induced tracheitis is prevented. Atelectasis and postoperative pneumonia are prevented. Venous stasis and its attendant phlebitis are markedly reduced because the patient contracts muscles during the operation. Bleeding from the epidural veins is markedly reduced because of the absence of positive pressure during the inspiratory phase of respiration.

Comfort

This technique reduces postoperative grogginess and nausea. The patient is able to ambulate, and eat and drink immediately following the procedure. The incisional pain is blocked for about 1 hour postsurgery. Powerful postoperative narcotics are normally not needed, leading to faster resumption of bowel function. A final, less tangible, but no less real advantage, is the fact that the patient feels as though he or she has been part of the therapeutic experience. This induces a form of postoperative euphoria that markedly reduces postoperative pain behavior and leads to faster recovery.

Other Advantages

This form of anesthesia allows the surgeon the opportunity to probe the surgical area and thereby confirm the presence or absence of painful tissues. The surgeon will soon learn, as the author has observed, that most of the spinal tissues are painless, and that the inflamed or compressed nerve is the only tissue that produces sciatica when gently manipulated. Similarly, the disc annulus is the only tissue that produces the deep, poorly localized, nauseating discomfort of mechanical low back pain. In certain cases, the facet joint capsule produces sharp, localized back pain (2,5). On rare occasions, the surgeon will note a painless nerve root at the target site. If this occurs, he or she should recheck the level and side of the operation, because it is likely that the wrong level or side has been exposed (3).

REFERENCES

1. Falconer MA, McGeorge M, Begg AC. Observations on the cause and mechanism of symptom production in sciatica and low back pain. *J Neurol Neurosurg Psychiatry* 1948;11:13–26.
2. Kuslich SD, Ulstrom CL. The tissue origin of low back pain and sciatica: a report of pain response to tissue stimulation during operations on the lumbar spine using local anesthesia. *Orthop Clin North Am* 1991;22(2): 181–187.
3. Kuslich SD. Microsurgical lumbar nerve root decompression utilizing progressive local anesthesia. In Williams RW, McCulloch, Young PH, eds. *Microsurgery of the lumbar spine*. Rockville, MD: Aspen, 1990:139–147.
4. Murphy F. Experience with lumbar disc surgery. *Clin Neurosurg* 1973;20:1–8.
5. Nystrom B. Open mechanical provocation under local anesthesia—a definitive method for locating the focus in painful mechanical disorder of the motion segment. Paper presented at: The Swedish Orthopaedic Society; September 9–11, 1992; Falun, Sweden.
6. Smyth MJ, Wright V. Sciatica and the intervertebral disc. An experimental study. *J Bone Joint Surg* 1958;40: 1401–1418.
7. Spurling GR, Granthum EG. Neurologic picture of herniations of the nucleus pulposus in the lower part of the lumbar spine. *Arch Surg* 1940;40(3):375–388.
8. Wiberg G. Back pain in relation to the nerve supply of the intervertebral disc. *Acta Orthop Scand* 1950;19: 211–221.

34

Outpatient Logistics and Day-Case Discectomy

C.G. Greenough

Back pain is one of the largest single causes of disability in the European Union. In the United Kingdom, disability caused by low back pain has increased eightfold in the past 14 years and has doubled in the last 8 years (3). Back pain treatment alone accounts for 1.5% of the entire NHS budget. It is now well accepted that low back pain is strongly influenced by socioeconomic factors and, especially in areas with high unemployment, low back pain represents a very significant problem. This has led to a steady increase in referrals of patients with low back pain to hospital services, in such numbers that waiting times for clinic appointments have grown to unacceptable levels.

For example, a specialist spinal clinic was inaugurated in Teesside (UK) in January 1991. Owing to demand, the waiting time for appointment rose from 0 to 62 weeks in 18 months. This delay jeopardized the results of treatment of patients requiring surgery, reduced the chance of returning to work, caused considerable frustration to general practitioners, and was the cause of much anxiety and suffering for the patients.

A working party comprising both general practitioners and representatives of specialities in hospital practice developed a new service to address these problems, the Spinal Assessment Clinic. This clinic was the first in the United Kingdom where diagnosis and treatment for low back pain was entirely undertaken by a nurse practitioner. This major innovation was made possible by careful and thorough training. It was recognized that this innovation carried some potential risks and careful arrangements were made for rigorous auditing of the results, and in particular, the accuracy of diagnosis.

The philosophy of the Spinal Assessment Clinic is to provide integrated coordinated treatment for patients with low back complaints in an environment where audit and research are an integral part of the program. The medical philosophy of the clinic is to provide timely access to assessment and treatment. The subsequent publication of the Clinical Standards and Advisory Group report (3) and report of the Royal College of General Practitioners (5) echoes this approach to treatment, and the current standards for the Spinal Assessment Clinic are modeled on these reports.

Underpinning the approach of the Spinal Assessment Clinic is a concept of the etiology of back pain that is moving away from the pathologic model. It is recognized that in the treatment of mechanical low back pain there are no structural differences detectable in the bones, joints, ligaments, or discs between patients with mechanical low back pain, and age- and sex-matched volunteers. The results of rapid early intervention together with the results of research into the function of the paraspinal muscles indicate that it is probable that the muscular control and support of the spine is of great significance. Treatment is therefore aimed at restoring functionality and reducing the emphasis on management of pain. Patients are encouraged to understand the mechanical nature of the pain, and to accept that management of the problem lies within themselves. Concentration on improving activities of daily living and returning to normal activities is paramount. The necessity for early active management is acknowledged.

For those patients with surgically remediable lesions (usually nerve root compression), the philosophy of the clinic is to provide the fastest possible route to definitive diagnosis, to reduce patients suffering, and also to improve results by providing treatment before spinal decompensation progresses too far.

It must be acknowledged that treatment of low back pain cannot be undertaken by provision of a single clinic. A consistent approach across primary and secondary care and in the community is absolutely essential. To this end the Spinal Assessment Clinic has always produced detailed discharge summaries, outlining the philosophy of management and the progress of the patients, on every patient. These discharge summaries have been designed to inform and educate general practitioners and since the time the clinic began, the general practitioners' changes in the attitude have been measured.

THE SPINAL ASSESSMENT CLINIC

The Spinal Assessment Clinic is run by nurse practitioners. Protocols are used for history taking and physical examination. Patients are referred by general practitioners using a pro forma referral system. An appointment is made and the patient is seen and examined by the nurse practitioner and a diagnosis is formed.

For the purpose of treatment the patients are divided into one of five different categories:

1. Mechanical low back pain.
2. Suspected nerve root entrapment (prolapsed disc, central, or lateral stenosis, etc.).
3. Potentially serious conditions (malignant disease, infection, etc.).
4. Diagnosis uncertain.
5. Potentially suitable for manipulative physiotherapy.

Mechanical Low Back Pain

These patients comprise the majority of the referrals (approximately 75%). The patients are treated within the Spinal Assessment Clinic with an educational and behavioral modification program. Each patient has an individual educational session with the nurse practitioner, who outlines the diagnosis and explains in detail the etiology and proposed treatment. The patient then attends two class sessions, 6 weeks following the initial individual education session. Following the class sessions, each patient then has a further individual session with the nurse practitioner some 6 weeks after the educational classes are complete. At these sessions the advice is recapitulated and the patient has an opportunity to clarify any questions. Follow-up after this session is geared to individual patient need with many patients being discharged at this stage. It should be noted that these patients will have been seen and treated only by a nurse practitioner.

Suspected Nerve Root Entrapment

Patients who are suspected of having neurologic entrapment either by prolapsed disc or by central or lateral stenosis are referred directly by the nurse practitioner for scanning.

Once the patient's scan has been completed, the patient is reviewed by a member of the medical team and surgery is recommended as appropriate.

Potentially Serious Conditions

Those patients with suspected serious pathology are referred for consultant opinion with an appropriate degree of urgency. The nurse practitioner has the option of admitting the patient straight to the ward or arranging an urgent outpatient follow-up within 4 weeks.

Diagnosis Uncertain

These patients are referred for specialist surgical opinion on an accelerated track in the outpatient clinic.

Potentially Suitable for Manipulative Physiotherapy

At the inception of the Spinal Assessment Clinic, discussions were held with the Department of Physiotherapy and agreement was reached on the type of patient most suitable for physiotherapy treatment. A close liaison has now been developed between the Spinal Assessment Clinic and the Physiotherapy Department and regular contact is maintained with a named physiotherapist to ensure smooth functioning and a seamless provision of care between the two departments.

RESULTS

Waiting Times

The waiting time for a routine appointment for the Spinal Assessment Clinic is now 4 weeks (Fig. 34.1). Urgent patients may be seen the same week following referral by telephone.

The waiting time for the specialist spinal clinic fell from a peak of 68 weeks to less than 20 weeks and the consultants' time is being more effectively used for more complex cases (Fig. 34.2). More recently, the increase in workload generated by the Spinal Assessment Clinic has increased the waiting time. It should be noted, however, that this figure represents the wait for a routine general practice referral and that patients from the Spinal Assessment Clinic and tertiary referrals are seen sooner than this.

The waiting time for surgical treatment fell significantly, the time taken to obtain a scan is now the longest part of the waiting time for a decision on surgery. At its worst, the time taken from a routine general practitioner referral to review of the patient with a scan and decision to undertake surgery was 85 weeks (64 weeks for an outpatient appointment, 12 weeks for the scan, and 9 weeks for review). This figure has been reduced to 24 weeks (16 weeks are accounted for by outpatient scanning). Acute referrals, such as prolapsed intervertebral disc, may now be seen on the week of referral, have a scan some 6 weeks later, and be reviewed 2 weeks after that. More urgent cases may be admitted for inpatient scanning.

As a further refinement, in the last year patients with a clinical diagnosis of nerve root entrapment in whom surgery is clinically indicated are counseled regarding surgery at the initial assessment appointment. If scanning confirms the clinical diagnosis, they are placed on the surgical waiting list without review. The surgeon will see the patient for the first time on the morning of admission. With highly trained nurse practitioners, this has proved very satisfactory.

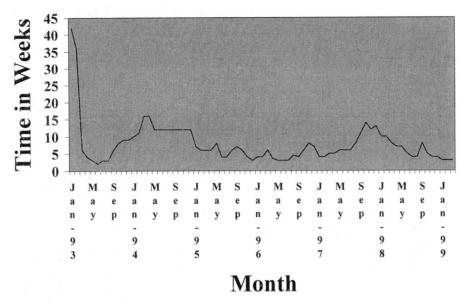

FIG. 34.1. Waiting time for appointment at the Spinal Assessment Clinic.

Patient Recovery

A formal audit of a sample of 90 patients with a diagnosis of mechanical back pain was undertaken with a minimum follow-up of 12 months. Ninety-six percent expressed satisfaction with the Spinal Assessment Clinic and 67% felt that the rehabilitation had been helpful. Low back outcome scores improved from 29 at presentation, to 35 at review

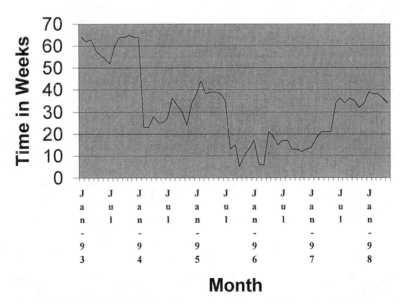

FIG. 34.2. Waiting time for an appointment with a specialist.

($P < 0. 01$). Eighteen patients reduced analgesia intake although five increased intake. Eleven patients returned to work while four left work during this period.

An audit of general practitioners was also undertaken and 94% of those questioned were satisfied with the clinic's function. The majority of general practitioners believed a reasonable time to obtain a routine appointment was between 4 and 8 weeks.

Integrated Audit

Clinical audit depends on reliable and valid data on clinical outcomes. The drawbacks of paper-based data collection are well known: failure to return the questionnaire, failure to complete all questions (particularly those involved in scoring systems), ambiguous answers, and the need to enter the data into a computer database. A light–pen interface allows any patient to complete the questionnaire by directly interacting with the computer without supervision, eliminating the need for data entry and also preventing omission of data items and eliminating ambiguous answers.

The patients complete a computer questionnaire at their initial appointment and also on their final review following the rehabilitation classes. Longer term follow-up is undertaken using questionnaires send through the mail that are suitable for input via an optical mark reader. This has achieved our aim of making audit and research an absolutely integral part of the treatment program.

Cost

The Spinal Assessment Clinic now sees and treats 1,500 patients each year. The cost of referral to a general practitioner is less than the standard outpatient appointment, and includes the educational program and all follow-up.

Acceptability to Patients

Audit of patient satisfaction with the Spinal Assessment Clinic has demonstrated ratings of better than 90%. The vast majority of patients seen only by the nurse practitioners do not return for medical evaluation in the spinal outpatient clinic or other clinics. Feedback to nurse practitioners has been very positive; nearly all patients appear to have confidence in their advice.

Training

Following the presentation of the results of the Spinal Assessment Clinic, both locally and nationally, considerable interest has been generated throughout the National Health Service. Representatives from many other health centers have visited the clinic in the last 5 years and a competency-based training program for nurse practitioners is now offered. Seven nurse practitioners have completed the formal training and 17 clinics have been set up in the UK based on this model.

Summary

The Spinal Assessment Clinic has provided an entirely new way of managing low back pain in secondary care and is now providing new insights into possible improvements in the management of low back pain within primary care and the community. It has allowed major improvements in the speed at which the service can be provided, and proven measurable benefit to patients. We believe the concept of total integration of audit and research within the clinical setting is of paramount importance to making progress in the treatment of this extremely difficult problem.

DAY-CASE CONVENTIONAL DISCECTOMY

Day surgery is developing rapidly and more patients are now being considered to undergo this type of treatment. The type of operations considered suitable is also increasing.

There are a number of reports of microdiscectomies undertaken as day cases (1,4,6,8). To the author's knowledge only one report exists examining the performance of conventional fenestration and discectomy (7).

Together with a colleague (Ms. A. Gonzalez-Castro, FRCS), the author undertook a study comparing conventional fenestration and discectomy performed either as a day case or on an inpatient basis.

Patients with prolapsed intervertebral disc were included in the trial based on the following criteria:

1. Leg pain as the main symptom.
2. Presence of at least one clinical sign.
   a. positive stretch test
   b. motor deficit
   c. sensory deficit
   d. absent reflex unilaterally
3. Clinical diagnosis confirmed by computed tomography or magnetic resonance imaging scan with correlating findings.
4. Failure to respond to conservative treatment for a minimum of 6 months.
5. Patients who required urgent surgical intervention due to cauda equina syndrome or progressive neurologic deficit were excluded from the study.

Patients also had to be eligible for day case management. These criteria are:

1. Less than 65 years old.
2. Absence of significant concurrent medical problems.
3. Adequate home support and a responsible adult to take the patient home after surgery.
4. Traveling time from hospital to home of less than 1 hour.

The patients were then randomized to day case care or to overnight admission. All the patients were admitted on the day of the operation. Patients and staff were aware of the inpatient or day case status.

Two patients had to be withdrawn from the study. One was later found to have sleep apnea and the other patient's sciatic symptoms resolved completely before surgery, thus treatment was no longer necessary. All patients had the same standard operation performed by the same surgeon (fenestration and discectomy) under general anesthesia. Curettage of the endplates was not undertaken.

All patients were assessed on the evening of the operation. The level of pain, amount of analgesia, and mobility status were recorded. Inpatients stayed overnight and day cases were assessed for discharge using the Post Anaesthetic Discharge Scoring System (2). They were given an information sheet with postoperative instructions and contact telephone numbers. They were encouraged to gradually increase their level of activity by walking regularly but avoiding lifting any weight.

TABLE 34.1. *Mobility after surgery*

	1a	1b	2
Unable to sit up		4	8
Able to sit or stand			2
Able to walk with or without help	13	1	3

1a vs. 2, $P < 0.001$.

TABLE 34.2. *Patients' opinion of length of stay*

	1a	1b	2
Too short	2	1	1
Adequate	11	4	8
Too long	0	0	4

TABLE 34.3. *Hours of sleep (first night)*

	1a	1b	2
None	2	1	5
Less than usual	4	4	6
Same as usual	5	0	1
More than usual	2	0	1

TABLE 34.4. *Daytime hours spent in bed on first postoperative day*

	1a	1b	2
Whole/most of the day	5	4	7
Half day/few hours	3	1	6
None	5	0	0

1a vs. 2, $P < 0.05$.

TABLE 34.5. *Walking distance at 2 weeks (compared to preoperative level)*

	1a	1b	2
Less	0	0	3
Same	6	3	8
More	7	2	2

1a vs. 2, $P < 0.05$.

TABLE 34.6. Ability to do housework at 2 weeks (compared to preoperative level)

	1a	1b	2
Less	1	2	5
Same	6	1	6
More	6	2	2

A total of 31 patients were studied; 18 were randomized to day case management and 13 to overnight stay. Age and sex distribution were similar (41.5, range 32 to 65 versus 42.5 range, 32 to 61; seven women and 11 men versus four women and nine men).

Of the 18 planned day cases, 5 (72%) patients could not be discharged. Two failed to mobilize, two had minor postanesthetic problems, and one did not have adequate pain control.

The patients therefore were categorized into three groups:

Group 1a. Patients discharged as day cases.
Group 1b. Planned day cases who required admission.
Group 2. Planned inpatients.

One patient in each group required readmission (one episode of syncope, two episodes a week after surgery for adjustment of analgesia).

Mobility after surgery, length of stay, hours of sleep, general practitioner or hospital contacted, adequate pain relief, walking distance, ability to do house work, and ability to exercise at 2 weeks were investigated (Tables 34.1 through 34.6).

Day cases were able to mobilize on the same evening of the operation but the majority of inpatients could not. There was a trend for day cases to sleep better than the inpatients on the first night. The day after the operation, the inpatients spent more hours in bed than the day cases.

No significant difference was noted in the number of patients seeking medical advice after discharge. Two weeks after the operation, the day cases had improved their walking distance compared with the inpatients. Ability to do house work tended to be better among the day cases.

It may be that the difference in the speed of recovery is due to the patient's expectations. Day cases may recover quicker because less emphasis is placed on the operation and more on mobilization. Postoperative pain control and postoperative advice are the key issues when planning day case discectomies. Interestingly, most resistance to day case surgery was found in the nursing staff. In this study, for one list day cases were admitted to a day case ward where for another list others were admitted to an inpatient ward. Most failures to discharge as day patients were on the inpatient ward, where other surgeons were admitting discectomies for 5 days. The results of this study convinced the nursing staff, and now day case discectomies are routine.

CONCLUSIONS

This randomized study supports other researchers in concluding that conventional discectomy is not only safe as a day case procedure but it may be also beneficial for the patients.

REFERENCES

1. Bookwalter JW, Bush H, Nicely D. Ambulatory surgery is safe and effective in radicular disease. *Spine* 1994;19(5):526–530.
2. Chung F. Discharge criteria—a new trend. *Can J Anaesth* 1995;42(11):1056–1058.
3. Clinical Standards Advisory Group. *Low back pain.* London: HMSO, 1994.
4. Griffiths HB. The 100th day case disc. *West Engl Med J* 1992;7(2):43–44.
5. *Guidelines for the management of low back pain.* London: Royal College of General Practitioners, 1996.
6. Kelly A, Griffith HB. Results of day case surgery for lumbar disc prolapse. *Br J Neurosurg* 1994;8:47–49.
7. Newman NM. Outpatient conventional laminotomy and disc excision. *Spine* 1995;20(3):353–355.
8. Zahrawi F. Microlumbar discectomy. Is it safe as an out-patient procedure? *Spine* 1994;19(9):1070–1074.

35

Outcome Measurements and Different Languages: An Introduction

Margareta Nordin

Standardized outcome measures are increasingly used in clinical daily practice. If we assume that language is an expression for culture, then cross-cultural issues must be addressed in health outcome measures. Can we use a perceived disability or health outcome measure in different languages and assume that the results are comparable? (1,2). Health outcome measures can be helpful in clinical practice to obtain perceived well being and/or perceived disability from the patient. They are essential to evaluate outcome in studies. The topic is also highly relevant in the globalization aspect of health care and research. Exclusion of certain population groups due to different cultures or languages may lead to a systematic bias (2).

The purpose of this chapter is to introduce the topic. The aim is also to provide some aspects on the development of an outcome instrument in different languages and what caution needs to be taken.

DEVELOPMENT OF A PATIENT SELF-ADMINISTERED OUTCOME MEASURE

Three approaches are used for the development of outcome measures in cross-cultural settings. They are the *sequential* approach, the *parallel* approach, and the *simultaneous* approach (2).

The Sequential Approach

The sequential approach consists of the translation and performance evaluation of an existing instrument. For example, a sequential approach may use one panel of multidisciplinary experts first to determine the appropriateness of the instrument. Thereafter, the instrument is submitted to a panel of lay people to elicit verbal expressions for the targeted population.

The Parallel Approach

The parallel approach uses translation and evaluation of the instrument in different cultures with adaptation to the cultures. For example, the content of the instrument in the development phase is decided by an international group of diverse professional and cultural background. The selection of this group ensures that the items proposed in the instrument are meaningful, relevant, and applicable across different cultural contexts. The instrument can then be tested to determine its performance in cross-cultural settings.

The Simultaneous Approach

The simultaneous approach focuses around the development of an international conceptualization of a construct, and each culture or nation develops its own content. This procedure has been used, for example, in developing quality of life instruments. The process involves developing and internationally operationalizing a set of items for quality of life. Each working group within specific cultures formulates relevant instrument content. From the pool of questions, core questions are used in the final instrument.

All above approaches can be combined, however, it is perhaps most important to recognize that the development of a questionnaire is a major undertaking. In cross-cultural settings the responses must yield cross-cultural meaningful answers.

Forward and Backward Translation

All approaches use forward and backward translation. Guidelines and recommendations have been developed to address this issue (1,2). The importance of forward and backward translation can be summarized as follows: the choice of linguistic competent translators, the cultural background of the translators, the translators' awareness of the objective of their role, structured evaluation of the translators, and the importance to have at least two independent translators. Furthermore, the recommendations bring up the review process, including cross-cultural equivalency and the field pretesting for comparison of the original questionnaire.

METHODOLOGIC PROBLEMS

Methodologic problems in cross-cultural outcome measures can be divided into *technical*, *conceptual*, and *linguistic* problems (2).

Technical Problems

One example of a technical problem is illiteracy. Using a self-administered instrument assumes a satisfactory level of literacy and familiarity with the method of data collection. Many populations still retain a high level of illiteracy particularly among older adults and certain ethnic minorities. In this case the use of a trained interviewer is necessary and may introduce a new set of problems.

Conceptual Problems

An example of a conceptual problem is the description of health. People of Afro-Caribbean descent describe health as being strong and fit, while Asian people define it as one's ability to perform everyday activities. Health beliefs differ extensively between populations and groups. The experience of an illness is a cultural phenomenon reflecting beliefs about etiology, illness behavior, and assigned role, as well as type of treatment and social system. Showing emotional distress, anxiety, or depression is discouraged in certain cultures, while in other cultures it is normal to meet with a psychologist to solve weekly problems.

Cultural status and cultural system can greatly affect outcome of care. Should patient and health care provider belong to two totally different culturally conceptual groups, conflict is unavoidable.

Cultural differences must be taken into account prior to adapting an existing instrument or in the development of a new instrument. If these aspects are not satisfactorily considered, the use of an instrument should be used with great caution.

Linguistic Problems

A linguistic problem can be illustrated through a question on depression (2). A European or American health care provider may ask a patient the following question: "Last week, were you depressed?" Among Africans, however, the same question might need to be rephrased as: "Recently, have you felt like a branch hanging from a tree?" An item in an instrument can be translated from one language to another language semantically, however, the translation may still have a different meaning in the target language. The item in one culture will not be representative of the same thing in another culture.

CROSS-CULTURAL EQUIVALENCY

Five items have been cited to judge the criteria for cross-cultural equivalency in the development on an instrument (1,2). These are: *content* equivalency (i.e., regarding different social or leisure activities in different cultures); *semantic* equivalency (i.e., more important to translate the meaning than a direct literal translation); *conceptual* equivalency (i.e., the concepts of social support and family may have very different meanings in different languages); *technical* equivalency (i.e., self-administered data collection versus structured interview); and *criterion* equivalency (i.e., reliability and validity in cross-cultural settings).

CONCLUSIONS

New studies are constantly being developed. The importance of the choice of outcome measures can never be emphasized enough. The use of outcome measures in cross-cultural settings need to follow minimum criteria development (i.e., some of the aspects outlined in this chapter need to be met). For maximum criteria development, all criteria cited in this chapter should be fulfilled.

REFERENCES

1. Beaton DE, Bombardier C, Guillemin F, et al. Guidelines for the process of cross-cultural adaptation of self-report measures. *Spine* 2000;25(24):3186–3191.
2. Hutchinson A, Bentzen N, Konig-Zahn C. *Cross-cultural health outcome assessment: a user's guide*. European Research Group on Health Outcomes, 1996.

Subject Index